Binge Eating Disorder: Clinical Assessment and Treatment

Binge Eating Disorder: Clinical Assessment and Treatment

Editor: Tiara Clanton

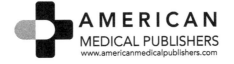

AMERICAN
MEDICAL PUBLISHERS
www.americanmedicalpublishers.com

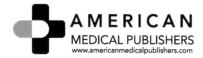

AMERICAN
MEDICAL PUBLISHERS
www.americanmedicalpublishers.com

Cataloging-in-Publication Data

Binge eating disorder : clinical assessment and treatment / edited by Tiara Clanton.
     p. cm.
Includes bibliographical references and index.
ISBN 978-1-63927-916-6
1. Compulsive eating. 2. Eating disorders--Diagnosis. 3. Eating disorders--Treatment. 4. Obesity--Psychological aspects.
5. Compulsive behavior. 6. Psychiatry. I. Clanton, Tiara.
RC552.C65 B56 2023
616.852 6--dc23

American Medical Publishers,
41 Flatbush Avenue,
1st Floor, New York,
NY 11217, USA

ISBN 978-1-63927-916-6 (Hardback)

Contents

Preface

This book has been a concerted effort by a group of academicians, researchers and scientists, who have contributed their research works for the realization of the book. This book has materialized in the wake of emerging advancements and innovations in this field. Therefore, the need of the hour was to compile all the required researches and disseminate the knowledge to a broad spectrum of people comprising of students, researchers and specialists of the field.

Binge eating disorder is an eating disorder characterized by frequent consumption of unusually large amounts of food and an inability to stop eating. Its common symptoms are eating large amounts of food without feeling hungry, eating alone due to feelings of embarrassment and shame, feelings of guilt or disgust with oneself, etc. There are multiple factors that can lead to an increased risk of developing binge eating disorder. Some of these factors are genetics, history of dieting, and psychological issues. Binge eating disorder is associated with complications, such as social isolation, obesity and poor quality of life. The clinical assessment of binge eating disorders is performed with the help of physical examination, blood tests, and urine tests. Its treatment involves psychotherapy, medications, and behavioral weight-loss programs. This book outlines the clinical assessment and treatment for binge eating disorders. A number of latest researches have been included to keep the readers up-to-date with the global concepts in this area of study. This book will provide comprehensive knowledge to the readers.

At the end of the preface, I would like to thank the authors for their brilliant chapters and the publisher for guiding us all-through the making of the book till its final stage. Also, I would like to thank my family for providing the support and encouragement throughout my academic career and research projects.

Editor

Patients' experiences from basic body awareness therapy in the treatment of binge eating disorder-movement toward health: A phenomenological study

Marit Nilsen Albertsen[1,2]* ⓘ, Eli Natvik[3] and Målfrid Råheim[4]

Abstract

Background: Binge Eating Disorder (BED) is the most common eating disorder. Patients with BED are often not diagnosed, nor offered adequate specific treatment. A great number of those who receive recommended treatment do not recover over time. More knowledge about central aspects of BED, and treatments that specifically target such aspects is needed. Previous research has linked body experience to the development and maintenance of eating disorders, as well as influencing treatment results and the risk of relapse. The aim of this study was to explore how patients with BED experience Basic Body Awareness Therapy (BBAT), which is a psychomotor physiotherapy treatment addressing body experience.

Method: In this phenomenological study, we interviewed two patients with BED in depth during and after treatment. Video observations of treatment sessions and logs written by the patients were used as supporting data. The analysis was guided by Van Manen's hermeneutic phenomenology.

Results: A meaning structure was identified: "On the way from the body as a problem to the body as a possibility." The two participants that besides BED also had a history of childhood trauma, perceived BBAT as a process of getting to know their own bodies in new ways, and described that the way they related to their own body changed as did aspects of their way of being. These changes were prominent when the participants described emotions, movement, pain, calmness, and self-experience, and interwoven with relational aspects as well as practices in everyday life.

Conclusion: The present results indicate that BBAT stimulated body experience in a way that opened new possibilities for two participants with BED, and hence that BBAT can improve the health status of BED patients also suffering from childhood trauma.

Keywords: Binge-eating disorder, Body-oriented therapy, Physiotherapy, Body experience, Phenomenology of the body

Plain English summary

Binge Eating Disorder is the most common eating disorder. Still, this disorder is often not addressed by the health care system, and current treatment shows poor results on a large group of these patients. Difficulties in relating to own body are linked to the development and maintenance of eating disorders in previous research, and seem to influence treatment results and the risk of relapse. Basic Body Awareness Therapy is a psychomotor physiotherapeutic treatment addressing the relation to one's own body. In this study, we have explored in-depth the experiences of two patients with Binge Eating Disorder during their treatment-process with Basic Body Awareness Therapy. This study indicates that changes in how these patients related to their own bodies during the treatment processes were meaningful to them, and

* Correspondence: albertsen@ipr.no
[1]Department of Global Health and Primary Care, University of Bergen, Bergen, Norway
[2]Present address: Department of Eating Disorders, Division of Psychiatry, Haukeland University Hospital, Institute of Psychological Counselling , Bergen, Norway
Full list of author information is available at the end of the article

implied a movement toward well-being and accepting one's own body. Findings from this study inspire more research on body awareness raising approaches in the treatment of patients with Binge Eating Disorder.

Highlights

- BBAT may contribute to meaningful change toward better health and well-being for patients with BED.
- BBAT stimulates body awareness and acceptance through simple movements and grounding oneself in one's own body.
- Being able to accept what feels unpleasant in the body may open new possibilities for the way in which patients with BED relate to themselves, others, and everyday life.

Introduction

Binge-eating disorder (BED) is reportedly the most-common eating disorder (Supina, Herman, Frye, & Shillington, 2016). Health-related quality of life is significantly worse in BED patients than in both individuals without BED and a population with extreme obesity (defined as BMI $\geq$40 kg/m^2) [3]. Patients with BED have more interaction with the health-care system than the general population, but research indicates that these patients are often not diagnosed nor offered adequate specific treatment [3, 17, 21, 50, 53, 61].

Psychotherapy is a recommended treatment for patients with eating disorders (Helsedirektoratet [The Norwegian Directorate of Health], [19]). The English guidelines recommend enhanced cognitive behavioural therapy (CBT-e) [12]. However, research shows that about 30% of patients with BED receiving the recommended treatment do not recover over time [12, 19, 29]. More knowledge about treatments that specifically target the central aspects of BED is needed.

Body image is a central aspect of eating disorders in general, and also in BED [8, 25]. Research has linked body-image disturbances to the development and maintenance of eating disorders. It has also been shown that such disturbances can influence treatment results and the risk of relapse to eating disorders generally [5, 6, 8, 13, 14, 18, 39, 40, 49, 51, 59]. Body image is a complex phenomenon that includes the evaluation and perception of one's own body, but also thoughts about, feelings for, and attitudes toward one's own body [8]. Body image is closely related to self-esteem, and body-image disturbances have long-term consequences on social, physical, and emotional development [60].

The need for more direct ways to address body image in treatment for eating disorders was emphasized in early studies [42]. Even though research in this area is scarce [8, 63], recent studies indicate promising results [16, 20, 24, 63]. Direct ways of addressing body image is still not systematized in therapy or in research. Physiotherapy is quite unusual to include in treatment of patients with eating disorders, even though physiotherapists have a wide array of approaches and techniques to address body image and body experience [38].

Basic Body Awareness Therapy (BBAT) is a type of psychomotor physiotherapy that falls between body-oriented treatment and psychotherapy. It is a physiotherapy approach within the movement awareness domain developed to bridge physical, mental, and relational health challenges [46]. BBAT is inspired by both Western and Eastern movement traditions [10, 11]. This body awareness training modality was first brought into physiotherapy by the Swedish physiotherapist Dr. Roxendal in the 1980s. It is further developed within the International Association of Teachers in Basic Body Awareness Therapy, and has since the 1990s been officially accepted and implemented in physiotherapy education in Scandinavia. BBAT has shown promising treatment results in psychiatry and mental health and is increasingly implemented in somatic health care such as rheumatology [32, 37]. The BBAT sessions create therapeutic learning situations for the patients that aim at exploring and integrating unity, flow and rhythm into daily-life movements such as lying, sitting, standing, walking and moving together [48]. Each exercise ends out by reflecting together with the therapist [32]. BBAT treatment is described in further detail in the method-section.

BBAT focuses on the whole person, enhancing body awareness and the quality of movements in attempting to promote health. Movement quality is seen as a unifying phenomenon and expression of health, representing a synthesis of biomechanical, physiological, psycho-socio-cultural, and existential aspects [48]. A systematic review of randomized controlled trials with different physical therapy interventions for patients with anorexia and bulimia nervosa found that the patients who received BBAT reported significant improvements in eating pathology and depressive symptoms [58]. There are many similarities between the main mechanisms in the different diagnoses of eating disorders [12], and body image disturbance is one of them [8, 25]. Therefore, gaining knowledge about body-oriented treatment approaches to BED is expected to be useful. To our knowledge no previous study has explored changes in body experience in patients with BED undergoing BBAT as part of their treatment. The purpose of this study is to explore how patients with BED experience BBAT, and in what ways and on what dimensions this body awareness therapy influenced them as described from their own perspective.

Theoretical foundation

The phenomenology of the body was developed by the philosopher Maurice Merleau-Ponty. His central contribution is the idea that how we perceive our body is our mode of access to the world, and hence the primary mode for knowing the world [27]. Humans are embodied minds and minded bodies, and as bodily beings we also inhabit the world. Meaning develops in the relationship between humans and the social world, primarily through noncognitive, often unconscious, preverbal bodily sensations and experiences. Our intentionality, an eternally to-from relationship with our world, is a bodily intentionality based on inhabiting the world [4, 26, 27, 41, 56, 62]. Our bodily being is also characterized by a kind of ambiguity that is existential in character [27]. We live in our bodies unreflectively, acting as agents inhabiting our world while simultaneously experiencing our bodies within the world. We reflect upon our own body and being in the world by objectifying it in different ways.

When the body changes dramatically, as in illness, our own relationship with the body and world also changes. Illness can be experienced as a split between the body as subject and object that changes our relationships with the practical and social world and thereby our self-experience and usual way of being in the world. Illness often generates resistance. A kind of strangeness replaces the familiar, reducing our comfort and pleasure in being in our own body and world. This sense of being is related to our inevitable perishability, in contrast to life being a spontaneous and meaningful interaction when we are healthy [54, 55].

Phenomenology is a philosophical discipline. Empirical research approaches inspired by phenomenology include a phenomenological attitude of openness and wonder, and thorough reflection on the basic structures of human experience [57].

Method

Methodology, design and methods

This qualitative, longitudinal study explored some of the impacts of BBAT on body experience in two participants who met DSM-5 [1] criteria for BED. This choice of design was deemed suitable for exploring the phenomenon of body experience in depth while searching for context and connections [4, 33]. We followed the participants over time during multiple periods of data collection [34]. In-depth interviews were chosen since, from a phenomenological perspective, they provide a privileged access to a person's experiences of his or her lifeworld [22, 57]. We also videoed one BBAT session with each participant. In addition, the participants wrote logs about the process, as is common in BBAT. In-depth interviews were the main data source, supported by video observations and patient logs.

Participants

The participants were recruited using a purposive sampling method called criterion sampling [33]. The two included participants had been diagnosed with BED and admitted for treatment at a specialized unit for eating disorders based on certain criteria. The number of participants was based on sufficient information being obtained to answer the research questions [34]; in-depth explorations can involve only a few participants if they provide rich material and are analysed thoroughly [33].

Two female participants with BED were included in the study: Participant A was in her twenties and Participant B was in her forties. Both reported a history of childhood trauma related to attachment, bullying and one of them being sexually abused. They suffered physical and mental health issues in addition to severe obesity and BED. Participant A was working, but participant B had not been working after having children. Both lived together with their children and the children's father. We have chosen Ann as pseudonym for participant A, and Claudia as pseudonym for participant B.

Treatment

The participants took part in treatment at a specialized unit for eating disorders, where CBT-e is the usual treatment. BBAT is offered as part of the treatment for patients who may especially benefit from it, when physiotherapists are available. Both participants took part in individual BBAT sessions in addition to CBT-e weekly from the start of the treatment process. The treatment trajectories were adjusted according to their individual needs throughout the process.

CBT-e consisted of sessions with a psychotherapist where they used daily written real-time recordings to become aware of eating-disorder behaviour. The participants were gradually able to eat more regularly by writing plans for what and when to eat during the day, stop gaining and stabilizing their weight. In CBT-e they also addressed processes maintaining their eating disorder, such as over-evaluation of shape and weight, dietary restraint and sensitivity to outside events and moods [12].

BBAT sessions involve the physiotherapist enhancing contact with "self" by focusing on basic movement principles when performing simple everyday movements (lying, sitting, standing, walking, and relational movements), use of the voice, and a special kind of massage. Postural balance, free breathing, and mental awareness are seen as inseparable key elements for improving movement quality. In a therapeutic environment, the patient is invited to explore and integrate flow, elasticity, rhythm, and intentionality in coordinated movement in relation to time, space, and energy. The sessions include reflections around the present experience. The therapist assists the bridging between the experiences from the sessions and everyday life [28, 37, 47, 48, 52].

The sessions often started with the participant lying down straight out on her back on a mat. The therapist sitting beside her at level with the abdomen. The therapist invited her to become aware of the contact between body and ground, becoming aware of the body, part by part by simply noticing without searching for anything in particular, starting with the legs, moving upwards with open curiosity. Then the therapist invited her to try to experience the whole body as one unity. To become aware of the breathing, the hands (of the patient) were resting on the abdomen, following this little movement with the fingertips, freeing the breathing by trying not to direct it in any way, and doing some small stretching movements from the centre, along the midline of the body. Ending this sequence very slowly, giving the body time, stretching and yawning, and in her own time sitting up. Then, together with the therapist reflecting upon her experience. In the next sequence sitting on a simple stool, facing each other, they usually did something quite similar, contacting the body with awareness. With accepting curiosity, noticing how they related to the ground with feet and pelvic area, adjusting to the midline, freeing the breathing, closing up very slowly and reflecting together. The same body awareness raising elements were usually performed when standing, where they also included some qi gong movements. Qi gong is traditional Chinese exercises from martial art, characterized as "meditative movements", that are widely practiced for their documented health benefits [2]. The BBAT-session often ended with a light massage, called BBAT-massage, with the participant in a lying down or sitting position.

Data production

Our plan was to follow each participant for 40 weeks, since the treatment was stipulated to take 20 weeks, with a follow-up session 20 weeks later. Since treatment for both participants lasted for more than 20 weeks, due to their individual needs, we followed Ann for 55 weeks and Claudia for 47 weeks. Before treatment started, the first author conducted individual in-depth interviews with both participants. Ann was interviewed again at the end of treatment, and at follow-up. Claudia was interviewed again 47 weeks into treatment. Since she received bariatric surgery, the ongoing treatment with CBT-e and BBAT was paused, and the second (and last) interview with her took place 1 week before surgery. Flexible designs are usual in qualitative research, being continually adjusted to ensure that it remains consistent with the objectives of a study [34].

Each interview lasted about 1.5 h. A guide developed for each interview revolved around themes relevant to the research question: experiences from BBAT, changes, relationship with one's own body, and possible relatedness between BBAT, body experience, and everyday life. With questions such as: "Can you tell me about your process with BBAT? Did you find it challenging in any way? Did you find aspects of the treatment especially useful or positive in any way?" Follow-up questions according to what the participants were telling, description of concrete situations to illustrate, as well as open questions were emphasized. The interviews were conducted in a treatment room of a specialized unit in calm and familiar surroundings. Each interview was audiotaped and transcribed verbatim. Figures 1 and 2 illustrate the timeline for each participant.

Analysis

The data material consisted of the transcriptions from five in-depth interviews. The purpose of phenomenological analysis is to capture and describe essential meanings of the phenomenon under investigation. Meaning is always multidimensional, involving several layers. This analytic process aimed to illuminate structural and thematic aspects of the lived experience of patients with BED receiving BBAT.

Van Manen [57] distinguished between holistic and selective reading. Holistic reading involves reading the text as a whole while trying to capture an overall essential phenomenological meaning from the participants' experiences, whereas selective reading involves reading the text several times, finding phrases or statements that seem particularly important for describing the phenomenon [57].

The first author wrote summaries after each interview, including descriptions of the mood and atmosphere. All of the authors read the interview material for each participant separately, using holistic reading, and then together discussed the core meanings. We then looked at the entire material from both participants, still using holistic reading, to determine an overall essential-meaning structure. A preliminary essential-meaning structure was identified. We then switched to selective reading, searching for phrases specific to the essential-meaning structure. Going back and forth between these two reading processes while reflecting and searching for meaning was the core part of the analysis.

The meaning structure that evolved and the five essential themes of the meaning structure are described in the Results.

Reflexivity

The first author is a physiotherapist, a trained BBAT therapist, and has a long clinical experience of working with patients with eating disorders. The other authors are physiotherapists and senior researchers, but are not BBAT therapists and do not have any clinical experience with this patient group. Therefore, repeated discussion with the other authors together with other reflective practices were practiced to maintain an analytic distance

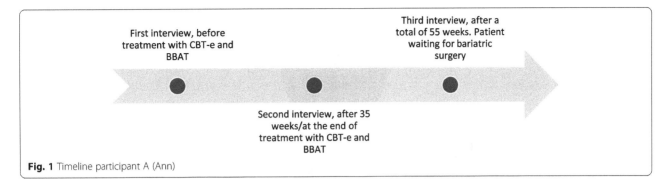

Fig. 1 Timeline participant A (Ann)

and avoid drifting away from the lived experience of the participants.

Results

The meaning structure "On the way from the body as problem to the body as possibility" is presented first. This is the overarching theme, a condensed description of the core content. This is followed by five sub-themes, "emotions", "movement", "pain", "calmness", and "self-experience", that describe important nuances and variations in the participants' treatment experiences and include quotes.

On the way from the body as problem to the body as possibility

In the first interview, the participants described their body as a problem. They used words such as fat, heavy, ugly, and felt that the body took up too much space, was painful, made them restless, and was problematic when moving. It was difficult to identify themselves with a body like this, and it was an obstacle to them participating fully in daily life. They described the body as an object, something strange, like something being experienced from a distance. They were ashamed of their big body, and saw fixing the body through bariatric surgery as the only way out of the misery they were experiencing.

The participants perceived BBAT as a process of getting to know their own bodies in new ways. When the participants were able to have new experiences in their own bodies, new possibilities were revealed. Changes occurred despite the body size, the wish to be thinner,

the pain, the difficult emotions, and the cultural stigma related to obesity not going away. They went from hating their own bodies to being more accepting. First and foremost, this was related to a shift from trying to avoid attending to their own bodies and ignoring bodily sensations and reactions, to being more present in their own bodies while moving and acting. This development meant being able to take in and experience sensations and bodily reactions, and implied being less overwhelmed or controlled by fatness, emotions, or pain. New body-based experiences and recognitions became available to them since they were now more in contact with their own body. Moments of calmness and well-being stood out as significant experiences, and an evolving experience of their body and self as more unified opened new ways of relating to others and acting in their everyday lives. As illustrated in Fig. 3, the changes they experienced were especially prominent when the participants described emotions, movement, pain, calmness, self-experience in relation to others, and practices in everyday life.

Emotions: from avoiding difficult emotions toward new emotional experiences

Both participants described that ever since they were small children they had used food to soothe themselves when experiencing uncomfortable emotions, which were often caused by difficulties in their lives. "I believe I have always done it. Like, when you are not fine, you can eat and then you will feel fine." Their body became gradually larger, which resulted in hating their own bodies

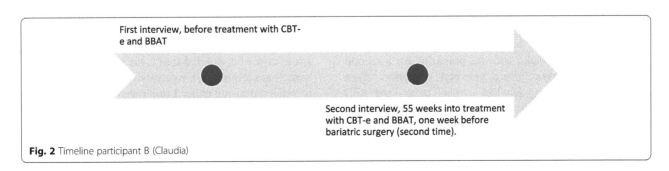

Fig. 2 Timeline participant B (Claudia)

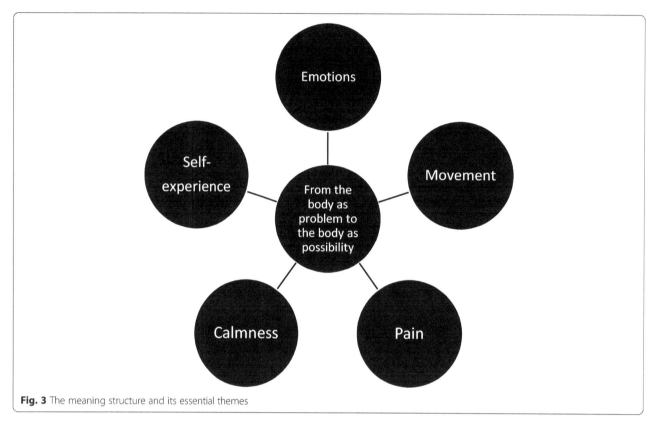

Fig. 3 The meaning structure and its essential themes

and made them feel ashamed and guilty. "I believe that I started to hate my own body when I was a little child." These uncomfortable emotions were avoided through more binge eating, which became a kind of automatic response that they had little awareness of. They described themselves as caught in a vicious circle.

> "My body is a result of how I have been through the years. So when I see my body, I think back on my past. Think of what made it this way. I walk around with a constant reminder of what happened."

They also described their large body as a manifestation of how they had failed to take care of themselves, a proof of self-hate.

They saw bariatric surgery as the only solution to their problems, and it was in consultations at the hospital preparing for bariatric surgery that they both were diagnosed with BED. "This was the first time *eating disorder* was mentioned. It had never been talked about before." Claudia had received bariatric surgery previously, but had regained the weight, and was preparing for a second operation. Ann was having her first operation. Even though it in one way felt like a relief to get the BED diagnosis, they were also afraid that the diagnose could become an empty excuse. Having to first receive conservative treatment with CBT-e and BBAT also led to disappointment and anger. "Afterwards I became a bit

angry. Why has nobody brought this up ever in my entire life?"

The CBT-e for BED helped them to gain more control over the binge eating, by making plans for the day and eating regularly. At the end of treatment, they had stopped gaining weight and their weight had stabilized, which is a goal in CBT-e. The CBT-e and BBAT made them more aware of the relationships between food, the body, and emotions. Even though the size of the body stayed the same, the emotions related to their body and the capability to experience emotions in general had started to change. Ann expressed less hate toward her body, while Claudia became aware how much she hated herself because of her size; she now realized that even though she sometimes had imagined that she loved her own body, it was not true. This was a painful recognition, but also a precondition and a motivation for future change.

> Then, I realized that what I say is just words. It is not the truth. … But I really want to, I hope, hope very much that I can change it. That I hope for. Because I am always a bit worried that I, my God I hate my body. I am a mother, a role model, and what I do will be reflected in my child. I don't want her to adopt my mistakes.

Both participants described how this treatment process had taught them more constructive ways to cope with difficult emotions: "...But now I have found things I can do instead of comfort eating." They could use elements from BBAT to calm down. Sometimes they started with listening to music, tidying the house, or talking to others before they could calm down through being present in the body here and now. This made it possible to endure emotional pain, and avoided turning to binge eating. However, sometimes they slipped back into old patterns with binge eating to avoid emotional pain. The ability of being present in their body facilitated more-positive emotions: "I feel a little in harmony, actually. I feel good, yes."

During the treatment process, both participants seemed to acknowledge that it was necessary to treat the eating disorder before receiving surgery. Becoming slimmer would not necessarily solve their problems:

> This was why I needed the operation so badly. To change it, to be able to be skinny. At the same time I thought "hallo," the problems won't go away, even though I become skinny. It is not in the head I will have an operation, it is actually in my stomach.

The participants did not believe that surgery and weight loss could solve all their difficulties. However, their current body size remained impossible for them to accept and live with, and both of them were still determined to receive surgery at the end of this process.

Movement: from guilt and discomfort toward joy and well-being

Both participants had suffered from negative experiences in gym classes at school and health clubs. They felt physical activity was something they ought to do, it was painful, they did not cope, and often they ended up avoiding it. Physical activity was associated with duty and guilt. Their associations with movement were different. They described finding joy in everyday movements like walking, dancing, swimming, and playing with their children. Moving more and differently became more integrated with their everyday lives during the BBAT process, both at work and at home. Ann made small changes to her physical activity, such as choosing to walk up stairs rather than taking the elevator, changing position more often, and going for small walks. Movement could improve well-being: "It is lovely to be back after having a walk outside, and feel that I have done something good for my body. Oooh yes, it makes me feel more comfortable with myself."

Ann also started to challenge herself in new ways, such as going hiking in the mountains because she felt a desire to do so. It was physically demanding, but she still got a lot of joy out of it:

> I struggled and wanted to give up on the way up. It was completely horrible. Oh my God, what have I started, what am I doing? I found out that I am in terrible shape (laughing). My physical condition is non-existent. But, I look at it with a bit of humor. I struggled and struggled and struggled. ...... And then, reaching the top...It was so delightful, damn (laughing)! It was so good! I think I have not been hiking in the mountains for at least 10 years. Since I finished secondary school. ...It was so good, hah, I made it!

Performing new movements opened new possibilities in everyday life, from intense physical activity (as described above) to greater awareness of muscle tension, relaxation, and body posture. Claudia described how she used to activate her muscles by simply tensing up when sitting down with others, believing that this would prevent the chair from collapsing under her weight. Once she became aware of this, she learned how to relax her muscle tension. Ann discovered that she could sit down on the floor with her child. She had previously considered this impossible and so had never tried it due to the potential for feeling embarrassed if she would need assistance getting back up. However, now she could sit there for a while when adjusting her position, playing with her daughter, and get back up again on her own. She could attend to her child in new ways. This change was deeply valuable to her as a mother, she had previously felt shameful for passively observing her child play. To get down on the floor and play was important for their contact and interaction.

Pain: from being controlled by pain toward living with pain through self-care

Both participants lived with pain, and worried that their body size could cause serious health problems. During the treatment process, they started to relate to pain in a different way that made them able to deal with it differently. Initially, they thought that there was nothing they could do when in pain other than taking painkillers. Now, they developed a different awareness of the pain, adjusting to it, trying to be more relaxed, and more able to cope with it. Claudia felt initially that the pain was her body telling her to take better care of herself. However, she ignored this even though she knew it was the wrong reaction. She found it difficult to take care of herself, which resulted in her pain intensifying. She slowly discovered that what she had learned in BBAT about adjusting her posture, letting go of muscle tension, breathing more freely, and being present and aware in her body reduced the pain: "I am actually constantly in pain. But, it is like when you do this (BBAT) it decreases. And, very often in these moments, it is actually really interesting, it feels as though the pain is letting go." She found new ways to relate to the pain, where the pain did not absorb her awareness. The way she related to her own body, the way she moved, was a way to take care of herself.

Coping with pain became gradually more integrated in their everyday lives. One of the participants related this to the necessity of learning to take care of herself more generally: "The BBAT therapist made me realize that I need to function well with myself, in order to function well around others. So, I need to take care of myself. I have not been good at that."

Calmness: toward finding calmness in the body even in demanding situations

Both participants reported that they had a trustful relationship with the BBAT therapist. They found her calm, which positively influenced the sessions. They especially enjoyed the massage, and the exercises they learned helped them to relax in a new way that encouraged bodily well-being. They described this as more than just a change in muscle tone, using words such as delightful and wonderful: "Oooh it is so good. It is so delightful. ... I get so relaxed." They described the calmness stemming from BBAT as a new way of anchoring themselves in their body, which influenced how they experienced themselves and the surroundings." My center, becoming aware of my breathing, being able to let go. A way of letting go of the outer world, while connecting to your inner world, if you might say it that way, actually my body." The contact with the body and the awareness of inner resources was inter-related.

Both participants had busy lives full of responsibilities and stress. Finding calmness became a useful strategy in demanding situations. Ann started to go to the restroom at work when she just needed to be with herself. Claudia had always experienced problems when trying to put her child to sleep. She discovered that doing a "lying down exercise" from BBAT when putting her daughter to bed helped both her child and herself to calm down, enabling the daughter to fall asleep quickly. The participant described it almost like magic. She started to do this regularly, including in situations when she needed to calm her daughter down. Ann too described how she could calm down others by finding her own calmness: "I feel more in control. I am somehow trying to calm them both down (partner and child). And I feel I succeed better than I used to."

Claudia described how she was able to take an MRI examination without taking valium for claustrophobia. She claimed that she would not have been able to do this without using what she had learned in BBAT about finding calmness in her body:

When having an MRI examination I would usually have said to my doctor that you have to give me

something for my claustrophobia...But I managed to get through it by landing my whole body on the MRI machine, to find my centre, to find my breathing. I was actually so incredibly proud. Even though I hated it...I did not need to take a Valium pill, and I managed to do it on my own with the tools she (the physiotherapist) has given me.

One of the participants also used elements from BBAT to calm down when being overwhelmed with flashbacks from traumas. Avoiding discomfort through eating was a major problem for both participants. Hence being able to find calmness from within was of great significance. Learning how to calm down was described as one of the most positive aspects of BBAT.

Self-experience: from self-hate toward finding strength from within

Initially the body size of the participants seemed to preoccupy their relationship with their own bodies. This influenced them when growing up, feeling limited by their body size in situations involving physical activity, not being able to dress as they wanted to, and avoiding certain social situations. During treatment, they seemed to open up to being more accepting of their own body. They were able to understand the body in new ways. One of the participants discovered that the hate toward her own body started after being sexually abused as a child. The other participant described how her body carried her history, and was a kind of reminder of difficulties from the past. One of the participants expressed how she started to relate to her body in a more accepting way: feeling safer and more familiar in her own body, and feeling more in balance. Both participants saw BBAT as a way of finding their true selves. They started to describe own body as part of their self, but still in a distanced language: "Him (my body) is not just there anymore. He has been included in me." There was a movement towards integration, but still a distance between herself and her experienced body.

Claudia who had realized the hate toward her own body longed for feeling proud in, and of, her own body. As her perspective on her own body changed, she was less preoccupied by its size. "My body is just a part of me. The way I look is a temporary situation. But I have value from being who I am. And I mean something to myself and for the people around me." In our last interview, she expressed that a more free and solid self-experience was related to letting go of the exclusively negative viewpoint of her body as being too big. Saying this out loud was an eureka moment for her. Gradually she felt more integrated with her own body, and this was associated with well-being and empowerment: "So I felt kind of ok, in here there is a lot like ...Him (my power), just have to be released again, if I can say it that way."

The participants felt like getting in touch with some kind of force from within. In these moments, the negativity toward their body size was less prominent. They felt more unified and stronger when opening up about their own body, and newly perceived their own body as a carrier of their life history, which increased their acceptance of their body:

> Previously I often thought that I could have just changed my whole body. It would not matter. I would gladly have done it. I would have done it on the day. But now, I get like no, no. Because this body, it influences me. In a way it proves what I have been through. I do not want to get rid of my body now. Its mine. I know it sounds all weird, but...

This participant talked about resisting the usual goals to change one's body, and that positive outcome usually is measured by this. Instead, she reclaims her body as part of the self – as having an energy of its own ("influences me"), holding and respecting her history as a survivor ("it proves what I have been through") and a reclaiming of her body as her own ("it is mine"). Finally, her qualification at the end "I know it all sounds weird" suggests that conceptualizing her body on these terms is a different discourse to what she has previously been positioned by – a shift from changing my/her body towards reclaiming my/her body to be me.

Their increasing ease with their own bodies opened up new possibilities in everyday life. One of the participants described how she now dared to do things that she used to hate, like wearing a bikini when going to a spa hotel with her husband. It was difficult, but she could do it. She was able to realize that people have different shapes and most of them have complexes. She was working on stopping comparing herself to others and accepting the way she was: "Everybody has different shapes, and almost everybody also has complexes."

Negative feelings toward her own body had previously prevented her from engaging socially. She started to put more effort into how she looked, and took up new activities and social engagements that she really enjoyed. In safe situations, it was easier to be themselves, especially with their children:

> Usually I will say that my body and myself are not there in a way. But I believe maybe that when I am with my daughter, then it melts together. Then it is just me. And then it is all ok...

Being a mother was a large part of the identity of both participants, something they felt proud about. They really wanted to be good role models for their children. They wanted their children to feel good about their own bodies, and focused on transferring this during the treatment process. But, even at the end of this process, one of the participants expressed worries and guilt about what she was still unable to offer her daughter. Her body prevented her from participating in activities commonly associated with being a mother, such as going on rides in an amusement park, jumping together on a trampoline, or going downhill on sledges during wintertime. She was afraid that her child could be bullied because of the size of her mother. She longed for strong self-confidence, realizing that it would be of great value to her daughter.

The five essential sub-themes and the meaning structure are integrated, meaning that the sub-themes both describe the meaning structure in depth and are part of it. The participants expressed how the treatment initiated change in relation to own body, to self, and to surroundings and others. They experienced feeling better, even though they still felt the need to lose weight.

Discussion

The findings of this study suggest that the participants experienced a change. They started out feeling fragmented, trying to avoid perceived unpleasant aspects about their body weight and shape, difficult emotions, own history, and pain, all rooted in the body, fighting themselves from within. Gradually they became able to accept these problems as part of who they had become, and started a process of feeling more integrated with their own bodies. We now discuss how this change was related to the treatment they received.

The participants described that in CBT-e they learned how to reduce the destructive eating patterns that they had previously used for coping with difficult emotions. Giving up habitual coping strategies, even destructive ones like binge eating, increases the need to receive training in new ways of coping, which in our case supports a synergistic combination of CBT-e and BBAT. In the BBAT sessions, the participants were encouraged to explore the sensations and reactions of their own bodies, and being present while performing simple movements with curiosity and acceptance. They reflected upon these experiences together with the therapist. Being aware of sensations, even when they are unpleasant, can be a new way of coping, as an alternative to avoidance. Instead of continuing to fight themselves from within, they started to get to know their bodies in new ways, by being more aware of aspects they previously had tried to avoid. As apparent in the participants' narratives, becoming aware through acceptance of one's own sensations may make a person able to get in touch with their own needs and resources.

From a phenomenological point of view, moving from avoidance to greater acceptance of one's own body is a crucial shift, since the body is understood as our mode of access to the world [26, 27]. From this perspective it is understandable that negative feelings for and problems with one's own body when performing practical tasks and socializing due to being overweight and experiencing pain and shame leads to experiencing a distance and alienation from the body and from certain dimensions of the everyday world. In this sense, discomfort and unpleasurable experience of being in their own body and world seemed to be the baseline condition in which the treatment process was started, which is how illness might be understood from a phenomenological point of view [55].

The female participants in this study had not suddenly fallen seriously ill, nor experienced a sudden marked bodily change. Instead, their habitual bodies were connected to different forms of objectifications and alienation that they had experienced. Objectification of one's own body can indicate a split in experience between body and self [55]. The participants initially judged themselves as having fat bodies, and were very sensitive to others judging them as being too big. They described their present body shape as a temporary state, something they wanted to get rid of, and a preoccupation with their body size seemed to grow alongside their self-hate. However, they were still able to perform their usual activities such as taking care of their children and participating in working life. The experienced split was related only to some aspects of their own body and the everyday world. These kind of challenges from being obese, such as overwhelming physical sensations and body shame is also described in other qualitative studies [7, 43]. This current study adds to the knowledge base in describing bodily experiences as a potential for change, a therapeutic access, and highlighting the central role of the body in BED.

The change the participants described represented a movement from an experience of fragmentation to feeling more unified and in harmony with their body. According to a phenomenological understanding, these opposing experiences are both rooted in the ambiguity of our bodily existence [27]. The process of the change that emerged from the participant's stories can also be understood as a movement from illness toward health.

BBAT is based on the clinical assumption that health issues may be related to a threefold lack of contact with the physical aspect of one's own body, physiological, and mental processes, and with the environment which includes both the physical reality and relationships with others ([10], 1997). From a phenomenological point of view, the lived body is mutually interrelated with the lived space, time, and relationships. Splits of different

kinds experienced between the body and self and the body and the world are anchored in this interrelationship [27]. In our context there seemed to be close links between experiencing integration between the body, self, and world, and increased contact with their own bodies. From a phenomenological perspective, the body has primacy in understanding and giving meaning to the world [26, 27]. Gendlin [15] emphasized how tuning in to one self or focusing inwards on one's own body may lead to a deeper and wiser self. Gendlin described this "felt sense" in the body as the physical experience of meaning in life [15].

Integrating parts of self into a more cohesive sense of identity is the goal in a diverse range of psychotherapies [36]. As a slow integration of parts of self became apparent in the process of the participants, they describe a calmer and more anchored way of being. Being aware of present sensations, making contact with own breathing, rhythms, and touch, and tuning into oneself and others—as participants practice in BBAT—are also ways of regulating activation in the nervous system [23, 35, 44, 45]. Turning off the defence-systems and achieving a more-optimal physiological activation, referred to as the window of tolerance, makes one able to take in and be aware of the situation, to explore, reflect, and learn, and stimulates social engagement [30, 35, 44, 45]. The experiences of the two participants in this study appeared to reveal a link between being in contact with their own bodies, integration of self and more-optimal neurophysiological regulation. Self-integration, regulation, and the window of tolerance are well known concepts within the field of trauma, developmental psychology and attachment theories [30, 31]. Both participants had troubled childhood experiences, and the treatment processes with BBAT seemed to be useful in addressing their experiences of some of the adverse consequences of childhood trauma. BBAT encouraged a greater acceptance and a new familiarity with their bodies that these participants initially wanted to get rid of, and avoid. They did not actually start to like these aspects, but they were able to relate to them and expressed that they were more able to live with them. They started to relate more to their current situation, to the here and now. Their experiences resonate with findings from other eating disorder research where an improved familiarity with one's own body was found to improve treatment outcomes [9].

Conclusions

Our study points to CBT-e and BBAT representing a synergistic combination of two treatment approaches in the treatment of patients with BED. Addressing the patients' relationships with their own bodies in therapy—BBAT in this study— may improve their health status. These insights indicate that bodily approaches such as BBAT might be useful for patients struggling with

BED and suffering from childhood trauma. The two participants` relation to own body was characterized by struggles with emotions, movement, pain, difficulties in relating to aspects of own history, body size, and shape.

Pragmatic validity refers to the relevance and usefulness of core findings and insights from qualitative studies in practice [22], for instance for clinicians treating these patients. Description of the essential dimensions of patients' experiences from two treatment processes in this study, combined with insights from the discussion, might encourage clinicians to become more curious about, and open to explore bodily awareness raising treatment approaches such as BBAT in the treatment of patients with BED also suffering from childhood trauma. This study indicates that contact with own body seems to facilitate a more integrated self and improved health for these patients, and more research in this area is needed.

Abbreviations
BBAT: Basic Body Awareness Therapy; BED: Binge Eating Disorder

Authors' contributions
MNA conducted the study under thorough supervision of EN and MR. All authors read and approved the final manuscript.

Authors' information
MNA is a physiotherapist, a trained BBAT therapist, and has a long clinical experience of working with patients with eating disorders. EN and MR are physiotherapists and senior researchers.

Competing interests
The authors declare that they have no competing interests.

Author details
[1]Department of Global Health and Primary Care, University of Bergen, Bergen, Norway. [2]Present address: Department of Eating Disorders, Division of Psychiatry, Haukeland University Hospital, Institute of Psychological Counselling , Bergen, Norway. [3]Department of Health and Caring Sciences, Western Norway University of Applied Sciences, Førde, Norway. [4]Department of Global Health and Primary Care, University of Bergen, Bergen, Norway.

References
1. American Psychiatric Association. (2013). Diagnostic and statistical manual of mental disorders (5th ed.). Washington, DC: Author.
2. Abbott R, Lavretsky H. Tai chi and Qigong for the treatment and prevention of mental disorders. Psychiatr Clin North Am. 2013;36(1):109–19. http://doi.org/. https://doi.org/10.1016/j.psc.2013.01.011.
3. Ágh T, Kovács G, Supina D, Pawaskar M, Herman BK, Vokó Z, Sheehan DV. A systematic review of the health-related quality of life and economic burdens of anorexia nervosa, bulimia nervosa, and binge eating disorder. Eat Weight Disord. 2016;21(3):353–64. https://doi.org/10.1007/s40519-016-0264-x.
4. Bengtsson J. Å forske i sykdoms- og pleieerfaringer: livsverdensfenomenologiske bidrag. Kristiansand: Høyskoleforlaget; 2006.
5. Bratland-Sanda S, Sundgot-Borgen J, Rø Ø, Rosenvinge JH, Hoffart A, Martinsen EW. Physical activity and exercise dependence during inpatient treatment of longstanding eating disorders: an exploratory study of excessive and non-excessive exercisers. Int J Eat Disord. 2010;43(3):266–73. https://doi.org/10.1002/eat.20769.
6. Cash TF, Deagle EA. The nature and extent of body-image disturbances in anorexia nervosa and bulimia nervosa: a meta-analysis. Int J Eat Disord. 1997;22(2):107–26. https://doi.org/10.1002/(SICI)1098-108X(199709)22:2<107::AID-EAT1>3.0.CO;2-J.
7. Christiansen B, Borge L, Solveig Fagermoen M. Understanding everyday life of morbidly obese adults-habits and body image. Int J Qual Stud Health Well Being. 2012;7(1):17255. https://doi.org/10.3402/qhw.v7i0.17255.
8. Danielsen M. Disturbed body image and compulsive exercise in female eating disorder patients (unpublished doctoral dissertation). Trondheim: Norwegian University of Science and Technology; 2016.
9. Danielsen M, Rø Ø. Changes in body image during inpatient treatment for eating disorders predict outcome. Eat Disord. 2012;20(4):261–75. https://doi.org/10.1080/10640266.2012.689205.
10. Dropsy J. Leva i sin kropp: kroppsuttryck och mänsklig kontakt. Stockholm: Aldus; 1997.
11. Dropsy J. Den harmoniska kroppen. Stockholm: Natur och Kultur; 1988.
12. Fairburn CG. Cognitive behavior therapy and eating disorders. London/New York: Guilford Press; 2008.
13. Fairburn CG, Peveler RC, Jones R, Hope R, Doll HA. Predictors of 12-month outcome in bulimia nervosa and the influence of attitudes to shape and weight. J Consult Clin Psychol. 1993;61(4):696–8.
14. Garner DM. Body image and anorexia nervosa. In: Cash TF, Pruzinski T, editors. Body image: a handbook of theory, research, and clinical practice. New York: Guilford Press; 2002. p. 295–303.
15. Gendlin ET. Focusing. 5th ed. New York: Bantam Books; 2007.
16. Griffen N, Hildebrandt. Mirror exposure therapy for body image disturbances and eating disorders: a review. Clinical Psychology Review. 2018;65:163–74 Web.
17. Grucza RA, Przybeck TR, Cloninger CR. Prevalence and correlates of binge eating disorder in a community sample. Compr Psychiatry. 2007;48(2):124–31. https://doi.org/10.1016/j.comppsych.2006.08.002.
18. Gummer R, Giel KE, Schag K, Resmark G, Junne FP, Becker S, et al. High levels of physical activity in anorexia nervosa: a systematic review. Eur Eat Disord Rev. 2015;23(5):333–44. https://doi.org/10.1002/erv.2377.
19. Helsedirektoratet (2017). Nasjonal faglig retningslinje for tidlig oppdagelse, utredning og behandling av spiseforstyrrelser. Retrieved from www.helsedirektoratet.no/retningslinjer/spiseforstyrrelser: Helsedirektoratet.
20. Keizer A, Engel MM, Bonekamp J, Van Elburg A. Hoop training: a pilot study assessing the effectiveness of a multisensory approach to treatment of body image disturbance in anorexia nervosa. Eat Weight Disord. 2018. https://doi.org/10.1007/s40519-018-0585-z.
21. Kessler RC, Berglund PA, Chiu WT, Deitz AC, Hudson JI, Shahly V, et al. The prevalence and correlates of binge eating disorder in the World Health Organization world mental health surveys. Biol Psychiatry. 2013;73(9):904–14. https://doi.org/10.1016/j.biopsych.2012.11.020.
22. Kvale S, Brinkmann S. Det kvalitative forskningsintervju. 2nd ed. Oslo: Gyldendal Norsk Forlag; 2009.
23. Levine PA. In an unspoken voice: how the body releases trauma and restores goodness. Berkeley: North Atlantic Books; 2010.
24. Lewer, M., Kosfelder, J., Michalak, J., Schroeder, D., Nasrawi, N., & Vocks, S. (2017). Effects of a cognitive-behavioral exposure-based body image therapy for overweight females with binge eating disorder: A pilot study. J Eat Disord, 5, 43. doi:http://dx.doi.org.pva.uib.no/https://doi.org/10.1186/s40337-017-0174-y
25. Lewer M, Nasrawi N, Schroeder D, Vocks S. Body image disturbance in binge eating disorder: a comparison of obese patients with and without binge eating disorder regarding the cognitive, behavioral and perceptual component of body image. Eat Weight Disord. 2016;21(1):115–25. https://doi.org/10.1007/s40519-015-0200-5.
26. Merleau-Ponty M. Kroppens fenomenologi. Danish translated ed. Oslo: Pax Forlag; 1994.
27. Merleau-Ponty M. Phenomenology of perception. English ed. New York: Routledge; 2012.
28. Norsk Institutt for Basal Kroppskjennskap (NIBK) (2017). Om: Hva er Basal Kroppskjennskap (BK). Retrieved from: www.nibk.org
29. National Institute for Health and Care Excellence (2017). NICE guideline, Eating disorders: recognition and treatment. Retrieved from: www.nice.org.uk.
30. Nordanger DØ, Braarud HC. Regulering som nøkkelbegrep og toleransevinduet som modell i en ny traumepsykologi. Tidsskrift for Norsk Psykologforening. 2014;51(7):530–6.

31. Ogden P, Fisher J. Sensorimotor Psychotherapy: interventions for trauma and attachment. New York: W. W. Norton & Company, Inc.; 2015.

32. Olsen AL, Skjaerven LH. Patients suffering from rheumatic disease describing own experiences from participating in basic body awareness group therapy: a qualitative pilot study. Physio Theory Pract. 2016;32(2):98–106.

33. Patton MQ. Qualitative research & evaluation methods. 3rd ed. Thousand Oaks: Sage Publications; 2002.

34. Polit DF, Beck CT. Nursing research: generating and assessing evidence for nursing practice. 9th ed. China: Wolters Kluwer Health / Lippincott Williams & Wilkins; 2012.

35. Porges SW. The polyvagal theory: neurophysiological foundation of emotions, attachment, communication and self-regulation. New York: W. W. Norton & Company; 2011.

36. Power MJ. The multistory self: why the self is more than the sum of its autoparts. J Clin Psychol. 2007;63:187–98. https://doi.org/10.1002/jclp.20341.

37. Probst M, Skjaerven LH. Physiotherapy in mental health and psychiatry. Poland: Elsevier Health Sciences; 2017.

38. Probst M, Majeweski ML, Albertsen MN, Catalan-Matamoros D, Danielsen M, De Herdt A, et al. Physiotherapy for patients with anorexia nervosa. Adv Eat Disord. 2013;1(3):224–38. https://doi.org/10.1080/21662630.2013.798562.

39. Probst M. Body experience in eating disorder patients, Unpublished doctoral dissertation. Leuven: K. U. Leuven; 1997.

40. Probst M, Vandereycken W, Van Coppenolle H, Pieters G. Body size estimation in eating disorder patients: testing the video distortion method on a life-size screen. Behav Res Ther. 1995;33(8):985–90. https://doi.org/10.1016/0005-7967(95)00037-X.

41. Rasmussen TH. Kroppens Filososf: Maurice Merleau-Ponty. Copenhagen: Semi-forlaget; 1996.

42. Rosen JC. Body image assessment and treatment in controlled studies of eating disorders. Int J Eat Disord. 1996;20(4):331–43. https://doi.org/10.1002/(SICI)1098-108X(199612)20:4<331::AID-EAT1>3.0.CO;2-O.

43. Rørtveit K, Åström S, Severinsson E. The feeling of being trapped in and ashamed of one's own body: a qualitative study of women who suffer from eating difficulties. Int J Ment Health Nurs. 2009;18(2):91–9. https://doi.org/10.1111/j.1447-0349.2008.00588.x.

44. Salvesen KT, Wæstlund M. Mindfulness og medfølelse: en vei til vekst etter traumer. Oslo: Paw Forlag; 2015.

45. Siegel DJ. The mindful brain: reflection and attunement in the cultivation of well-being. New York: W.W. Norton & Company; 2007.

46. Skjaerven LH, Mattsson M, Catalan-Matamoros D, Parker A, Gard G, Gyllensten AL. Consensus on core phenomena and statements describing Basic Body Awareness Therapy within the movement awareness domain in physiotherapy. Physiother Theory Pract. 2019;35(1):80-93. https://www.tandfonline.com/doi/abs/10.1080/09593985.2018.1434578?journalCode=iptp20.

47. Skjaerven LH, Gard G, Sundal MA, Strand LI. Reliability and validity of the body awareness rating scale (BARS), an observational assessment tool of movement quality. Eur J Phys. 2015;17(1):19–28. https://doi.org/10.3109/21679169.2014.992470.

48. Skjaerven LH, Kristoffersen K, Gard G. An eye for movement quality: a phenomenological study of movement quality reflecting a group of physiotherapists' understanding of the phenomenon. Physiother Theory Pract. 2008;24(1):13–27. https://doi.org/10.1080/01460860701378042.

49. Stice, E. (2002). Body image and bulimia nervosa. In T. F. Cash & T Pruzinsky, T., Body image: a handbook of theory, research, and clinical practice (pp. 304–321). New York: Guilford Press.

50. Striegel-Moore RH, Cachelin FM, Dohm F-A, Pike KM, Wilfley DE, Fairburn CG. Comparison of binge eating disorder and bulimia nervosa in a community sample. Int J Eat Disord. 2001;29(2):157–65. https://doi.org/10.1002/1098-108X(200103)29:2<157::AID-EAT1005>3.0.CO;2-8.

51. Striegel-Moore RH, Franko DL. Body image issues among girls and women. In: Cash TF, Pruzinsky T, editors. Body image: a handbook of theory, research, and clinical practice. New York: Guilford Press; 2002. p. 183–91.

52. Sundal M-A. Bevegelseskvalitet - et utrykk for helse og velvære (master's thesis). Bergen: University of Bergen; 2007.

53. Supina D, Herman BK, Frye CB, Shillington AC. Knowledge of binge eating disorder: a cross-sectional survey of physicians in the United States. Postgrad Med. 2016;128(3):311–6. https://doi.org/10.1080/00325481.2016.1157441.

54. Svenaeus F. The body uncanny – further steps towards a phenomenology of illness. Med Health Care Philos. 2000;3(2):125–37.

55. Svenaeus F. Sykdommens mening -og møtet med det syke mennesket. Oslo: Gyldendal Akademiske; 2005.

56. Thornquist E. Kommunikasjon: teoretiske perspektiver på praksis i helsetjenesten. 2nd ed. Oslo: Gyldendal Norsk Forlag; 2009.

57. Van Manen M. Phenomenology of practice. New York: Routledge; 2014.

58. Vancampfort D, Vanderlinden J, De Hert M, Soundy A, Adámkova M, Skjaerven LH, et al. A systematic review of physical therapy interventions for patients with anorexia and bulimia nervosa. Disabil Rehabil. 2014;36(8):628–34. https://doi.org/10.3109/09638288.2013.808271.

59. Vocks S, Wächter A, Wucherer M, Kosfelder J. Look at yourself: can body image therapy affect the cognitive and emotional response to seeing oneself in the mirror in eating disorders? Eur Eat Disord Rev. 2008;16(2):147–54. https://doi.org/10.1002/erv.825.

60. WHO. (2009/10). Health behaviour in school-aged children: World Health Organization Collaborative Cross-National Survey. Retrieved from www.hbsc.org/publications/datavisualisations/body_image.html

61. Wonderlich SA, Gordon KH, Mitchell JE, Crosby RD, Engel SG. The validity and clinical utility of binge eating disorder. Int J Eat Disord. 2009;42(8):687–705.

62. Zahavi D. Faeomenologi. Fredriksberg, Copenhagen: Roskilde Universitetsforlag; 2003.

63. Ziser K, Mölbert SC, Stuber F, Giel KE, Zipfel S, Junne F. Effectiveness of body image directed interventions in patients with anorexia nervosa: a systematic review. Int J Eat Disord. 2018;51(10):1121–7. https://doi.org/10.1002/eat.22946.

2

Validation of the arabic version of the binge eating scale and correlates of binge eating disorder among a sample of the Lebanese population

Rouba Karen Zeidan[1,2,3†], Chadia Haddad[4,5†], Rabih Hallit[6], Marwan Akel[2,7], Karl Honein[6], Maria Akiki[6], Nelly Kheir[8], Souheil Hallit[2,6*†] ⓘ and Sahar Obeid[2,4,9*†]

Abstract

Objectives: To test the psychometric properties of the Arabic version of the Binge Eating Scale (BES), a self-questionnaire assessing binge eating, in a sample of the Lebanese population. The secondary objective was to evaluate factors associated with binge eating.

Methods: This cross-sectional study, conducted between January and May 2018, enrolled 811 adult participants from all districts of Lebanon. The BES was administered to study its psychometric properties. The sample was divided into two separate samples (405 for sample 1 and 406 for sample 2). An exploratory factor analysis was executed on Sample 1, followed by a confirmatory factor analysis on Sample 2 using the structure obtained in Sample 1. Three hierarchical stepwise linear regressions were conducted to assess factors associated with binge eating.

Results: The factor analysis suggested a two-factor structure for the BES explaining a total of 41.4% of the variance. All items could be extracted from the list. The internal consistency of the measurement was adequate (Cronbach's alpha = 0.86). The confirmatory factor analysis revealed an adequate fit to the model with satisfactory Maximum Likelihood Chi-Square/Degrees of Freedom (χ^2/df), Steiger-Lind RMSEA, Joreskog GFI, and AGFI. Higher BMI, depression, anxiety, emotional eating, greater body dissatisfaction, and more pressure from media to lose weight were associated with higher binge eating. Higher expressive suppression facet score was associated with lower binge eating.

Conclusion: The Arabic version of BES could be a useful tool for screening and assessing the binge eating behaviors in clinical practice and research. Also, being dissatisfied with one's body size, having a history of sexual abuse, family history of binge eating, increased depressive/anxiety symptoms, and lower self-esteem seem to be associated with higher BES scores.

Keywords: Binge eating disorder, Psychometrics properties, Depression, Body dissatisfaction, Emotions, Anxiety

* Correspondence: souheilhallit@hotmail.com; saharobeid23@hotmail.com
†Rouba Karen Zeidan and Chadia Haddad are first co-authors.
†Souheil Hallit and Sahar Obeid are last co-authors.
²INSPECT-LB: Institut National de Santé Publique, Epidemiologie Clinique et Toxicologie, Beirut, Lebanon
Full list of author information is available at the end of the article

Plain English summary

The Binge Eating Scale in its Arabic version is a suitable instrument to screen for binge eating among the Lebanese population. Some factors (body dissatisfaction, having a history of sexual abuse, a family history of binge eating, greater depressive/anxiety symptoms, and lower self-esteem) seem to be associated with higher binge eating.

Introduction

Binge eating disorder (BED) is an eating disorder (ED) characterized by recurrent episodes of binge eating (BE) without subsequent compensatory behaviors, such as self-induced vomiting or over-exercising [1]. Diagnosis of BED according to the Diagnostic and Statistical Manual of Mental Disorders, Fifth Edition (DSM-5), is based on the occurrence of at least one BE episode per week for three consecutive months; these episodes are characterized by the consumption of larger amounts of food in a short period when compared to the typical amounts for most people under similar circumstances, accompanied by a sense of loss of control over eating and a marked distress during these episodes [2]. A large study, pooling results from different community surveys done across 14 countries (high, upper-middle, and lower-middle income countries), revealed an average lifetime prevalence estimate of 1.9% [0.2–4.7%] for BED, making it the most common ED [3, 4]. Previous reviews showed that ED most frequently afflict young Western females within high-income and industrialized Western Europe and North America, but do also occur in diverse countries and cultures worldwide [5, 6]. While there is a stabilization - even a lowering -of the incidence rates of eating disorders in Caucasian North American and Northern European groups, increased rates appear in Arab and Asian countries [7]. In fact, as Lebanon and other countries in the Middle Eastern and North African region continue to develop and undergo epidemiologic transition and cultural change, the burden of ED in these countries is rising [8, 9].

Binge eating correlates

The disorder was found to be more common in the population suffering from obesity [3], and it has been associated with several psychiatric (anxiety, depression, obsessive–compulsive disorder) and physical comorbidities (diabetes, hypertension) [3, 6, 10]. Previous findings showed that adverse childhood experiences (i.e. sexual/physical abuse, other parental problems), parental depression, negative self-evaluation, vulnerability to obesity, and repeated exposure to negative comments about shape, weight, or eating were associated with BED. These findings support the hypothesis that risk factors associated with BED are similar to those with psychiatric disorders and obesity [11]. Furthermore, researchers have found BED to share characteristics with substance use and addictive disorders [12, 13]. In addition to other similarities, BED and substance use can both be induced by stress and major life events, childhood trauma, neglect, and abuse [14–16].

Arabic countries and Lebanon

BED research remains limited in the Arab-speaking countries, despite overweight and obesity being important public health issues. Older studies done in Egypt [17, 18] first showed evidence for BE, without reporting any prevalence rates. Other findings revealed that 82% of females and 76% of males (mean age = 20 years) had experienced at least one BE episode [19]. In Jordan, results showed that 16.9% of females (mean age = 13) reported BE and 1.8% were considered as suffering from BED [20]. The prevalence of BE in Saudi Arabia females was 68.8% [21], whereas it ranged between 24 to 36% in the United Arabic Emirates [22].

In Lebanon, previous research revealed that 21.2% of one-university students were vulnerable to developing an ED, whereas 11.4% had already been diagnosed with an ED. The same paper showed that anxiety was the most important associated factor with ED, followed by stress, body image and depression [23]. Another Lebanese study published in 2017, done on patients suffering from ED and comparing BED to anorexia nervosa and bulimia nervosa, concluded that outpatients were mostly single, female, young adults coming from middle and high socio-economic backgrounds, suffering from severe ED symptoms and depression [24].

The binge eating scale (BES)

Due to the high prevalence of BE, its comorbidities and outcomes, there was a need to establish instruments for its measurement. The BES, developed by Gormally et al. [25], is an interesting tool both in terms of evaluation and monitoring of these patients, because it can be used for the purposes of screening, evaluation of severity or monitoring of the disorder. The BES has been found to demonstrate a very good internal consistency (between 0.85 and 0.90) and a good construct validity [25, 26].

The scale has previously been validated in many populations, including but not limited to, French [27], Italian [28], Spanish [29], Persian [30] and Malay [31]. The BES was found to have good validity and internal consistency in the original normative samples, consisting of overweight women seeking behavioral treatment for obesity [25]. A study done by Imperatori et al. that evaluated the dimensionality and psychometric properties of the Italian version of the BES had found that the scale had good internal consistency (α = 0.89), with a moderate mean inter-item correlation [28]. A study done among a sample of 1008 women from the general population confirmed that the BES presents a one-dimensional factorial structure, with very good construct reliability and convergent validity, and with a very good retest reliability [32]. In the French version, one factor was obtained that explained 61% of the total variance [27]. Timmerman had also found a good test-retest reliability r = 0.87 for the total BES score. However, its factor structure is still controversial. Although Gormally et al. originally proposed a two-dimensional structure, dividing the items into cognitive and behavioral BE, results on its dimensionality are contradictory. In a Mexican [33] and a Malay study [31], results showed a two-factor structure through exploratory factor analyses; they also found the unidimensional structure to be relevant as well. A study done on Portuguese women found the BES to have a good fit for a one-factor structure using a confirmatory factor analysis [32]. This was also supported by a French study done in non-clinical and clinical samples using an exploratory factor analysis [27]. A recent Spanish study targeting a sample of Spanish college students reported that a one-factor model fit the data best [34].

To our knowledge, no publication has reported the validation and the psychometric properties of the BES in the Arabic-speaking population. In addition, there is a need for more evidence about the factor structure of the scale in non-clinical samples, because most research has tested the validity of BES in specific populations (sufferers of overweight/obesity and bariatric surgery patients). Also, no study has been previously done on the Lebanese general population in order to study BED and its correlates when compared to healthy individuals. Hence, the aim of this work was to test the psychometric properties of an Arabic version of the BES, by establishing the factorial structure, its internal consistency and its construct validity in a sample of the Lebanese population. Another objective was to study BED's associated sociodemographic and clinical factors.

Methods

Participants

This study was cross-sectional, conducted between January and May 2018. Out of 1000 distributed questionnaires, 811 (81.1%) were completed and collected. Enrollment of participants was done using a proportionate random sample from all Lebanese Mohafazat (Beirut, Mount Lebanon, North, South and Bekaa). Each Mohafaza is divided into Caza (stratum). In each Caza, two villages were randomly selected from the list of villages provided by the Central Agency of Statistics in Lebanon. Participants were randomly selected from each village. In each selected village, the questionnaire was distributed randomly to the households, based on random sampling technique to select the included house. Houses were assigned identification numbers and

randomized according to an online software, Research Randomizer (www.randomizer.org). All members in the household, if eligible, were invited to participate in the study; those who accepted our invitation were asked to fill out the questionnaire. The same methodology was used in previous papers [35–38].

Prior to participation, individual subjects were briefed on the study objectives and methodology, and were assured of the anonymity of their participation. Individuals agreeing to participate in the study were then asked to read through and sign off on a written, informed consent form. Individual participants had the right to accept or refuse participation in the study with no financial compensation provided in exchange for individual participation. All participants above 18 years of age were eligible to participate. Excluded participants were those suffering from a clinical mental impairment affecting cognition and their ability to comprehend participation in the study and/or their ability to answer the questionnaire. The sample was divided into two separate samples for the validation of the BES (Study 1: $n = 406$ for the exploratory analysis; Study 2: $n = 405$ for the confirmatory analysis; therefore, $406/16 = 25$ participants per item were included in study 1 and $405/16 = 25$ per item in study 2 as well). However, the whole sample ($n = 811$) was used to study the factors correlated with BE.

The mean age of the participants in the first sample was 27.96 ± 11.83 years, with 67.6% females. The majority (73.3%) had a university level of education, single (66.1%), with a low monthly income (76.4%). Almost all participants drank caffeine (90.5%), 31.7% were smokers and 3.1% were drank alcohol. The majority practice physical activities (63.6%). More than half of the participants had normal weight (52.4%), 27.2% were overweight and only 11.1% suffered from obesity, with a mean BMI of 24.10 ± 4.98 Kg/m^2. The majority of the participants (82.8%) had no binge eating, 15.9% had moderate BE and 1.3% had severe BE.

In sample 2, the mean age of the participants was 27.19 years, 65.4% were females, 67.8% were single, and 79.2% had low monthly income. The majority had a university degree (73.1%) and 61.3% practice physical activities. More than half of the participants had normal weight (53.8%), 26.5% had overweight and only 12.4% suffered from obesity, with a mean BMI of 24.60 ± 5.55. No significant difference was found between the two samples ($p > 0.05$) (Table 1).

Minimal sample size calculation

Comrey and Lee suggested that a minimum of 10 observations per item is necessary in order to avoid computational difficulties [39]. Since the BES questionnaire contains 16 questions, a minimal sample of 160 patients was needed to conduct an exploratory factor analysis.

Table 1 Characteristics of the study sample

	Total Frequency (%)	Sample 1 Frequency (%)	Sample 2 Frequency (%)	p-value
Gender				
Male	270 (33.5%)	131 (3.4%)	139 (34.6%)	0.518
Female	536 (66.5%)	273 (67.6%)	263 (65.4%)	
Marital status				
Single	533 (67.0%)	263 (66.1%)	270 (67.8%)	0.395
Married	230 (28.9%)	120 (30.2%)	110 (27.6%)	
Widowed	11 (1.4%)	7 (1.8%)	4 (1.0%)	
Divorced	22 (2.8%)	8 (2.0%)	14 (3.5%)	
Education level				
Primary	24 (3.1%)	11 (2.8%)	13 (3.3%)	0.760
Complementary	61 (7.8%)	34 (8.7%)	27 (6.9%)	
Secondary	125 (15.9%)	60 (15.3%)	65 (16.6%)	
University	574 (73.2%)	288 (73.3%)	286 (73.1%)	
Monthly income				
No income	340 (45.1%)	168 (44.4%)	172 (45.7%)	0.140
< 1000 USD	247 (32.8%)	121 (32.0%)	126 (33.5%)	
1000–2000 USD	117 (15.5%)	56 (14.8%)	61 (16.2%)	
> 2000 USD	50 (6.6%)	33 (8.37%)	17 (4.5%)	
Smoking				
Yes	246 (30.8%)	127 (31.7%)	119 (29.8%)	0.572
No	554 (69.2%)	274 (68.3%)	280 (70.2%)	
Alcohol				
Yes	32 (4.2%)	12 (3.1%)	20 (5.4%)	0.124
No	724 (95.8%)	372 (96.9%)	352 (94.6%)	
Caffeinated beverages				
Yes	721 (90.0%)	362 (90.5%)	359 (89.5%)	0.646
No	80 (10.0%)	38 (9.5%)	42 (10.5%)	
Practicing sport activities				
Yes	490 (62.4%)	248 (63.6%)	242 (61.3%)	0.501
No	295 (37.6%)	142 (36.4%)	153 (38.7%)	
BMI categories				
Underweight	65 (8.3%)	36 (9.3%)	29 (7.3%)	0.733
Normal	417 (53.1%)	204 (52.4%)	213 (53.8%)	
Overweight	211 (26.9%)	106 (27.2%)	105 (26.5%)	
Obese	92 (11.7%)	43 (11.1%)	49 (12.4%)	
	Mean ± SD	Mean ± SD	Mean ± SD	
Age (in years)	27.59 ± 11.76	27.96 ± 11.83	27.19 ± 11.68	0.354
BMI (Kg/m^2)	24.35 ± 5.28	24.10 ± 4.98	24.60 ± 5.55	0.182

Procedure

Data collection was performed through personal interviews with participants by trained clinical psychologists, independent of this study, who clinically evaluated the level of psychiatric illness to exclude those who have psychiatric problems.

Materials

The questionnaire used during the interview was in Arabic, the native language of Lebanon. The first part assessed the sociodemographic details and other characteristics of the participants (i.e. age, gender, monthly income, education level, details about alcohol and caffeine intake, drug addiction, smoking status, and the physical activity). The monthly income was divided into four levels: no income, low income < 1000 USD; intermediate income 1000–2000 USD; and high income > 2000 USD. Afterward, the monthly income was categorized in three groups: low (no income with income < 1000 USD), intermediate (1000–2000 USD) and high (> 2000 USD) income, since the majority of the participants were university students and they have no real income. The heights and weights of participants were measured to calculate the Body Mass Index (BMI) (kg/m^2). The BMI was classified into four categories: underweight (< $18.5\,kg/m^2$), normal ($18.5.24.9\,kg/m^2$), overweight ($25.0.29.9\,kg/m^2$), and obese ($30.0\,kg/m^2$) [40]. The Total Physical Activity Index was calculated by multiplying the intensity, duration, and frequency of daily activity, with higher scores indicating better physical activity.

The second part of the questionnaire consisted of behavioral practices of certain eating habits among participants. Questions about eating disorders were identified from previous articles [41–43]. Questions included: "Do you take your weight daily?", "Do you follow a diet to lose weight?", "Do you exercise to lose weight?", "Do you take diet pills to lose weight?", "Do you take laxatives or vomit to lose weight?", "Do you starve yourself to lose weight?"

Binge eating scale (BES)

The BES was originally developed to identify participants with binge eating within people suffering from obesity [25]. It does not specify a time frame and presents a series of differently weighted statements for each item, from which respondents select the statement that best describes their attitudes and behaviors. This yields a continuous measure of BE pathology of 0–46. Scores of ≥27 have conventionally served as a cutoff value for identifying the presence of severe BE and 17 as a cutoff value for mild or no BE [44]. The BES has good test-retest reliability (r = 0 .87, p < 0 .001). The Arabic version can be found at the end of this manuscript (Additional file 1: Appendix 1).

Body dissatisfaction subscale of the eating disorder inventory-second version (EDI-2)

In the present study, the body dissatisfaction score was measured from the eating disorder inventory (EDI-2) subscale since the body dissatisfaction could cause restraint eating which in turn causes susceptibility to loss of control over eating. The scale assesses the levels of dissatisfaction with the overall body shape and specific body parts. The body dissatisfaction subscale consists of nine items, measured in 4-point Likert scales, ranging from 0 (sometimes, rarely, never) to 3 (always). Five questions were reversed

while doing the score calculation. The total score was calculated by summing the nine items. The total score ranged from 0 to 27. Higher scores are indicative of greater body dissatisfaction [45]. In this study, the Cronbach's alpha was 0.779.

Self-esteem scale

The Rosenberg Self-Esteem10-item scale is used to assess beliefs and attitudes regarding general self-worth by using 4-point scales ranging from 1 (strongly disagree) to 4 (strongly agree). Five questions (3, 5, 8, 9, and 10) were reversed while doing the score calculation. Higher scores indicated a more negative self-esteem [41]. In this study, the Cronbach's alpha was 0.759.

Perceived stress scale (PSS)

The questions in the PSS ask about feelings and thoughts during the last month [42]. The PSS is a ten-item scale with answers ranging from never (0) to almost always (4). Items 4, 5, 7, and 8 are reversed items. The total score is calculated by summing the 10 items with higher scores indicating more perceived stress [42]. In this study, the Cronbach's alpha was 0.709.

HAM-A scale

The Hamilton Anxiety Rating Scale (HAM-A), recently validated in Lebanon [43], consists of 14 symptom-defined elements, and targets both psychological and somatic symptoms. Each item is scored on a basic numeric scoring of 0 (not present) to 4 (severe). Higher scores indicating higher anxiety. In this study, the Cronbach alpha's was 0.912. The Arabic version can be found at the end of this manuscript (Additional file 1: Appendix 2).

HAM-D scale

The Hamilton Scale for Depression (HAM-D), validated in Lebanon [46], is a multiple item questionnaire used to provide an indication of the severity of depression and is widely used in research. The 17-item version was used in this study, with each item rated on either a 3- or 5-point scale and summed to obtain the total score. Higher scores indicated higher depression. In this study, the Cronbach's alpha was 0.879. The Arabic version can be found at the end of this manuscript (Additional file 1: Appendix 3).

Emotion regulation questionnaire (ERQ)

The ERQ is used to measure respondents' tendency to regulate their emotions in two ways: (1) Cognitive Reappraisal and (2) Expressive Suppression. The cognitive reappraisal facet is a way of managing and controlling attention and cognitively changing the meaning of emotionally stimulating stimuli. It is considered a healthy emotion regulation strategy [47]. The expressive suppression involves inhibition of emotionally expressive behavior, thereby changing the emotional impact of a situation [48]. It is considered a less healthy emotion regulation strategy [48]. A 10-item scale ranging from 1 (strongly disagree) to 7 (strongly agree). Items 1, 3, 5, 7, 8, 10 make up the Cognitive Reappraisal facet and items 2, 4, 6, 9 make up the Expressive Suppression facet. Each facet's scoring is kept separate. The higher the scores, the greater the use of the emotion regulation strategy [49]. In this study, the Cronbach's alpha values for the Cognitive Reappraisal facet and for the Expressive Suppression facet were 0.764 and 0.658 respectively.

Emotional eating scale (EES)

The EES scale is composed of twenty-five items, with three derived subscales: anger, anxiety and depression. Participants rate the extent to which certain feelings lead to the urge to eat, using a five-point Likert scale ranging from 0 (no desire to eat) to 4 (an overwhelming urge to eat). Higher scores indicate a reliance on using food to help manage emotions [50]. The original EES scale had a good test-retest reliability (r = 0.79, $p < 0.001$) and an acceptable internal consistency Cronbach alpha = 0.81 [51]. In this study, the Cronbach's alpha was 0.957.

State adult attachment measure (SAAM)

The SAAM measures 3 different aspects of adult attachment: security, anxiety, and avoidance. A secure attachment style is characterized by the confidence in the emotional balance in times of distress and need [52]. The attachment anxiety is characterized by a perceived failure to handle threats, which intensifies need for interpersonal closeness, love, and support [53]. The attachment avoidance is characterized by discomfort with interpersonal intimacy, hesitancy to trust others, and preventing the emotions evoked by rejection by others [54]. It consists of 21 Likert style questions ranging from 1 (strongly disagree) and 7 (strongly agree). Higher scores indicate high features of attachment [55]. In this study, the Cronbach's alpha was 0.827.

Dutch restrained eating scale

The Dutch Restrained Eating Scale, recently validated in Lebanon [35], is a ten-item scale that assesses the frequency of dieting behaviors by using a five-point Likert scale, ranging from 1 (never) to 5 (always). The score for this scale was obtained by dividing the total items score by the total number of items. A higher score would indicate a higher degree of restrained eating. In this study, the Cronbach's alpha was 0.928. The Arabic version can be found at the end of this manuscript (Additional file 1: Appendix 4).

Translation procedure

The forward and backward translation method was conducted in all the scales except for the HAMD, HAMA and Dutch restrained eating scales (the Arabic versions of these scales can be found in Additional file 1: Appendices 2, 3 and 4). The forward translation was done by a single bilingual translator, a health professional familiar with the terminology of the scales, whose native language is Arabic and is fluent in English. An expert committee formed by healthcare professionals and a language professional verified the Arabic translated version. A backward translation was then performed by a native English speaker translator, fluent in Arabic, and unfamiliar with the concepts of the scales. All translators were informed of the purpose of the study prior to translation. The back-translated English questionnaire was subsequently compared to the original English one, by the expert committee, aiming to discern discrepancies and to solve any inconsistencies between the two versions. Revisions of problematic questions were communicated with the translators involved for version updating. The process of forward-back translation was repeated until all ambiguities disappeared.

Statistical analysis

The SPSS software version 23 was used to conduct data analysis. Descriptive analyses were done using counts and percentages for categorical variables, mean, standard deviation for continuous measures. As for the reduction of data, an exploratory factor analysis was first executed to detect groups of factors that are reported together and are associated with BE in the sample. After confirming sample adequacy with the Kaiser–Meyer–Olkin (KMO) index and Bartlett's Chi-square test of sphericity, factors (groups of items) were extracted using a principal component analysis method and a promax rotation since factors were correlated. We retained factors with an Eigenvalue higher than one; we confirmed their adequacy with a Scree plot, taking into account interpretability of the results. Items with factor loading > 0.4 were considered as loading on a factor. We also checked the reliability using Cronbach's alpha values for different factors and the total scale.

Second, a confirmatory factor analysis was carried out in Sample 2 using the maximum likelihood method for discrepancy function to assess the structure of the instrument. We also reported several goodness-of-fit indicators: the Relative Chi-square (χ^2/df), the Root Mean Square Error of Approximation (RMSEA), the Goodness of Fit Index (GFI) and the Adjusted Goodness of Fit Index (AGFI). The value of χ^2 divided by the degrees of freedom (χ^2/df) has a low sensitivity to sample size and may be used as an index of goodness of fit (cut-off values:< 2–5). The RMSEA tests the fit of the model to the covariance matrix. As a guideline, values of< 0.05 indicate a close fit and values below 0.11 an acceptable fit. The GFI and AGFI are Chi-square-based calculations independent of degrees of freedom. The recommended thresholds for acceptable values are ≥ 0.90 [56].

The Student T-test was used to compare continuous variables in two groups. Pearson correlation was used for linear correlation between continuous variables. For categorical variables, the Chi-square and Fisher exact tests were used. The ANOVA F tests were used when comparison involved three or more groups. A post-hoc analysis, Bonferroni test was used to compare the mean difference between groups. Three hierarchical stepwise linear regressions were conducted, taking the BES as the dependent variable. All variables that showed a $p < 0.1$ in the bivariate analysis were considered as important variables to be entered in the model in order to eliminate potentially confounding factors as much as possible. These three models were built by adding variables to the previous model at each step in order to determine that the newly added variables would improve the proportion of explained variance of the dependent variable by the model (improve in adjusted R^2). In the first model the sociodemographic were considered as predictor factors, in the second model the eating behaviors were added, and in the third models the emotion scales were added. The stepwise method was used to simultaneously remove variables that were weakly correlated to the dependent variable. Thus, the final variables kept in the model better explain the distribution. A P-value of less than 0.05 was considered significant.

Results
Study 1
Exploratory factor analysis
None of the BES items were removed. All items could be extracted from the list since no items over-correlated to each other (r > 0.9), had a low loading on factors (< 0.3) or because of a low communality (< 0.3). The factor analysis for the BES was run over the first sample (Total $n = 406$). The BES items converged over a solution of two factors that had an Eigenvalue over 1, explaining a total of 41.40% of the variance. A Kaiser-Meyer-Olkin measure of sampling adequacy of 0.925 was found, with a significant Bartlett's test of sphericity ($p < 0.001$). According to the promax rotated matrix, the first factor accounted for 34.59% of the variance and the second factor accounted for 6.81%. Table 2 displays the items and factor loadings for the factors. The first factor, which seems to index behavioral manifestations of BED, had strong loadings on 12 items. The second factor, which seemed to index feelings/cognitions, had high loadings on the remaining four items. Moreover, a Cronbach's alpha of 0.862 was found for the full scale, 0.826 for Factor 1 and 0.682 for Factor 2.

Table 2 Promax rotated matrix of the Arabic version of the Binge Eating Scale

BES Items	Factor loadings	
	Factor 1	Factor 2
BES 4	0.750	
BES 15	0.677	
BES 10	0.619	
BES 9	0.588	
BES 13	0.586	
BES 5	0.581	
BES 11	0.553	
BES 7	0.552	
BES 16	0.544	
BES 2	0.516	
BES 8	0.508	
BES 3	0.433	
BES 1		0.877
BES 6		0.775
BES 14		0.664
BES 12		0.475
Cronbach alpha	0.826	0.682
Percentage of variance explained	34.59%	6.81%

Cronbach alpha of the whole scale = 0.862
Factor 1: Behavioral manifestations; Factor 2: Feelings/Cognitions

Correlation factors
Table 3 displays the correlation factors between each item of the BES and the whole scale. The correlation factors ranged between 0.459 and 0.660 for an individual item. To note that all factors were highly significantly correlated with the whole scale with $p < 0.001$ for all of them.

Study 2
Confirmatory factor analysis
A confirmatory factor analysis was run on sample 2 ($n = 405$), using the two-factor structure obtained in Sample 1. The following results were obtained: the Maximum Likelihood Chi-Square = 257 and Degrees of Freedom = 104, which gave a $\chi^2/df = 2.4$. For non-centrality fit indices, the Steiger-Lind RMSEA was 0.12 [0.104–0.155]. Moreover, the Joreskog GFI equaled 0.799 and AGFI equaled 0.706.

Bivariate analysis conducted on the whole sample
A significantly higher mean of BES was found in participants with primary education compared to university education (13.04 vs. 8.65, $p = 0.022$). A significantly higher mean of BES was found in patients following a diet (10.75 vs. 8.23, $p < 0.001$), patients who exercised to lose weight (10.26 vs. 8.20, $p < 0.001$), patients who vomited or took laxatives to lose weight (13.37 vs. 8.51, $p < 0.001$), taking

Table 3 Correlation for each item and the total score of the Binge eating scale (BES)

Item	Pearson Correlation coefficient[a]	p-value
BES 4	0.620	< 0.001
BES 15	0.579	< 0.001
BES 10	0.660	< 0.001
BES 9	0.559	< 0.001
BES 13	0.570	< 0.001
BES 5	0.526	< 0.001
BES 11	0.648	< 0.001
BES 7	0.616	< 0.001
BES 16	0.575	< 0.001
BES 2	0.584	< 0.001
BES 8	0.548	< 0.001
BES 3	0.602	< 0.001
BES 1	0.562	< 0.001
BES 6	0.583	< 0.001
BES 14	0.629	< 0.001
BES 12	0.584	< 0.001

[a]Corrected item-total correlations were reported

diet pills (13.00 vs. 8.57, p < 0.001), starving self to lose weight (12.20 vs. 8.19, p < 0.001), weighing daily (10.75 vs. 8.58, $p = 0.005$) compared to those who don't follow these eating habits. Also, a significantly higher mean of BES was found in participants that have been insulted (12.40 vs. 8.53, $p < 0.001$), experienced physical abuse (11.26 vs. 8.80, $p = 0.014$) and sexual abuse (15.37 vs. 8.74, $p = 0.003$), felt pressure from media to lose weight (12.80 vs. 8.18, $p < 0.001$), and have a family history of eating disorders (11.86 vs. 8.17, p < 0.001) compared to those who do not agree with these statements.

In addition, more BE was significantly associated with more body dissatisfaction (r = 0.245, p < 0.001), more restrained eating (r = 0.096, $p = 0.008$), higher BMI (r = 0.200, p < 0.001), higher perceived stress (PSC score) (r = 0.194, p < 0.001), higher anxiety (HAMA) (r = 0.344, p < 0.001), higher depression (HAMD) (r = 0.399, p < 0.001), higher state adult attachment scale-avoidance (r = 0.083, $p = 0.021$), and higher emotional eating (EES scale) (r = 0.259, p < 0.001). However, higher emotional regulation cognitive reappraisal facet, expressive suppression facet (r = − 0.113, p = 0.003 and r = − 0.095, $p = 0.013$ respectively), and a more secure adult attachment (r = − 0.173, p < 0.001) were significantly associated with less BE (Table 4). No significant association was found between BES and gender ($p = 0.758$).

Multivariable analysis conducted on the whole sample

The results of a first linear regression, considering the BES to be the dependent variable and the sociodemographic as independent variables, showed that a primary level of education compared to illiteracy (Beta = 4.203) was associated with more BE.

A second linear regression, taking the BES as the dependent variable and the opinion about eating habits as independent variables, showed that a higher BMI (Beta = 0.252), starving self to lose weight (Beta = 1.618), pressure from media to lose weight (Beta = 3.036), sexual abuse (Beta = 4.991), receiving comments from the family concerning losing weight (Beta = 1.162) and family history of eating disorders (Beta = 1.582) were associated with more BE.

A third linear regression, taking the BES as dependent variable and the scales and opinion about eating habits as independent variables, showed that higher BMI (Beta = 0.185), higher depression (Beta = 0.298), higher anxiety (Beta = 0.070), higher emotional eating (Beta = 0.072), greater body dissatisfaction (Beta = 0.198) and greater pressure from media to lose weight (Beta = 2.010), were associated with higher BE. Higher expressive suppression facet (Beta = − 0.108) was associated with lower BE (Table 5).

Discussion

Although there are numerous studies on BE behavior worldwide, studies on this behavior in Lebanon remain limited. Therefore, this cross-sectional study aimed to evaluate the psychometric properties of an Arabic version of the BES and to determine the correlates of BED among a sample of the Lebanese population. The results demonstrated that the Arabic version of this tool had a very good internal consistency and a good construct validity. Our results also showed that higher BMI, starving self to lose weight, feeling pressure from media to lose weight, a history of sexual abuse, a family history of eating disorders, higher depression and anxiety scores, higher emotional eating, and greater body dissatisfaction were associated with higher BE scores. A low monthly income compared to no income and a higher expressive suppression facet score were associated with lower BE scores.

Validation of the BES

The factor structure of the Arabic version revealed two main factors, in line with the Malay study [31]. Also, another study done among a sample of bariatric surgery candidates on the replication and evaluation of BES found that a two-factor model improved significantly the model fit, supporting the presence of a higher-order severity factor accounting for a significant amount of variance [57]. The internal consistency of our results was similar to the original scale [25] and to the other versions (Cronbach alpha ranged from 0.85 [30] to 0.93 [27]).

Table 4 Bivariate analysis of the factors associated with the Binge Eating Scale (BES) score

	BES Mean ± SD	p-value
Education level[+]		
Primary	13.04 ± 9.36	0.022
Complementary	8.65 ± 6.86	
Secondary	9.95 ± 8.25	
University	8.65 ± 7.43	
Monthly income		
Low	8.69 ± 7.44	0.459
Intermediate	9.64 ± 8.84	
High	9.26 ± 7.75	
Dieted to lose weight (past 30 days)		
Yes	10.75 ± 7.74	< 0.001
No	8.23 ± 7.47	
Exercised to lose weight (past 30 days)		
Yes	10.26 ± 7.72	< 0.001
No	8.20 ± 7.47	
Vomited or taken laxatives to lose weight (past 30 days)		
Yes	13.37 ± 7.29	< 0.001
No	8.51 ± 7.53	
Taken diet pills to lose weight (past 30 days)		
Yes	13.00 ± 7.69	< 0.001
No	8.57 ± 7.53	
Starving self to lose weight (past 30 days)		
Yes	12.20 ± 8.20	< 0.001
No	8.19 ± 7.30	
Daily weighing		
Yes	10.75 ± 7.92	0.005
No	8.58 ± 7.53	
Receiving comments from the family concerning losing weight		
Yes	10.90 ± 8.03	< 0.001
No	8.12 ± 7.32	
Have you been insulted		
Yes	12.40 ± 8.46	< 0.001
No	8.53 ± 7.34	
Have you been physically abused		
Yes	11.26 ± 8.68	0.014
No	8.80 ± 7.53	
Have you been		

Table 4 Bivariate analysis of the factors associated with the Binge Eating Scale (BES) score (Continued)

	BES Mean ± SD	p-value
sexually abused		
Yes	15.37 ± 10.26	0.003
No	8.74 ± 7.44	
Have you been in a bad romantic relationship		
Yes	10.44 ± 8.10	0.001
No	8.38 ± 7.38	
Family history of eating disorders		
Yes	11.86 ± 8.08	< 0.001
No	8.17 ± 7.33	
Pressure from TV, magazine to lose your weight		
Yes	12.80 ± 8.07	< 0.001
No	8.18 ± 7.31	
	Pearson correlation coefficient	p-value
Body dissatisfaction score	0.245	< 0.001
Restrained eating scale	0.096	0.008
Body Mass Index	0.200	< 0.001
Perceived stress scale	0.194	< 0.001
Anxiety	0.344	< 0.001
Depression	0.399	< 0.001
ERQ cognitive reappraisal facet	−0.113	0.003
ERQ expressive suppression facet	−0.095	0.013
State Adult attachment scale-security	−0.173	< 0.001
State Adult attachment scale-avoidance	0.083	0.021
EES scale	0.259	< 0.001

ERQ Emotional Regulation Questionnaire, EES Emotional Eating Scale
[+]One-way analysis of variance (ANOVA): post hoc analysis for education level: primary vs. complementary (13.04 vs. 8.65, p = 0.111); primary vs. secondary (13.04 vs. 9.95, p = 0.449); primary vs. university (13.04 vs. 8.65, p = 0.04); complementary vs. secondary (8.65 vs. 9.95, p = 1.000); complementary vs. university (8.65 vs. 8.65, p = 1.000); secondary vs. university (9.95 vs. 8.65, p = 0.536)

All BES items positively correlated above 0.5, indicating good predictive value. This was similar to a study done by Grupski et al. that found nearly half of the items correlated positively [58], but conflicted with the study done by Greeno et al., which found very low correlations for most items [44]. The inconsistency in results between the studies might be due to methodological differences and/or sample characteristics. The results obtained in Sample 1

Table 5 Multivariable analysis

	Unstandardized Beta	Standardized Beta	p-value	Confidence interval	
				Lower Bound	Upper Bound
Model 1: Linear regression taking the Binge Eating Scale (BES) as dependent variable and the sociodemographic characteristics as independent variables.					
Primary vs illiterate* level of education	4.203	0.093	0.009	1.039	7.376
Variables entered: Education level.					
Model 2: Linear regression taking the Binge Eating Scale (BES) as dependent variable and the opinion about eating habits as independent variables.					
Pressure from TV, magazine to lose your weight (yes vs no*)	3.036	0.151	< 0.001	1.522	4.549
Body Mass Index (BMI)	0.252	0.173	< 0.001	0.149	0.356
History of sexual abuse (yes vs no*)	4.991	0.103	0.005	1.505	8.478
Receiving comments from the family concerning losing weight	1.162	0.071	0.061	−0.052	2.376
Starving self to lose weight (past 30 days) (yes vs no*)	1.618	0.083	0.029	0.167	3.069
Family history of eating disorders (yes vs no*)	1.582	0.083	0.030	0.153	3.012
Variables entered = BMI, education level, Exercised to lose weight (past 30 days), Dieted to lose weight (past 30 days), Vomited or taken laxatives to lose weight (past 30 days), Taken diet pills to lose weight (past 30 days), Starving self to lose weight (past 30 days), Daily weighing, Receiving comments from the family concerning losing weight, Have you been insulted, Have you been physically abused, Have you been Sexually abused, Have you been in a bad romantic relationship, family history of eating disorders, Pressure from TV, magazine to lose your weight.					
Model 3: Linear regression taking the Binge Eating Scale (BES) as dependent variable and the eating disorders and emotion scales and opinion about eating habits as independent variables.					
Depression	0.298	0.298	< 0.001	0.216	0.380
Body dissatisfaction	0.198	0.157	< 0.001	0.103	0.292
Emotional eating	0.072	0.192	< 0.001	0.046	0.098
Body Mass Index (BMI)	0.185	0.131	< 0.001	0.082	0.288
Pressure from TV, magazine to lose your weight (yes vs no*)	2.010	0.102	0.005	0.610	3.410
Anxiety	0.070	0.094	0.025	0.009	0.131
Emotional regulation expressive suppression facet	−0.108	−0.072	0.038	−0.210	−0.006
Variables entered in the model: BMI, education level, Exercised to lose weight (past 30 days), Dieted to lose weight (past 30 days), Vomited or taken laxatives to lose weight (past 30 days), Taken diet pills to lose weight (past 30 days), Starving self to lose weight (past 30 days), Daily weighing, Receiving comments from the family concerning losing weight, Have you been insulted, Have you been physically abused, Have you been Sexually abused, Have you been in a bad romantic relationship, family history of eating disorders, Pressure from TV, magazine to lose your weight, Body dissatisfaction score, Restrained eating scale, Perceived stress scale, HAMA, HAMD, ERQ cognitive reappraisal facet, ERQ expressive suppression facet, State Adult attachment scale and EES scale					

*Reference group

were confirmed later on a second sample, which further solidify the validation of the scale in its Arabic form. The findings of this study demonstrate that the Arabic version of the BES is a valid scale for the assessment of BED the Lebanese general population. This easy-to-administer 16-item scale can be used to provide relevant information about the symptoms and the severity of the BED.

Binge eating correlates

The results of our study showed that increased depression scores were associated with higher scores on the BES. In fact, comorbid depression has been found in 30–50% of patients suffering from BE [59, 60]. The association between these two disorders has been the subject of many studies and predicts symptoms of BE in white women [61], middle school students [62] and adolescent girls [63]. In a recent meta-analysis, previous authors [55, 64] have shown a reciprocal relationship between depression and BED; in fact depression can be a risk factor for BED, or a result of it. This dual relationship would emphasize the presence of common predisposing factors between the two disorders. Another possible explanation presented in previous studies is that exposure to a food with a pleasant taste is able to cause the activation of brain regions involved in feelings of reward in patients with a high level of negative emotions (such as depression) [65].

Moreover, the multivariable analysis indicates that higher anxiety was associated with more pronounced BE, in line with previous studies [66–69]. The comorbidity rate between BED and anxiety disorders is high, with a lifetime prevalence of 37% among patients suffering from BED [70]. In fact, anxiety disorders are the second most common comorbidity in BED subjects [70]. On the one hand, some studies suggest that anxiety may be secondary to overeating [71]; some genetic data has shown that people with BED have an increased risk of anxiety symptoms, regardless of BMI [72]. On the other hand, retrospective studies have shown that anxiety has been identified as a risk factor for various eating disorders, including BED [73, 74]; more specifically, anxiety disorders generally precede eating disorders, with early onset during childhood [75, 76]. Whether anxiety is a risk factor for BED or a consequence, the literature suggests that BE and anxiety can be linked through common vulnerability factors such as distal stress (for example, during childhood), proximal stress, and childhood stressors (teasing and bullying) [76].

More body dissatisfaction was also associated with greater BE, according to our results. In addition to the risk factors, the triggering and sustaining factors of the BED have been identified and integrated into a recent Tuschen-Caffier and Hilbert model [77]. Based on this model, the authors pointed out that there are different external and internal stressors (relationship conflicts, exposure to food, impulsivity, low self-esteem, tensions) that can trigger BE. In addition, they add that over concentration on weight and shape, as well as body dissatisfaction, are risk factors for the etiology, maintenance and relapse of BED. This model is in line with other studies [78, 79]. Other studies have shown that subjects with BED exhibited negative emotions and had more negative body-related cognitions when examining their own bodies than healthy controls [80, 81]. This disturbed perception of body size and shape may be related to a biased treatment of information, which is now considered an important factor in the development and maintenance of body image disruption in the pathology of the BED [82, 83]. Therefore, this erroneous treatment

of information will be an important aspect of psychotherapeutic work in BED subjects [84, 85].

In our study, higher expressive suppression facet was associated with lower BE. Strategies for regulating inappropriate negative emotions (such as disappointment, suffering, loneliness, etc.) have been shown to play a role in the appearance and maintenance of BED [86, 87]. More particularly, people with BED tend to suppress and ruminate on their undesirable emotions, resulting in an increase in psychopathological beliefs and symptoms [88, 89]. Emotional eating was found to be positively related to BE. In fact, overeating just for emotional reasons and cravings may turn quickly into BED [90].

According to our results, a positive and significant correlation was found between a history of sexual abuse and BED, in line with several studies [91, 92]. A correlation was found between traumatic events and eating disorders used as a means of self-management of feelings and experiences related to trauma. Specifically, previous findings [91, 93] have found that 30% of children with an eating disorder have been sexually abused, with BED, in particular, being linked to trauma as a means of self-protection. The cycle of frenzy/overeating behaviors seems to reduce awareness of thoughts and emotions as a way of evading negative emotions that accompany traumatic experiences [94].

As for BMI, our results showed that a higher BMI was associated with higher BED. Previous findings [95] have focused on the significant correlation between obesity and BED and hypothesize that these conditions may potentially contribute to one another and/or exacerbate each other. The co-existence between obesity and BED is of concern due to the medical and psychosocial risks [96].

As for pressure from media, our results indicated a positive correlation between BE and pressure from media to lose weight. Few studies exist specifically on BED and media, but different studies have shown a direct relationship between media exposure, media pressure, eating disorders, body dissatisfaction, and negative affect [97].

Finally, results of our study indicate that a family history of eating disorders was associated with higher BE. BED was found to aggregate strongly within families, which may reflect genetic influences [98, 99]. Also, a population-based twin study found a considerable heritability estimate (41%) for the BED, thus supporting the heritable nature of this syndrome [72]. Although family and twin studies have suggested the role of genetics in BED, gene studies have not confirmed the involvement of a particular gene or genetic pathway. Both genetic and environmental factors are now hypothesized to work together in order to influence the risk for eating disorders. Studies have not yet reached a definitive measure of the extent of relative importance of each component due to the difficulty in statistically distinguishing between the genetic and environmental factors involved in the association [100].

Limitations

There are many limitations in this study. First, we relied on participants to provide us with information on BE, depression, anxiety, emotion regulation, body dissatisfaction and others using self-report questionnaires. Second, the study has a cross sectional design and causality cannot be proved. Third, although the sample was randomly selected across Lebanese regions, the majority was young, single, with a university degree, which hinders the generalizability of the results. Fourth, test-retest reliability was not assessed. Finally, many scales used were not validated in Lebanon. Nonetheless the authors believe that their findings are noteworthy, since they are consistent with other recent studies.

Conclusion

The results showed that the Arabic version of the BES could be used as an appropriate measure for assessing BE behaviors in clinical practice and research. The findings suggest that the scale is bi-factorial. The study also found that having higher BES scores is associated with being dissatisfied with one's body size, having a history of sexual abuse, a family history of BE, increased depressive/anxiety symptoms, and lower self-esteem.

Comprehensive treatments should address the psychological antecedents and consequences of this behavior, as they are critically important to the syndromal nature of BED. It is in this context that the role of mental health professionals is essential in providing interventions for long-term BE episodes and dealing with negative emotions and related psychological factors. Moreover, this study suggests putting into action certain behaviors aimed at preventing individuals from engaging in excessive food consumption: 1) an increase and improvement in family and relational interactions, 2) the promotion of a positive body image, and better self-esteem by professionals and in media 3) prevention of depression and anxiety. These recommendations must be incorporated into intervention programs on eating behavior. Psychologists, counselors, and nutritionists should also work together to improve people's eating habits, nutritional status, and mental health.

Abbreviations

AGFI: Adjusted Goodness of Fit Index; ANOVA: Analysis of variance; BE: Binge eating; BED: Binge eating disorder; BES: Binge Eating Scale; BMI: Body Mass Index; DSM-5: Diagnostic and Statistical Manual of Mental Disorders, Fifth Edition; DSM-IV: Fourth Edition of the Diagnostic and Statistical Manual of Mental Disorders; ED: Eating disorder; EDI-2: Body dissatisfaction subscale of the Eating Disorder Inventory-second version; EDNOS: Eating disorder not otherwise specified; EES: Emotional eating scale; ERQ: Emotion Regulation Questionnaire; GFI: Goodness of Fit Index; HAM-A: Hamilton Anxiety Rating Scale; HAM-D: Hamilton Scale for Depression; KMO: Kaiser–Meyer–Olkin; PSS: Perceived Stress Scale; RMSEA: Root Mean Square Error of Approximation; SAAM: State adult attachment measure

Acknowledgments

Cloe Zeidan for proofreading the article. All participants who helped us filling the questionnaire.

Authors' contributions

SO and SH conceived and designed the survey. MA, KH, MA and NK performed the data collection and entry. CH and SH were involved in the statistical analysis and data interpretation. RZ and CH wrote the manuscript. All authors read the manuscript, critically revised it for intellectual content, and approved the final version.

Competing interests

The authors declare that they have no competing interests.

Author details

[1]Faculty of Public Health, Lebanese University, Fanar, Lebanon. [2]INSPECT-LB: Institut National de Santé Publique, Epidemiologie Clinique et Toxicologie, Beirut, Lebanon. [3]CERIPH: Center for Research in Public Health, Pharmacoepidemiology Surveillance Unit, Faculty of Public Health, Lebanese University, Fanar, Lebanon. [4]Psychiatric Hospital of the Cross, P.O. Box 60096, Jall-Eddib, Lebanon. [5]Univ. Limoges, UMR 1094, Neuroépidémiologie Tropicale, Institut d'Epidémiologie et de Neurologie Tropicale, GEIST, 87000 Limoges, France. [6]Faculty of Medicine and Medical Sciences, Holy Spirit University of Kaslik (USEK), Jounieh, Lebanon. [7]School of Pharmacy, Lebanese International University, Beirut, Lebanon. [8]Faculty of Pedagogy, Holy Family University, Batroun 5534, Lebanon. [9]Faculty of Arts and Sciences, Holy Spirit University (USEK), Jounieh, Lebanon.

References

1. Dingemans AE, Bruna MJ, van Furth EF. Binge eating disorder: a review. Int J Obes Relat Metab Disord. 2002;26:299–307.
2. American Psychiatric Association, editor. Diagnostic and statistical manual of mental disorders. 5th ed: American Psychiatric Association; 2013. Available from: https://psychiatryonline.org/doi/book/10.1176/appi.books.9780890425596
3. Kessler RC, Berglund PA, Chiu WT, Deitz AC, Hudson JI, Shahly V, et al. The prevalence and correlates of binge eating disorder in the World Health Organization world mental health surveys. Biol Psychiatry. 2013; 73:904–14.
4. Myers LL, Wiman AM. Binge eating disorder: a review of a new DSM diagnosis. Res Soc Work Pract. 2014;24:86–95.
5. Hoek HW. Epidemiology of eating disorders in persons other than the high-risk group of young Western females. Curr Opin Psychiatry. 2014; 27:423–5.
6. Smink FR, van Hoeken D, Hoek HW. Epidemiology of eating disorders: incidence, prevalence and mortality rates. Curr Psychiatry Rep. 2012;14:406–14.
7. Pike KM, Hoek HW, Dunne PE. Cultural trends and eating disorders. Curr Opin Psychiatry. 2014;27:436–42.
8. Erskine HE, Whiteford HA, Pike KM. The global burden of eating disorders. Curr Opin Psychiatry. 2016;29:346–53.

9. Popkin BM, Adair LS, Ng SW. Global nutrition transition and the pandemic of obesity in developing countries. Nutr Rev. 2012;70:3–21.

10. Agh T, Kovacs G, Pawaskar M, Supina D, Inotai A, Voko Z. Epidemiology, health-related quality of life and economic burden of binge eating disorder: a systematic literature review. Eat Weight Disord. 2015;20:1–12.

11. Fairburn CG, Doll HA, Welch SL, Hay PJ, Davies BA, O'Connor ME. Risk factors for binge eating disorder: a community-based, case-control study. Arch Gen Psychiatry. 1998;55:425–32.

12. Gearhardt AN, White MA, Potenza MN. Binge eating disorder and food addiction. Curr Drug Abuse Rev. 2011;4:201–7.

13. Schulte EM, Grilo CM, Gearhardt AN. Shared and unique mechanisms underlying binge eating disorder and addictive disorders. Clin Psychol Rev. 2016;44:125–39.

14. Allison KC, Grilo CM, Masheb RM, Stunkard AJ. High self-reported rates of neglect and emotional abuse, by persons with binge eating disorder and night eating syndrome. Behav Res Ther. 2007;45:2874–83.

15. Harrington EF, Crowther JH, Henrickson HC, Mickelson KD. The relationships among trauma, stress, ethnicity, and binge eating. Cultur Divers Ethnic Minor Psychol. 2006;12:212–29.

16. Naish KR, Laliberte M, MacKillop J, Balodis IM. Systematic review of the effects of acute stress in binge eating disorder. Eur J Neurosci. 2018.

17. Nasser M. Comparative study of the prevalence of abnormal eating attitudes among Arab female students of both London and Cairo universities. Psychol Med. 1986;16:621–5.

18. Nasser M. The psychometric properties of the eating attitude test in a non-Western population. Soc Psychiatry Psychiatr Epidemiol. 1994;29:88–94.

19. Dolan B, Ford K. Binge eating and dietary restraint: a cross-cultural analysis. Int J Eat Disord. 1991;10:345–53.

20. Mousa TY, Al-Domi HA, Mashal RH, Jibril MA-K. Eating disturbances among adolescent schoolgirls in Jordan. Appetite. 2010;54:196–201.

21. Rabie MA, Abo-El-Ezz NF, El-din M. Anxiety and social anxiety symptoms among overweight females seeking treatment for obesity. Curr Psychiatr Ther. 2010;17:13–20.

22. Schulte SJ. Predictors of binge eating in male and female youths in the United Arab Emirates. Appetite. 2016;105:312–9.

23. Doumit R, Khazen G, Katsounari I, Kazandjian C, Long J, Zeeni N. Investigating vulnerability for developing eating disorders in a multi-confessional population. Community Ment Health J. 2017;53:107–16.

24. Zeeni N, Safieddine H, Doumit R. Eating disorders in Lebanon: directions for public health action. Community Ment Health J. 2017;53:117–25.

25. Gormally J, Black S, Daston S, Rardin D. The assessment of binge eating severity among obese persons. Addict Behav. 1982;7:47–55.

26. Hood MM, Grupski AE, Hall BJ, Ivan I, Corsica J. Factor structure and predictive utility of the binge eating scale in bariatric surgery candidates. Surg Obes Relat Dis. 2013;9:942–8.

27. Brunault P, Gaillard P, Ballon N, Couet C, Isnard P, Cook S, et al. Validation of the French version of the binge eating scale: examination of its factor structure, internal consistency and construct validity in a non-clinical and a clinical population. Encephale. 2016;42:426–33.

28. Imperatori C, Innamorati M, Lamis DA, Contardi A, Continisio M, Castelnuovo G, et al. Factor structure of the binge eating scale in a large sample of obese and overweight patients attending low energy diet therapy. Eur Eat Disord Rev. 2016;24:174–8.

29. Partida O, Garcia R, Cardenas A, Agraz F. Evaluation of the binge eating scale in Mexican population: translation and psychometric properties of the Spanish version. Psiquiatria. 2006;22:6.

30. Mootabi F, Moloodi R, Dezhkam M, Omidvar N. Standardization of the binge eating scale among Iranian obese population. Iran J Psychiatry. 2009;4:143–6.

31. Robert SA, Rohana AG, Suehazlyn Z, Maniam T, Azhar SS, Azmi KN. The validation of the malay version of binge eating scale: a comparison with the structured clinical interview for the DSM-IV. J Eat Disord. 2013;1:28.

32. Duarte C, Pinto-Gouveia J, Ferreira C. Expanding binge eating assessment: validity and screening value of the binge eating scale in women from the general population. Eat Behav. 2015;18:41–7.

33. Zúñiga O, Robles R. Validez de constructo y consistencia interna del Cuestionario de Trastorno por Atracón en población mexicana con obesidad. Psiquis. 2006;15:126–34.

34. Escrivá-Martínez T, Galiana L, Rodriguez-Arias M, Baños RM. The binge eating scale: structural equation competitive models, invariance measurement

between sexes, and relationships with food addiction, impulsivity, binge drinking, and body mass index. Front Psychol. 2019;10:530.

35. Saade S, Hallit S, Haddad C, Hallit R, Akel M, Honein K, et al. Factors associated with restrained eating and validation of the Arabic version of the restrained eating scale among an adult representative sample of the Lebanese population: a cross-sectional study. J Eat Disord. 2019;7:24.

36. Haddad C, Hallit R, Akel M, et al. Validation of the Arabic version of the ORTO-15 questionnaire in a sample of the Lebanese population. Eat Weight Disord. 2019. https://doi.org/10.1007/s40519-019-00710-y.

37. Haddad C, Zakhour M, Akel M, Honein K, Akiki M, Hallit S, et al. Factors associated with body dissatisfaction among the Lebanese population. Eat Weight Disord. 2019;24:507–19. https://doi.org/10.1007/s40519-018-00634-z.

38. Haddad C, Obeid S, Akel M, Honein K, Akiki M, Azar J, et al. Correlates of orthorexia nervosa among a representative sample of the Lebanese population. Eat Weight Disord. 2019;24:481–93. https://doi.org/10.1007/s40519-018-0631-x.

39. Comrey AL, Lee HB. A first course in factor analysis: Psychology press; 2013.

40. Weary-Smith KA. Validation of the physical activity index (PAI) as a measure of total activity load and total kilocalorie expenditure during submaximal treadmill walking: University of Pittsburgh; 2007.

41. Rosenberg M. Rosenberg self-esteem scale (RSE). Acceptance and commitment therapy Measures package, vol. 61; 1965.

42. Cohen S, Kamarck T, Mermelstein R. Perceived stress scale. Measuring stress: a guide for health and social scientists, vol. 10; 1994.

43. Hallit S, Haddad C, Hallit R, Akel M, Obeid S, Haddad G, et al. Validation of the Hamilton anxiety rating scale and state trait anxiety inventory a and B in Arabic among the Lebanese population. Clin Epidemiol Glob Health. 2019;7:464–70. https://doi.org/10.1016/j.cegh.2019.02.002.

44. Greeno CG, Marcus MD, Wing RR. Diagnosis of binge eating disorder: discrepancies between a questionnaire and clinical interview. Int J Eat Disord. 1995;17:153–60.

45. Garner DM. The Eating Disorder Inventory-2. Professional manual. Odessa: Psychological Assessment Resources, Inc; 1991.

46. Obeid S, Abi Elias Hallit C, Haddad C, Hany Z, Hallit S. Validation of the Hamilton depression rating scale (HDRS) and sociodemographic factors associated with Lebanese depressed patients. Encephale. 2018;44:397–402.

47. Gross JJ. Emotion regulation: affective, cognitive, and social consequences. Psychophysiology. 2002;39:281–91.

48. Gross JJ, Levenson RW. Emotional suppression: physiology, self-report, and expressive behavior. J Pers Soc Psychol. 1993;64:970–86.

49. Gross JJ, John OP. Individual differences in two emotion regulation processes: implications for affect, relationships, and well-being. J Pers Soc Psychol. 2003;85:348–62.

50. Beaton DE, Bombardier C, Guillemin F, Ferraz MB. Guidelines for the process of cross-cultural adaptation of self-report measures. Spine (Phila Pa 1976). 2000;25:3186–91.

51. Arnow B, Kenardy J, Agras WS. The emotional eating scale: the development of a measure to assess coping with negative affect by eating. Int J Eat Disord. 1995;18:79–90.

52. Bowlby J. A secure base: parent-child attachment and healthy human development: Basic books; 2008.

53. Griffin DW, Bartholomew K. Models of the self and other: fundamental dimensions underlying measures of adult attachment. J Pers Soc Psychol. 1994;67:430.

54. Bartholomew K. Avoidance of intimacy: an attachment perspective. J Soc Pers Relat. 1990;7:147–78.

55. Puccio F, Fuller-Tyszkiewicz M, Ong D, Krug I. A systematic review and meta-analysis on the longitudinal relationship between eating pathology and depression. Int J Eat Disord. 2016;49:439–54.

56. Marsh HW, Hau K-T, Wen Z. In search of golden rules: comment on hypothesis-testing approaches to setting cutoff values for fit indexes and dangers in overgeneralizing Hu and Bentler's (1999) findings. Struct Equ Modeling. 2004;11:320–41.

57. Marek RJ, Tarescavage AM, Ben-Porath YS, Ashton K, Heinberg LJ. Replication and evaluation of a proposed two-factor binge eating scale (BES) structure in a sample of bariatric surgery candidates. Surg Obes Relat Dis. 2015;11:659–65.

58. Grupski AE, Hood MM, Hall BJ, Azarbad L, Fitzpatrick SL, Corsica JA. Examining the binge eating scale in screening for binge eating disorder in bariatric surgery candidates. Obes Surg. 2013;23:1–6.

59. Hudson JI, Hiripi E, Pope HG Jr, Kessler RC. The prevalence and correlates of eating disorders in the National Comorbidity Survey Replication. Biol Psychiatry. 2007;61:348–58.

60. Swanson SA, Crow SJ, Le Grange D, Swendsen J, Merikangas KR. Prevalence and correlates of eating disorders in adolescents. Results from the national comorbidity survey replication adolescent supplement. Arch Gen Psychiatry. 2011;68:714–23.

61. Mitchell KS, Mazzeo SE. Binge eating and psychological distress in ethnically diverse undergraduate men and women. Eat Behav. 2004;5:157–69.

62. Pearson CM, Zapolski TC, Smith GT. A longitudinal test of impulsivity and depression pathways to early binge eating onset. Int J Eat Disord. 2015;48: 230–7.

63. Skinner HH, Haines J, Austin SB, Field AE. A prospective study of overeating, binge eating, and depressive symptoms among adolescent and young adult women. J Adolesc Health. 2012;50:478–83.

64. Culbert KM, Racine SE, Klump KL. Research review: what we have learned about the causes of eating disorders - a synthesis of sociocultural, psychological, and biological research. J Child Psychol Psychiatry. 2015;56: 1141–64.

65. Bohon C, Stice E. Negative affect and neural response to palatable food intake in bulimia nervosa. Appetite. 2012;58:964–70.

66. Azarbad L, Corsica J, Hall B, Hood M. Psychosocial correlates of binge eating in Hispanic, African American, and Caucasian women presenting for bariatric surgery. Eat Behav. 2010;11:79–84.

67. Jones-Corneille LR, Wadden TA, Sarwer DB, Faulconbridge LF, Fabricatore AN, Stack RM, et al. Axis I psychopathology in bariatric surgery candidates with and without binge eating disorder: results of structured clinical interviews. Obes Surg. 2012;22:389–97.

68. Peterson CB, Thuras P, Ackard DM, Mitchell JE, Berg K, Sandager N, et al. Personality dimensions in bulimia nervosa, binge eating disorder, and obesity. Compr Psychiatry. 2010;51:31–6.

69. Fandiño J, Moreira RO, Preissler C, Gaya CW, Papelbaum M, Coutinho WF, et al. Impact of binge eating disorder in the psychopathological profile of obese women. Compr Psychiatry. 2010;51:110–4.

70. Grilo CM, White MA, Masheb RM. DSM-IV psychiatric disorder comorbidity and its correlates in binge eating disorder. Int J Eat Disord. 2009;42:228–34.

71. Tanofsky-Kraff M, Shomaker LB, Olsen C, Roza CA, Wolkoff LE, Columbo KM, et al. A prospective study of pediatric loss of control eating and psychological outcomes. J Abnorm Psychol. 2011;120:108.

72. Reichborn-Kjennerud T, Bulik CM, Tambs K, Harris JR. Genetic and environmental influences on binge eating in the absence of compensatory behaviors: a population-based twin study. Int J Eat Disord. 2004;36:307–14.

73. Pallister E, Waller G. Anxiety in the eating disorders: understanding the overlap. Clin Psychol Rev. 2008;28:366–86.

74. Bulik CM, Sullivan PF, Carter FA, Joyce PR. Lifetime anxiety disorders in women with bulimia nervosa. Compr Psychiatry. 1996;37:368–74.

75. Kaye WH, Bulik CM, Thornton L, Barbarich N, Masters K, Group P.F.C. Comorbidity of anxiety disorders with anorexia and bulimia nervosa. Am J Psychiatry. 2004;161:2215–21.

76. Godart NT, Flament MF, Curt F, Perdereau F, Lang F, Venisse JL, et al. Anxiety disorders in subjects seeking treatment for eating disorders: a DSM-IV controlled study. Psychiatry Res. 2003;117:245–58.

77. Tuschen-Caffier B, Hilbert A. Binge-Eating-Störung [Binge Eating Disorder]. Göttingen: Hogrefe; 2016.

78. Lammers MW, Vroling MS, Ouwens MA, Engels RC, van Strien T. Predictors of outcome for cognitive behaviour therapy in binge eating disorder. Eur Eat Disord Rev. 2015;23:219–28.

79. Jacobi C, Hayward C, de Zwaan M, Kraemer HC, Agras WS. Coming to terms with risk factors for eating disorders: application of risk terminology and suggestions for a general taxonomy. Psychol Bull. 2004;130:19.

80. Bauer A, Schneider S, Waldorf M, Cordes M, Huber TJ, Braks K, et al. Visual processing of one's own body over the course of time: evidence for the vigilance-avoidance theory in adolescents with anorexia nervosa? Int J Eat Disord. 2017;50:1205–13.

81. Vocks S, Legenbauer I, Wächter A, Wucherer M, Kosfelder J. What happens in the course of body exposure?: emotional, cognitive, and physiological reactions to mirror confrontation in eating disorders. J Psychosom Res. 2007;62:231–9.

82. Aspen V, Darcy AM, Lock J. A review of attention biases in women with eating disorders. Cognit Emot. 2013;27:820–38.

83. Rodgers RF, DuBois RH. Cognitive biases to appearance-related stimuli in body dissatisfaction: a systematic review. Clin Psychol Rev. 2016;46:1–11.

84. Delinsky SS, Wilson GT. Mirror exposure for the treatment of body image disturbance. Int J Eat Disord. 2006;39:108–16.

85. Vocks S, Legenbauer T, Troje N, Schulte D. Body image therapy in eating disorders. Influencing of perceptive, cognitive-affective, and behavioral components of the body image. Zeitschrift fur klinische Psychologie und Psychotherapie-Gottingen. 2006;35:286.

86. Zerwas S, Larsen JT, Petersen L, Thornton LM, Mortensen PB, Bulik CM. The incidence of eating disorders in a Danish register study: associations with suicide risk and mortality. J Psychiatr Res. 2015;65:16–22.

87. Keski-Rahkonen A, Mustelin L. Epidemiology of eating disorders in Europe: prevalence, incidence, comorbidity, course, consequences, and risk factors. Curr Opin Psychiatry. 2016;29:340–5.

88. Svaldi J, Griepenstroh J, Tuschen-Caffier B, Ehring T. Emotion regulation deficits in eating disorders: a marker of eating pathology or general psychopathology? Psychiatry Res. 2012;197:103–11.

89. Nolen-Hoeksema S, Blair E, Sonja L. Rethinking rumination. Pers Psychol Sci. 2008;3:400–24.

90. Svaldi J, Caffier D, Tuschen-Caffier B. Emotion suppression but not reappraisal increases desire to binge in women with binge eating disorder. Psychother Psychosom. 2010;79:188–90.

91. Dunkley DM, Masheb RM, Grilo CM. Childhood maltreatment, depressive symptoms, and body dissatisfaction in patients with binge eating disorder: the mediating role of self-criticism. Int J Eat Disord. 2010;43:274–81.

92. Eating Disorders and Trauma / PTSD (Post Traumatic Stress Disorder) Co-Occurring Eating Disorder Hope. Eating disorder help treatment, recovery articles, facts & Statistics on anorexia and bulimia eating disorder Hope; 2012. Available from: http://www.eatingdisorderhope.com/treatment-for-eating-disorders/co-occurring-dualdiagnosis/trauma-ptsd#Connection-and-Relationship-between-Trauma-and-Eating-Disorders

93. Johnson JG, Cohen P, Kasen S, Brook JS. Childhood adversities associated with risk for eating disorders or weight problems during adolescence or early adulthood. Am J Psychiatry. 2002;159:394–400.

94. Cash TF, Smolak L. Body image: a handbook of science, practice, and prevention. New York: Guilford Press; 2011.

95. Palavras MA, Kaio GH, Mari JJ, Claudino AM. A review of Latin American studies on binge eating disorder. Braz J Psychiatry. 2011;33(Suppl 1):S81–108.

96. Poli R, Maninetti L, Bodini P, Agrimi E. Obesity, binge eating, obstruction sleep apnea and psychopathological features. Clin Neuropsychiatry. 2012;9:166–71.

97. Utter J, Neumark-Sztainer D, Wall M, Story M. Reading magazine articles about dieting and associated weight control behaviors among adolescents. J Adolesc Health. 2003;32:78–82.

98. Hudson JI, Lalonde JK, Berry JM, Pindyck LJ, Bulik CM, Crow SJ, et al. Binge-eating disorder as a distinct familial phenotype in obese individuals. Arch Gen Psychiatry. 2006;63:313–9.

99. Javaras KN, Laird NM, Reichborn-Kjennerud T, Bulik CM, Pope HG Jr, Hudson JI. Familiality and heritability of binge eating disorder: results of a case-control family study and a twin study. Int J Eat Disord. 2008;41:174–9.

100. Trace SE, Baker JH, Peñas-Lledó E, Bulik CM. The genetics of eating disorders. Annu Rev Clin Psychol. 2013;9:589–620.

3

Patient descriptions of loss of control and eating episode size interact to influence expert diagnosis of ICD-11 binge-eating disorder

Laura A. Berner[1]* iD, Robyn Sysko[1], Tahilia J. Rebello[2], Christina A. Roberto[3] and Kathleen M. Pike[2]

Abstract

Background: Although data suggest that the sense of "loss of control" (LOC) is the most salient aspect of binge eating, the definition of LOC varies widely across eating disorder assessments. The WHO ICD-11 diagnostic guidelines for binge eating do not require an objectively large amount of food, which makes accurate LOC diagnosis even more critical. However, it can be especially challenging to assess LOC in the context of elevated weight status and in the absence of compensatory behaviors. This ICD-11 field sub-study examined how descriptions of subjective experience during distressing eating episodes, in combination with different eating episode sizes, influence diagnoses of binge-eating disorder (BED).

Method: Mental health professionals with eating disorder expertise from WHO's Global Clinical Practice Network (N = 192) participated in English, Japanese, and Spanish. Participants were asked to select the correct diagnosis for two randomly assigned case vignettes and to rate the clinical importance and ease of use of each BED diagnostic guideline.

Results: The presence of LOC interacted with episode size to predict whether a correct diagnostic conclusion was reached. If the amount consumed during a typical distressing eating episode was only subjectively large compared to objectively large, clinicians were 23.1 times more likely to miss BED than to correctly diagnose it, and they were 9.7 times more likely to incorrectly diagnose something else than to correctly diagnose BED. In addition, clinicians were 10.8 times more likely to make a false positive diagnosis of BED when no LOC was described if the episode was objectively large. Descriptions of LOC that were reliably associated with correct diagnoses across episodes sizes included two that are similar to those already included in proposed ICD-11 guidelines and a third that is not. This third description of LOC focuses on giving up attempts to control eating because perceived overeating feels inevitable.

Conclusions: Results highlight the importance of detailed clarification of the LOC construct in future guidelines. Explicitly distinguishing LOC from distressing and mindless overeating could help promote consistent and accurate diagnosis of BED versus another or no eating disorder.

Keywords: Binge eating, Loss-of-control eating, Overeating, Binge-eating disorder, Diagnosis and classification, ICD-11

* Correspondence: laura.berner@mssm.edu
[1]Department of Psychiatry, Icahn School of Medicine at Mount Sinai, New York, NY, USA
Full list of author information is available at the end of the article

Plain English summary

A sense of "loss of control" (LOC) is the feature that distinguishes binge eating from other kinds of overeating. LOC definitions vary widely, and this study aimed to examine how different descriptions of LOC influence whether a diagnosis of binge-eating disorder (BED) will be assigned. An internet-based vignette study was conducted through the World Health Organization's Global Clinical Practice Network; 192 mental health professionals with self-reported expertise in eating disorders participated. The size of the eating episode interacted with the presence of LOC to affect whether a correct diagnosis was given to the hypothetical patients. For episodes in which the amount eaten was within normal limits (i.e., only subjectively large) and LOC was described, clinicians were 23.1 times more likely to miss BED and 9.7 times more likely to incorrectly assign another diagnosis than to correctly diagnose BED. If the amount eaten was objectively large but there was no LOC, clinicians were 10.8 times more likely to make a false positive diagnosis of BED. Thus, how LOC is described is important to promote consistent and accurate diagnosis of BED versus another or no eating disorder.

Introduction

The behavioral disturbance of binge eating has been defined by two essential dimensions in the *Diagnostic and Statistical Manual of Mental Disorders* (DSM) and International Classification of Diseases (ICD). Beginning with the *DSM-III*, the presence of binge eating required the consumption of an objectively large amount of food (e.g., unusually large for the circumstances) coupled with the experience of loss of control (LOC). However, in clinical practice, descriptions of the amount of food eaten during binge eating episodes (i.e., episode size) is highly variable [1]. Individuals who report subjective binge eating, or consuming an amount of food that is within normal limits but is perceived as large while experiencing LOC, describe comparable levels of distress and indicators of psychopathology as individuals who report objective binge eating [2–5]. Thus, in the 11th Revision of the ICD (ICD-11), the guidelines for defining a binge episode were updated such that the critical characteristic of binge eating is a sense of LOC [6]. The guidelines specifically note that "binge eating episodes may be 'objective,' in which the individual eats an amount of food that is larger than most people would eat under similar circumstances, or 'subjective,' which may involve eating amounts of food that might be objectively considered to be within normal limits but are subjectively experienced as large by the individual." [6]. These differ from *DSM-5* criteria for binge eating, which still require both the consumption of an objectively large amount of food and a sense of LOC [7] (see Table S1).

Regardless of the amount of food consumed, the sense of LOC during eating episodes predicts significant distress, impairment, and clinical outcome, including the development of eating disorders, weight gain, and less weight loss when LOC persists or develops after bariatric surgery [8, 9]. Measures have been developed to dimensionally assess LOC severity [10, 11]; however their language and constructs vary, and no clinical "cutoff scores" are provided. As such, there is no standard method to diagnose LOC. Accurate assessment of LOC is particularly critical because, as aforementioned, the recently adopted ICD-11 guidelines do not require an objectively large amount of food in the diagnosis of binge eating.

Although supported by research and clinical practice, the omission of a large episode size guideline could increase the risk of binge eating misdiagnosis. One specific concern is that clinicians unfamiliar with updates in ICD-11 may underdiagnose binge eating in individuals who experience LOC during eating episodes that are not objectively large. This is problematic because LOC strongly contributes to more negative psychosocial, behavioral, and weight outcomes. Individuals with high LOC who could benefit significantly from receiving appropriate care may not be referred for treatment. In an initial field study, even clinicians with expertise in eating disorders from around the globe were significantly less accurate in diagnosing ICD-11 bulimia nervosa (BN) when subjectively large LOC episodes rather than objectively large LOC episodes were described [12]. As binge-eating disorder (BED) excludes the compensatory behaviors seen in BN that may more obviously signal an eating disorder, and it does not require the presence of any other maladaptive eating behaviors besides regular LOC eating in order to be diagnosed, clarifying the definition of LOC is particularly important for the prevention of BED underdiagnosis.

A second major concern is that other kinds of distressing eating could be conflated with LOC eating, leading to binge eating overdiagnosis. For example, among adults with overweight or obesity, several maladaptive eating behaviors that are not characterized by LOC are commonly reported, including grazing, chaotic or disorganized eating, stress-related or emotional eating, eating much more rapidly than normal, and mindless eating [13, 14]. The ICD-11 guidelines note that individuals with obesity who report overeating patterns that do not meet the definition of binge eating should not be diagnosed BED. However, it may be difficult to distinguish individuals who are binge eating from those who are only distressed by maladaptive eating behaviors.

Overall, accurate LOC diagnosis has significant implications for BED diagnostic sensitivity and specificity, and additional guidance on the diagnosis of LOC may be helpful for both clinical practice and research studies. The current study aimed to examine the influence of LOC and size of the eating episode on how clinicians assigned a diagnosis of BED, another diagnosis, or no eating disorder, according to ICD-11 guidelines. In addition, because accurate clinical detection of LOC is essential for the diagnosis of all eating disorders characterized by binge eating, we explored which descriptions of LOC most often promoted correct vs. incorrect diagnostic conclusions, across episode sizes. Mental health professionals with eating disorder expertise from the World Health Organization's (WHO's) Global Clinical Practice Network completed a survey with two randomized clinical vignettes and associated diagnostic questions. Vignettes were identical for all participants, except for the description of LOC eating, or lack thereof, and whether the episode size was objectively or subjectively large. We hypothesized that LOC and episode size would interact to predict diagnosis. Specifically, we predicted that vignettes that did not include descriptions of LOC would be more likely to be incorrectly associated with a BED diagnosis in the context of an objectively large amount of food, whereas quantity of food consumed would have less influence on BED diagnosis for vignettes that included clear descriptions of LOC.

Method

Participants

Participants were recruited globally from a pool of health professionals (the "Global Clinical Practice Network," or GCPN, http://gcp.network) who had previously registered and provided detailed demographic and professional information using an online Qualtrics software-based survey [15]. Clinicians in the GCPN who endorsed expertise in Feeding or Eating Disorders and indicated that they were an advanced speaker in English, Spanish, or Japanese ($n = 644$) were invited to participate in this sub-study. Of those eligible, 208 (32.3%) responded to the survey link and began the study.

Procedure

Participants were first presented with and asked to review an abbreviated version of proposed ICD-11 clinical diagnostic guidelines for BED and BN as of January 2018: For both disorders, definitions of LOC and any phrases related to episode size were omitted from the provided guidelines (see Table S1 for a summary of the language removed from the proposed guidelines in the version that was presented to raters). As such, the essential (required) feature of "Frequent, recurrent episodes of binge eating (e.g., once a week or more over a period of three months)" was described only as follows: "Binge eating is defined as a distinct period of time during which the individual experiences a loss of control over his or her eating behaviour. Other characteristics of binge eating episodes may include eating alone because of embarrassment, or eating foods that are not part of the individual's regular diet."

Next, in a repeated-measures design, participants were presented with two cases from a pool of 28 vignettes that varied based on the adult presenting for treatment (the "vignette base"; see Supplement for the two vignette bases used in this study), distressing eating episode size (objectively or subjectively large), and experience during distressing eating episodes (seven descriptions of LOC or no LOC; see Table 1). Across the two presented cases, each participant saw the two vignette bases, one paired with a subjectively large episode and one paired with an objectively large episode, and two different experience descriptors. The order of the vignette bases and episode sizes were independently randomized, and

Table 1 Descriptions of experiences during LOC and non-LOC eating episodes

Non-LOC Descriptors	Based on
"I'll be watching TV while I'm eating, so I don't really taste the food or notice what's happening, but I just keep going back for more. Before I know it, all the food is gone, and I've eaten more than I planned."	• Chen & Safer, 2010 [16] • Mindful Eating Questionnaire [17]
"I've never tried to stop myself; I like the taste of it, so I just keep eating."	Clinical descriptions from adults seeking weight loss treatment

LOC Descriptors	Based on
"During times like those, I feel helpless to control my urges to eat."	Binge Eating Scale [18]
"I feel this drive to keep eating once I get started."	Eating Disorder Examination [19]
"It's hard for me to stop eating when I eat like that."	• Eating Disorder Inventory-3 [20] • Three-Factor Eating Questionnaire [21] • Eating Disorder Examination [19]
"I feel like I can't stop or limit the amount of food or the type of food I'm eating."	• Questionnaire on Eating and Weight Patterns-5 [22] • DSM-5 [7]
"I don't really try to control my eating anymore. Eating like that is pretty much inevitable."	Eating Disorder Examination [19]

LOC loss of control

the experience descriptors were assigned using random selection without replacement.

The two vignette bases both described adult women with body mass indices (BMI) over $25 \, kg/m^2$ who self-reported high levels of distress about their weight and episodes of what they called "binge eating." Both case examples denied compensatory behaviors. The vignettes had been validated by eight independent eating disorder expert raters who confirmed that, if actual LOC was described, the individuals in both vignettes met all ICD-11 guidelines for BED diagnosis.

These raters also confirmed the classification of the two episode size descriptions. The episode characterized as within normal limits (i.e., subjectively large) was described as "5 small caramel candies with 2 standard-size scoops (i.e., approximately 1 cup or 214 g total) of ice cream." The episode characterized by an objectively large amount of food was described as "6 slices of regular-crust, cheese pizza and 2 large orders of French fries."

Five LOC descriptors were created based on items from well-validated measures of binge eating (see Table 1). In addition, we included two descriptions of distressing eating experiences that are not LOC. One specifically focused on mindless eating. As described by Chen & Safer [16], mindless eating is "not attending to one's eating (e.g., eating popcorn while watching TV and finding that one has finished the bowl without being aware of this occurring). Unlike binge eating, a loss of control is not experienced in mindless eating" (p. 303). Based on this description, and the items of the Mindful Eating Questionnaire [17], we developed a description of mindless eating without LOC. Finally, we included a description of no past attempt to control eating behavior. This was informed by descriptions of overeating from the co-authors' clinical experiences treating and assessing adults seeking weight loss treatment (Table 1).

For each vignette, participants were asked to select a diagnosis from a list of BN, BED, another feeding or eating disorder, no diagnosis, or a different diagnosis not on the list (in which case they could specify which diagnosis they selected in a text box). Participants were able to review the diagnostic guidelines and vignette while making their selection. After diagnostic selection, participants were asked to indicate whether each essential feature of their chosen diagnosis was present in the specific case vignette. After reviewing the essential features, participants had the option to change their response and select a different final diagnosis. Participants then reviewed a second clinical vignette and repeated the process. After viewing both vignettes, participants were asked to rate the clinical importance and ease of use of each of the five main BED diagnostic guidelines on a scale of 1–4 (1 = not at all, 4 = extremely) and provide additional information about how often they encounter individuals with BED through direct clinical contact.

Statistical analysis

Given the non-independence of our categorical data (each clinician made diagnostic decisions about two vignettes), we tested our hypotheses about the prediction of a correct or incorect diagnosis using binomial logit link generalized estimating equations (GEE) with subject as a repeating factor in R. An autoregressive correlation structure best fit the data ranked by QIC [23]. Multinomial GEEs examined the prediction of specific diagnostic conclusions. Vignette base was unrelated to whether a diagnosis was correct or whether the final diagnosis was BED ($ps > 0.05$). However, BED was more likely to be diagnosed on the first vignette than the second ($B = 0.84$, $SE = 0.25$, $p = 0.0007$), and specifically, BED was more likely to be correctly diagnosed than missed on the first vignette than the second ($B = 0.99$, $SE = 0.37$, $p = 0.008$). Therefore, all subsequent models included vignette number as a covariate.

We ran the following models to test our main hypotheses: (1) an overall model testing whether size (subjectively large, objectively large) and experience descriptor (LOC, no LOC) interact to predict whether a correct diagnosis is made, (2) a model testing whether size (subjectively large, objectively large) predicts specific diagnostic decisions when LOC is present (correct diagnosis of BED [reference category], missed BED diagnosis, or incorrect other diagnosis) and (3) a model testing whether size (subjectively large, objectively large) predicts specific diagnostic decisions when LOC is absent (correct conclusion of no diagnosis [reference category], false positive BED diagnosis, false positive other diagnosis). A fourth model examined whether patients' descriptions of their subjective experience (7 possibilities) and size (subjectively large, objectively large) interact to predict whether a correct diagnosis is made. Alpha was set at 0.0125 to Bonferroni correct for four tests. Finally, exploratory repeated-measures analyses of variance compared ratings of importance and ease of use of each of the BED guidelines.

Results

Of the 208 clinicians who began the survey, 192 completed questions about at least one vignette and were included in analyses. A total of 188 completed questions about two vignettes. Participant characteristics are shown in Table 2. Most were physicians or psychologists and were from Europe or North America. Participants mostly identified as female (66.1%) with a mean age of 49.2 ($SD = 10.8$) and roughly 18 years of clinical experience. Of note, the modal frequency of encountering patients with subthreshold or threshold BED was less than once per month (34.4% of the sample).

Table 2 Participant Characteristics (N = 192)

WHO Global Region	N (%)
Africa	2 (1.0)
USA and Canada	47 (24.5)
Latin America/Caribbean	16 (8.3)
Eastern Mediterranean	5 (2.6)
Europe	93 (48.4)
Southeast Asia	1 (0.5)
Western Pacific—Asia	20 (10.4)
Western Pacific—Oceania	8 (4.2)
Demographics	**N (%) or Mean (SD)**
Female:Male	127:65 (66.1:33.9)
Age	49.2(10.8)
Clinical Profession	**N (%)**
Medicine	72 (37.5)
Psychology	99 (51.6)
Nursing	3 (1.6)
Social Work	7 (3.6)
Other	4 (2.1)
Counseling	6 (3.1)
Occupational Therapy	1 (0.5)
Clinical Experience	**Mean (SD)**
Years of Experience	18.0 (10.4)
Frequency of encountering individuals with subthreshold or threshold BED (scale of 1–5, 1 = never, 5 = very frequently, multiple times per week)[a]	3.0 (1.1)

WHO World Health Organization; [a]*n* = 187

Does the influence of LOC presence or absence on correct diagnosis depend on episode size?

LOC presence interacted with episode size to predict whether a correct diagnostic conclusion was reached ($p < 0.0001$; Table 3). When LOC was present, correct diagnoses were most often reached in the context of large episodes (i.e., BED was correctly diagnosed when episodes were large). The most frequent incorrect diagnoses were made when the episode was subjectively large and LOC was present (i.e., BED was missed or incorrectly diagnosed as something else).

Table 3 LOC presence and size interact to predict correct diagnosis

Parameter	B	SE	Wald
Intercept	−0.47	0.31	2.26
Vignette Number	−0.77**	0.27	7.86
LOC Presence	1.00**	0.37	7.45
Episode Size	−1.76**	0.58	9.09
LOC Presence x Episode Size	4.34***	0.70	38.23

**$p < 0.01$, ***$p < 0.0001$; LOC = loss of control

Does episode size predict specific diagnostic decisions when LOC is present?

When one of the five true LOC descriptors was presented (see Table 1), episode size predicted specific diagnostic decisions (overall model $p < 0.0001$; Table 4). If the episode was subjectively large compared to objectively large, clinicians were 23.1 times more likely to miss BED than to correctly diagnose it, and they were 9.7 times more likely to incorrectly diagnose something else than to correctly diagnose BED (Table 4).

Does episode size predict specific diagnostic decisions when LOC is absent?

When one of the two non-LOC descriptors was used, episode size also predicted specific diagnostic decisions (overall model $p = 0.0001$). Specifically, clinicians were 10.8 times more likely to make a false positive diagnosis of BED than no diagnosis if the episode was objectively large compared to subjectively large (Table 4).

Does the influence of LOC description (or lack thereof) on correct diagnosis depend on episode size?

The description of the patient's experience during the eating episode interacted with episode size to predict whether a correct diagnostic conclusion was reached ($p = 0.014$; Table 5). As shown in Fig. 1, the only "true LOC" descriptors that were consistently associated with more correct than incorrect diagnostic conclusions across episode sizes were "It's hard for me to stop eating when I eat like that," "I feel like I can't stop or limit the amount of food or the type of food I'm eating," and "I don't really try to control my eating anymore. Eating like that is pretty much inevitable." In contrast, across both objectively large and subjectively large episode sizes, experts almost always made incorrect diagnoses when mindless eating was described, and they made more incorrect than correct diagnoses when no attempt to control eating was described.

Exploratory analyses: how important and easy to use is each diagnostic guideline for BED?

A total of 187 experts provided ratings on the importance and ease of use of the five ICD-11 BED diagnostic guidelines. Importance ($F (3.56, 186) = 15.04$, $p < 0.0001$) and ease ratings ($F(3.68, 185) = 17.47$, $p < 0.001$) differed across guidelines. Post-hoc pairwise comparisons indicated that importance ratings were significantly higher for the sense of LOC over eating than for episode size, binge episode frequency, and distress ($ps < 0.005$). However, experts rated the sense of LOC over eating guideline as the least easy (i.e., most difficult) to apply in a valid and/or reliable way, and these ease ratings were statistically significantly lower than those for binge episode frequency ($p < 0.001$) and the lack of compensatory behaviors guideline ($p = 0.005$).

Table 4 Episode size is linked to specific diagnostic decisions when LOC is present and absent

Parameter	B	SE	B	SE
LOC is Present	**Logit 1 (Incorrect Other Dx vs. Correct BED)**		**Logit 2 (BED Miss vs. Correct BED)**	
Intercept	−1.62***	0.31	−1.35***	0.30
Vignette Number	1.04**	0.38	1.52***	0.43
Episode Size	−2.27***	0.45	−3.14***	0.60
LOC is Absent	**Logit 1 (False Positive Other Dx vs. Correct No Dx)**		**Logit 2 (False Positive BED vs. Correct No Dx)**	
Intercept	−0.66	0.57	0.84*	0.39
Vignette Number	0.59	0.71	−1.15	0.66
Episode Size	0.40	0.77	2.38**	0.77

*$p < 0.05$, **$p < 0.01$, ***$p < 0.0001$; *BED* binge-eating disorder, *LOC* loss of control, *Dx* diagnosis; reference categories were correct BED diagnosis and a subjectively large episode

Discussion

The results of this study are important for the future diagnosis of BED. Because the ICD serves as the diagnostic system for all WHO member nations, and the 11th ICD revision is the first to include BED, ICD diagnostic guidelines regarding the behavioral disturbance of binge eating require significant attention. The current proposed ICD-11 guidelines explicitly indicate that binge-eating episodes can be comprised of small, normal, or large quantities of food, leaving LOC as their core defining feature. However, because this is a change from the ICD-10 description of binge eating (in BN guidelines) and is distinct from the *DSM-5* definition of binge eating, focused education will likely be necessary to ensure reliability of diagnosis.

Our findings indicate that experienced clinicians are best at recognizing BED when binge-eating episodes are characterized by both LOC and an objectively large amount of food. Although there is great cultural and contextual variation in the definition of an objectively large amount of food, at the extreme, consensus exists. Our results also suggest that experienced clinicians are likely to miss BED when binge-eating episodes are characterized by LOC and a subjectively large amount of food. As individuals with subjectively large LOC episodes experience levels of distress, associated psychopathology, and impairment comparable to those with objectively large LOC episodes [2–5], it is important that these individuals get diagnosed and referred for treatment.

Table 5 Specific LOC description (or lack thereof) and size interact to predict correct diagnosis

	B	SE	Wald
Intercept	−0.21*	0.81	0.06
Vignette Number	−0.60**	0.22	7.09
Descriptor	0.26***	0.08	11.85
Episode Size	−0.02	0.47	0.01
Descriptor x Episode Size	0.30*	0.12	5.99

*$p < 0.05$; **$p < 0.01$; ***$p < 0.001$; *LOC* loss of control

The change in the ICD-11 will allow for appropriate detection and referral; however, our findings highlight that clinician training may be vital to ensure that such individuals receive care.

Given the prioritization of LOC in defining a binge eating episode, establishing standard clinical descriptions of LOC is essential. Prior work provides some examples of detailed LOC descriptions and case examples that could be helpful to include in diagnostic training materials (e.g., [24]). Our results suggest that three descriptions of LOC were most reliably associated with correct diagnoses across episode sizes: "It's hard for me to stop eating when I eat like that," "I feel like I can't stop or limit the amount of food or the type of food I'm eating," and "I don't really try to control my eating anymore. Eating like that is pretty much inevitable." These findings may importantly inform future research studies examining BED and other eating disorders characterized by binge eating. The working definition of LOC proposed by Latner and colleagues [11], *DSM-5* diagnostic features for BN and BED, and the proposed ICD-11 guidelines for BN and BED (Table S1 and S2) include the first two of these three LOC descriptors. In addition, the diagnostic features sections of *DSM-5* note that "abandoned efforts" to control inevitable eating should be considered LOC [7]. Familiarity with these standard definitions of LOC may have increased clinicians' abilities to correctly diagnose these descriptions. Adding all three of these example descriptions to future drafted ICD guidelines could provide valuable supporting detail for diagnosticians.

In addition to clinical guidance on reliable descriptions of LOC, it will also be essential for clinical training and research to provide guidance on what LOC is not. In particular, it is important to maintain a boundary between binge eating and overeating. Our results suggest that a high percentage of even expert clinicians confuse binge eating with mindless overeating without LOC and overeating without any attempt to stop or LOC. To reduce this confusion, it may be helpful for guidelines to explicitly note that these patterns of overeating do not meet the definition of binge eating.

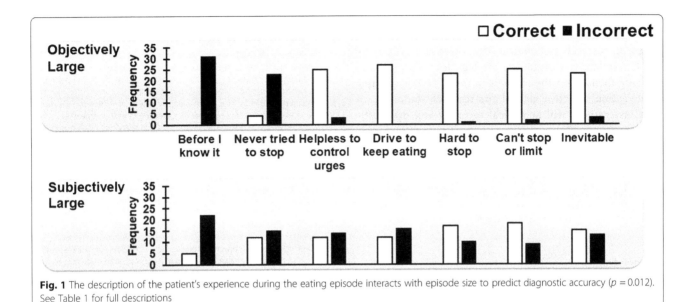

Fig. 1 The description of the patient's experience during the eating episode interacts with episode size to predict diagnostic accuracy (*p* = 0.012). See Table 1 for full descriptions

Of note, previous studies have suggested that subjective binge episodes are clinically meaningful, but have low reliability [25–27]. Improved diagnostic guidelines, assessment tool instructions, and new measures (e.g., the Eating Loss of Control Scale and the Loss of Control over Eating Scale) may help increase reliability and improve diagnosis and severity assessment across disorders characterized by binge eating [10, 11, 28, 29]. Our findings could help inform the refinement of these assessment tools to measure LOC. For example, although eating disorder experts who contributed to the development of the Loss of Control over Eating Scale (LOCES [11];) highly rated items describing mindless eating as "covering or reflecting" LOC, these mindless eating items had lower corrected item-total correlations [11], and one study found that the LOCES-Brief, which excludes these mindless eating items, provided a better fit to data from both clinical and non-clinical samples [28]. The current results more explicitly suggest that conflation of mindless and LOC eating may be a common cause of binge eating misdiagnosis. As such, diagnostic and research tools that clearly distinguish LOC from the mindlessness that it can sometimes co-occur with may be particularly helpful.

Strengths and limitations

The multilingual, global sample is significant strength of the study. Prior research has asked clinical and expert populations to explicitly define and describe LOC; however, our vignette-based, repeated-measures design mimicked real-world diagnostic decisions clinicians and researchers face when assessing what individuals describe as a "binge." As such, this first examination of the interacting influences of LOC and episode size on eating disorder diagnosis has implications directly relevant for clinical and research training and practice.

Several study limitations also should be noted. First, both patient vignettes were women, limiting the generalizability of our findings. BED is the most common eating disorder among men [30], and the influences of episode size and LOC descriptions on diagnosis may be even more complicated in men or other genders [31]. Second, as this study was focused on BED, both vignettes explicitly excluded compensatory behaviors. However, larger binge eating episodes may be linked to a stronger relationship between LOC and purging frequency (Forney et al., 2016), suggesting that the influence of LOC description and size on diagnostic conclusions may be more complex with the addition of purging to the clinical picture. Third, clinicians with eating disorder expertise were asked to make decisions in the context of brief vignettes, not a real clinical sample, and explorations of variation by country or world region were not possible with our modest sample size. Results may not generalize to non-expert clinicians or to individual patients or specific local populations or languages. Unexpectedly, participants diagnosed BED more frequently in the first vignette, regardless of the size or episode description included. As such, future research is needed to determine whether order effects exist in clinical or research diagnostic practice (e.g., whether the first patient of the day may be more likely to receive a correct than a missed diagnosis of BED).

Conclusions

Accurate and reliable assessment of binge eating is crucial for the diagnosis of BED and other eating disorders. The ICD-11 prioritizes the role of LOC over the amount of food consumed in the behavioral disturbance of binge eating. Although this guideline was established based on research and clinical data, there is currently no brief, standardized diagnostic strategy for LOC. Clinical training focused on the changes in the ICD-11 regarding binge eating and clear clinical and research standards for LOC assessment will be critical to increasing diagnostic consensus.

Abbreviations

BED: Binge-eating disorder; BN: Bulimia nervosa; DSM-5: Diagnostic and Statistical Manual of Mental Disorders, 5th Edition; ICD: International Classification of Diseases and Related Health Problems; LOC: Loss of control; WHO: World Health Organization; GEE: Generalized estimating equations

Acknowledgments

We are grateful to Sherin Asiimwe for assisting with survey programming and Chihiro Matsumoto and Tecelli Dominguez for translating our survey into Japanese and Spanish. In addition, we thank Geoffrey M. Reed and the members of the FSCG for their participation in discussions that helped improve this study design, and the experts who participated in this study for their time.

Authors' contributions

LAB and CAR conceived of the study; LAB, CAR, RS, and KMP designed the study; TR and KMP coordinated translation of the survey; TR supervised survey programming, monitored data collection, and supervised database management; LAB analyzed the data; LAB, RS, and KMP developed the manuscript draft, and all authors reviewed the draft and provided comments. All authors read and approved the final manuscript.

Competing interests

KMP was a member of the ICD-11 Feeding and Eating Disorders Working Group and the Field Studies Coordination Group for ICD-11 Mental and Behavioral Disorders (FSCG). TJR was a consultant to the FSCG. KMP and RS were supported by funds from Shire Pharmaceuticals. The authors alone are responsible for the views expressed in this paper and they do not necessarily represent the decisions, policy, or views of the WHO. The other authors declare that they have no competing interests.

Author details

[1]Department of Psychiatry, Icahn School of Medicine at Mount Sinai, New York, NY, USA. [2]Department of Psychiatry, Columbia University Irving Medical Center, New York, NY, USA. [3]Department of Medical Ethics and Health Policy, Perelman School of Medicine, University of Pennsylvania, Philadelphia, PA, USA.

References

1. Wolfe BE, Baker CW, Smith AT, Kelly-Weeder S. Validity and utility of the current definition of binge eating. Int J Eat Disord. 2009;42(8):674–86.
2. Watson HJ, Fursland A, Bulik CM, Nathan P. Subjective binge eating with compensatory behaviors: a variant presentation of bulimia nervosa. Int J Eat Disord. 2013;46(2):119–26.
3. Palavras MA, Morgan CM, Borges FMB, Claudino AM, Hay PJ. An investigation of objective and subjective types of binge eating episodes in a clinical sample of people with co-morbid obesity. J Eat Disord. 2013;1:26.
4. Brownstone LM, Bardone-Cone AM, Fitzsimmons-Craft EE, Printz KS, Le Grange D, Mitchell JE, et al. Subjective and objective binge eating in relation to eating disorder symptomatology, negative affect, and personality dimensions. Int J Eat Disord. 2013;46(1):66–76.
5. Fitzsimmons-Craft EE, Ciao AC, Accurso EC, Pisetsky EM, Peterson CB, Byrne CE, et al. Subjective and objective binge eating in relation to eating disorder symptomatology, depressive symptoms, and self-esteem among treatment-seeking adolescents with bulimia nervosa. Eur Eat Disord Rev. 2014;22(4):230–6.
6. Reed GM, First MB, Kogan CS, Hyman SE, Gureje O, Gaebel W, et al. Innovations and changes in the ICD-11 classification of mental, behavioural and neurodevelopmental disorders. World Psychiatry. 2019;18(1):3–19.
7. American Psychiatric Association. Diagnostic and Statistical Manual of Mental Disorders: Fifth Edition (DSM-5). Washington. D.C: American Psychiatric Association; 2013.
8. Goldschmidt AB. Are loss of control while eating and overeating valid constructs? A critical review of the literature. Obes Rev. 2017;18(4):412–49.
9. Devlin MJ, King WC, Kalarchian MA, White GE, Marcus MD, Garcia L, et al. Eating pathology and experience and weight loss in a prospective study of bariatric surgery patients: 3-year follow-up. Int J Eat Disord. 2016;49(12):1058–67.
10. Blomquist KK, Roberto CA, Barnes RD, White MA, Masheb RM, Grilo CM. Development and validation of the eating loss of control scale. Psychol Assess. 2014;26(1):77–89.
11. Latner JD, Mond JM, Kelly MC, Haynes SN, Hay PJ. The loss of control over eating scale: development and psychometric evaluation. Int J Eat Disord. 2014;47(6):647–59.
12. Claudino AM, Pike KM, Hay P, Keeley JW, Evans SC, Rebello TJ, et al. The classification of feeding and eating disorders in the ICD-11: results of a field study comparing proposed ICD-11 guidelines with existing ICD-10 guidelines. BMC Med. 2019;17(1):93.
13. Heriseanu AI, Hay P, Corbit L, Touyz S. Grazing in adults with obesity and eating disorders: a systematic review of associated clinical features and meta-analysis of prevalence. Clin Psychol Rev. 2017;58:16–32.
14. Tuomisto T, Tuomisto MT, Hetherington M, Lappalainen R. Reasons for initiation and cessation of eating in obese men and women and the affective consequences of eating in everyday situations. Appetite. 1998;30(2):211–22.
15. Reed GM, Rebello TJ, Pike KM, Medina-Mora ME, Gureje O, Zhao M, et al. WHO's global clinical practice network for mental health. Lancet Psychiatry. 2015;2(5):379–80.
16. Chen EY, Safer DL. Dialectical behavior therapy for bulimia nervosa and binge-eating disorder. In: Grilo CM, Mitchell JE, editors. The treatment of eating disorders: a clinical handbook. New York: Guilford Press; 2010. p. 294–316.
17. Framson C, Kristal AR, Schenk JM, Littman AJ, Zeliadt S, Benitez D. Development and validation of the mindful eating questionnaire. J Am Diet Assoc. 2009;109(8):1439 44.
18. Gormally J, Black S, Daston S, Rardin D. The assessment of binge eating severity among obese persons. Addict Behav. 1982;7(1):47–55.
19. Fairburn CG, Cooper Z, O'Connor M. Eating disorder examination (Edition 16.0D). In: Fairburn CG, editor. Cognitive behavior therapy and eating disorders. New York: Guilford Press; 2008.
20. Garner DM. Eating disorder Inventory-3. Professional manual. Lutz: Psychological Assessment Resources, Inc.; 2004.
21. Stunkard AJ, Messick S. The three-factor eating questionnaire to measure dietary restraint, disinhibition and hunger. J Psychosom Res. 1985;29(1):71–83.
22. Yanovski SZ, Marcus MD, Wadden TA, Walsh BT. The questionnaire on eating and weight Patterns-5: an updated screening instrument for binge eating disorder. Int J Eat Disord. 2015;48(3):259–61.

23. Pan W. Akaike's information criterion in generalized estimating equations. Biometrics. 2001;57(1):120–5.

24. Goldfein JA, Devlin MJ, Kamenetz C. Eating disorder examination-questionnaire with and without instruction to assess binge eating in patients with binge eating disorder. Int J Eat Disord. 2005;37(2):107–11.

25. Rizvi S, Peterson C, Crow S, Agras W. Test-retest reliability of the eating disorder examination. Int J Eat Disord. 2000;28(3):311–6.

26. Grilo C, Masheb R, Lozano-Blanco C, Barry D. Reliability of the eating disorder examination in patients with binge eating disorder. Int J Eat Disord. 2004;35(1):80–5.

27. Grilo CM, Masheb RM, Wilson GT. Different methods for assessing the features of eating disorders in patients with binge eating disorder: a replication. Obes Res. 2001;9(7):418–22.

28. Bodell LP, Forney KJ, Chavarria J, Keel PK, Wildes JE. Self-report measures of loss of control over eating: psychometric properties in clinical and non-clinical samples. Int J Eat Disord. 2018;51(11):1252–60.

29. Vannucci A, Ohannessian CM. Psychometric properties of the brief loss of control over eating scale (LOCES-B) in early adolescents. Int J Eat Disord. 2018;51(5):459–64.

30. Hudson JI, Hiripi E, Pope HG, Kessler RC. The prevalence and correlates of eating disorders in the National Comorbidity Survey replication. Biol Psychiatry. 2007;61(3):348–58.

31. Striegel-Moore RH, Rosselli F, Perrin N, DeBar L, Wilson GT, May A, et al. Gender difference in the prevalence of eating disorder symptoms. Int J Eat Disord. 2009;42(5):471–4.

4

The feasibility of emotion-focused therapy for binge-eating disorder: a pilot randomised wait-list control trial

Kevin Glisenti[1]*[iD], Esben Strodl[1], Robert King[1] and Leslie Greenberg[2]

Abstract

Background: Research into psychotherapy for binge-eating disorder (BED) has focused mainly on cognitive behavioural therapies, but efficacy, failure to abstain, and dropout rates continue to be problematic. The experience of negative emotions is among the most accurate predictors for the occurrence of binge eating episodes in BED, suggesting benefits to exploring psychological treatments with a more specific focus on the role of emotion. The present study aimed to explore the feasibility of individual emotion-focused therapy (EFT) as a treatment for BED by examining the outcomes of a pilot randomised wait-list controlled trial.

Methods: Twenty-one participants were assessed using a variety of feasibility measures relating to recruitment, credibility and expectancy, therapy retention, objective binge episodes and days, and binge eating psychopathology outcomes. The treatment consisted of 12 weekly one-hour sessions of EFT for maladaptive emotions over 3 months. A mixed model approach was utilised with one between effect (group) using a one-way analysis of variance (ANOVA) to test the hypothesis that participants immediately receiving the EFT treatment would demonstrate a greater degree of improvement on outcomes relating to objective binge episodes and days, and binge eating psychopathology, compared to participants on the EFT wait-list; and one within effect (time) using a repeated-measures ANOVA to test the hypothesis that participation in the EFT intervention would result in significant improvements in outcome measures from pre to post-therapy and then maintained at follow-up.

Results: Recruitment, credibility and expectancy, therapy retention outcomes indicated EFT is a feasible treatment for BED. Further, participants receiving EFT demonstrated a greater degree of improvement in objective binge episodes and days, and binge eating psychopathology compared to EFT wait-list control group participants. When participants in the EFT wait-list control group then received treatment and outcomes data were combined with participants who initially received the treatment, EFT demonstrated significant improvement in objective binge episodes and days, and binge eating psychopathology for the entire sample.

Conclusions: These findings provide further preliminary evidence for the feasibility of individual EFT for BED and support more extensive randomised control trials to assess efficacy.

(Continued on next page)

* Correspondence: kevin.glisenti@hdr.qut.edu.au
[1]School of Psychology and Counselling, Queensland University of Technology, Faculty of Health, Brisbane, Queensland, Australia
Full list of author information is available at the end of the article

(Continued from previous page)
Keywords: Emotion-focused therapy, Binge-eating disorder, Feasibility, Emotion regulation, Pilot randomised control trial

Plain English summary

Research into psychotherapy for binge-eating disorder (BED) has focused mainly on cognitive-behavioural therapies, but efficacy, failure to abstain, and dropout rates continue to be problematic. The experience of negative emotions is among the most accurate predictors for the occurrence of binge eating episodes in BED, suggesting benefits to exploring psychological treatments with a more specific focus on the role of emotion. This pilot randomised wait-list control trial aimed to investigate the feasibility of emotion-focused therapy (EFT) for BED using a variety of measures relating to recruitment, credibility and expectancy, therapy retention, objective binge episodes and days, and binge eating psychopathology outcomes.. Initially, participants were randomly allocated to an immediate EFT treatment or EFT wait-list control group. The treatment consisted of 12 weekly one-hour sessions of EFT over 3 months with 21 participants. Recruitment, credibility and expectancy, and therapy retention outcomes indicated EFT is a feasible treatment for BED. Further, participants immediately receiving the EFT demonstrated a greater degree of improvement in binge episodes, the number of days on which binge episodes occurred, and binge eating symptoms compared to participants in EFT the wait-list control group. Participants in the EFT wait-list control group then received treatment and outcomes data were combined with participants who initially received the treatment. EFT resulted in significant improvements in binge episodes and the number of days on which binge episodes occur, and binge eating psychopathology for the entire sample. These findings provide further preliminary evidence for the feasibility of individual EFT for BED, and support for more extensive randomised control trials to assess efficacy.

Binge-eating disorder (BED) is the most prevalent of all the eating disorders [1]. There is an estimated prevalence rate of 2.5 to 4.5% in females and 1.0 to 3.0% in males based on international data [2] and a 3-month prevalence rate of 5.58% based on Australian data [3]. The core symptoms include recurrent episodes of binge eating while experiencing a sense of lack of control in the absence of compensatory strategies [4]. Not surprisingly, many individuals with BED also have comorbid emotional disorders [5] including anxiety [6, 7] and depression [8, 9]. For BED, both The National Institute of Clinical Excellence (NICE) in the United Kingdom and the American Psychiatric Association guidelines suggest that cognitive behaviour therapy (CBT) is the psychological treatment of choice, with interpersonal therapy (IPT) and dialectical behaviour therapy (DBT) serving as second-line interventions [10, 11].

In a recent meta-analysis, Hilbert et al. [12] explored the efficacy of psychological treatments for BED. Psychological therapy, mostly CBT, demonstrated large effect sizes for the reduction of binge episodes and abstinence from binge eating in RCTs with inactive control groups, followed by structured self-help with medium-to-large effects when compared with wait-list. There was limited evidence for the of one treatment approach over another in RCTs with active control groups, and more extensive research with a focus on longer-term maintenance of therapy gains, efficacy, mechanisms of change and complex models of care was recommended [12]. In another more recent meta-analysis, Linardon [13] estimated the prevalence of patients with BED who achieved binge-eating abstinence following psychological or behavioural treatments. The most common treatment delivered was CBT (either in a clinician-led or guided self-help format), and other interventions include behavioural weight loss, behavioural weight loss combined with CBT, IPT, DBT, behaviour therapy, non-specific supportive therapy, mindfulness, psychodynamic therapy, and a combined psychotherapy approach. The total weighted percentage of treatment-completers who achieved abstinence at posttreatment was 50.9 and 50.30% at follow-up. The highest abstinence rate was observed in IPT, and clinician-led group treatments produced significantly higher posttreatment (but not follow-up) abstinence estimates than guided self-help treatments. The meta-analysis demonstrated that 50% of patients with BED do not fully respond to treatment, and there is, therefore, a need to explore other psychotherapies to improve outcomes [13].

Individuals with BED often experience difficulties with deficits in emotion regulation which can be defined as the "… attempt to influence which emotions we have, when we have them, and how these emotions are experienced or expressed." ([14], p. 224). Several emotion regulation theories have been proposed to explain eating-related problems. For example, emotional eating theory conceptualises eating as a coping strategy in response to emotional distress [15, 16]; escape theory presumes a reduction of negative affect while bingeing [17]; affect regulation theory [18] assumes an improvement in negative affect after bingeing; and emotional arousal theory conceptualises overeating as being evoked by emotional arousal in order to reduce the level of arousal [19]. Given each of these theories includes negative emotions as a trigger for binge eating (i.e., trigger component) and/or down-regulation of negative emotions (i.e., relief component) while or after binge eating, [20] proposes an 'emotion regulation model' of binge eating which incorporates both components and includes the whole emotion regulation process. Binge eating occurs in response to intolerable emotional experiences in the absence of more adaptive coping mechanisms [21] and represents an effort by an individual to regulate emotion by numbing, avoiding or soothing negative or overwhelming affect [22]. It occurs in the absence of effective regulation skills related to experiencing and differentiating as well as attenuating and modulating emotions [23], and individuals with BED experience more intense emotions and more significant difficulties in emotion regulation than individuals without BED [24].

Given that the experience of negative emotions is amongst the best predictors for the occurrence of binge eating episodes in BED [25], outcomes could be improved by psychological treatments with a more specific focus on the role of emotion. Indeed, innovative treatments for BED with a more specific focus on emotion are emerging, including integrative cognitive-affective therapy [26] and emotion-focused cognitive-behavioural therapy [27]. Emotion-focused therapy (EFT) is a compelling treatment for eating disorders and offers a unique framework for understanding the pathogenesis of emotional difficulties (either under-regulating or over-regulating affect) in this population [28]. The goal of EFT is to assist clients in 1) identifying and accepting primary emotions (their very first emotional response to a stimulus situation) from secondary emotions (a response that obscures their primary response) 2) processing primary maladaptive negative emotions by attending to and increasing awareness and expression of these primary maladaptive emotions; learning to tolerate and regulate painful underlying experience; reflecting upon and make meaning of emotion by symbolising emotional experience in words; and transforming maladaptive emotions by activating healthy, adaptive emotions together with their associated needs and action tendencies [29].

According to the EFT model, emotion organises experience through emotion schemes, which are constructed from lived emotional experience [30]. Central mechanisms of change in EFT include 1) identifying primary maladaptive emotion that are obscured by secondary symptomatic emotions and having arrived at these emotions, the use of adaptive emotion to transform maladaptive emotion schemes that are understood to generate chronic enduring pain and maintain secondary symptomatic behaviour and rigid and maladaptive modes of responding to experience [31], and a successful therapeutic relationship, in which the client feels empathically heard, understood, supported and safe [32]. The feasibility and efficacy of EFT have been established in various disorders including depression (e.g., [33–35]); complex trauma (e.g., [36–38]); and are emerging for anxiety [39–41]. While there is a growing body of literature exploring the use of EFT for eating disorders (e.g., [28, 29, 42–45]), this literature has generally included mixed samples of BED, Anorexia Nervosa (AN) and BN with limited research focusing specifically on BED.

To date, only one study has examined the feasibility and efficacy of EFT specifically for BED; however, this was group therapy based. In a non-randomised observational study, Compare and Tasca [46] compared the outcome of 20 weeks of emotionally focused group therapy (EFGT), aimed at helping clients change how they experienced and used their emotions, with combined therapy (CT) of EFGT plus dietary counselling, which sought to lower energy-dense food intake in 118 obese adults with BED. Participants were assigned to EFGT or CT based on consensus among clinicians. Binge episodes and weight significantly declined during both treatments; however, compared to EFGT, CT resulted in more rapid weight loss across the weeks of therapy. The dropout rate for EFGT was only 6%. Further, to date, only one study to date has examined the feasibility of individual therapy based EFT for BED [47]. This study involved the use of a multiple baseline case series design in which individual EFT over 12 weeks, was applied to six female adult participants with BED, with follow-ups at 2, 4- and 8-weeks posttreatment. All cases experienced reliable recovery from binge-eating psychopathology and also a significant decrease in binge-eating frequency. There was reliable improvement or recovery for eating and shape concerns for all cases, and improvement on weight concern for the majority of cases; and all cases experienced reliable recovery or improvement in overall emotion regulation. Most cases that were in the clinical range for anxiety at pre-treatment recovered and all cases experienced reliable improvement in, or recovery from, depression. Three of the six cases experienced reliable recovery or improvement in alexithymia. There were no treatment dropouts.

While there is emerging preliminary evidence for the use of EFT for BED, a pilot trial to further test feasibility is required. Arain, Campbell, Cooper and Lancaster [48] provide a useful model upon which the feasibility of a pilot study can be assessed. This model suggests that feasibility studies incorporate research conducted before the main study in order to identify important parameters needed to design the main study. These can include participant willingness to be randomised, the number of eligible participants, and other aspects such as therapy retention rates. Further, it has been proposed that the purpose of a pilot study is to examine the feasibility of an approach intended to be used in a larger-scale study, through evaluating recruitment, randomisation and retention, in addition to assessment procedures, new methods, and implementation of novel interventions [49]. The current study presents results from a pilot randomised wait-list control trial to assess the feasibility of individual EFT for BED. It was hypothesised that:

1 Participants would be willing to be randomised, and an appropriate number of participants would be deemed eligible for the research.

2 Participation in EFT would result in higher participant treatment credibility and expectancy for improvement scores.

3 There would be a lower dropout rate using EFT for BED compared to more commonly used psychological treatment approaches.

4 Immediate EFT treatment group participants would demonstrate a significantly greater degree of improvement in objective binge episodes, the number of days on which objective binge episodes occurred, and binge eating psychopathology, compared to participants in an EFT wait-list control group who had not received the treatment.

5 The total sample (i.e. the immediate EFT treatment group who initially received treatment, and also EFT wait-list group post receiving treatment), would experience significant improvements in objective binge episodes, the number of days on which objective binge episodes occurred, and binge eating psychopathology.

Method
Design
This study is a pilot randomised wait-list control trial designed to explore the feasibility of individual emotion-focused therapy (EFT) as a treatment for BED. It builds upon findings from an initial multiple baseline case series design of EFT for BED [47]. The sample size for the current study was calculated using the outcome measure of changes in binge eating episodes from the initial case series as a basis. This showed an effect size of Cohen's d = 2.91. Using GPower with this effect size, alpha at .05, power at .95, using repeated measures ANOVA between groups design with 3 time points, yielded a required total sample size of just 6 participants. Binge eating disorder treatment pilot study sample sizes vary, e.g., 7 [27], 10 [50], 36 [51], and 41 [52]. We chose a sample size clearly larger than what was required by

our power analysis from the initial case series, and at the mid-point of the aforementioned pilot studies.

Participants were initially randomly allocated to either an immediate EFT treatment group (12 weekly EFT sessions) or an EFT wait-list control group (12-week clinical monitoring preceding 12 weekly EFT sessions) using a block randomisation method [53]. This is a commonly used technique in clinical trial design which reduces bias and achieves sample size balance when allocating participants to treatment groups. It is particularly useful for smaller sample sizes and increases the probability that each allocation arm will contain an equal number of individuals by sequencing participant assignments by block. This project was approved by the Queensland University of Technology (QUT) University Human Research Ethics Committee (UHREC) and met the requirements of the National Statement on Ethical Conduct in Human Research (2007). The UHREC Reference number is 1700000986, and all participants provided written informed consent. Consolidated Standards of Reporting Trials (CONSORT) guidelines were fully adhered to – See Fig. 1.

Participants
Participants were recruited from local General Practitioners/Primary Care Physicians. Inclusion criteria included the following: being between 18 and 65 years of age, meeting the Diagnostic and Statistical Manual of Mental Disorders: DSM-V American Psychiatric Association – DSM-5 [4] diagnostic criteria for BED, and possessing sufficient English language skills to provide informed consent and participate in the study without translation. The exclusion criteria included current psychosis, intellectual disability, high suicide risk, drug or alcohol abuse, concurrent treatment for obesity, pregnancy, and the presence of AN or BN. The total sample consisted of 21 participants, of whom 17 were female, and 4 were male. The average age was 44.52 (SD = 11.89) years and the average age at first binge 18.23 (SD = 8.07) years. Ten participants were married or living with someone as married, 5 separated, 3 never married, 2 divorced and 1 widowed. Six participants had graduated four-year college, 5 graduated two-year college or trade school, 4 completed grades 7–12 (without graduating high school), 3 graduated high school or high school equivalent, 2 partially completed college/trade school and 1 postgraduate/professional school. Eleven participants were employed full-time, 5 part-time employment, 2 keeping house or caregiving full time, 2 in school/training and 1 disabled.

Measures
Pretherapy assessment measures
Pretherapy diagnostic assessment of BED was based on the Structured Clinical Interview for DSM-5-Research

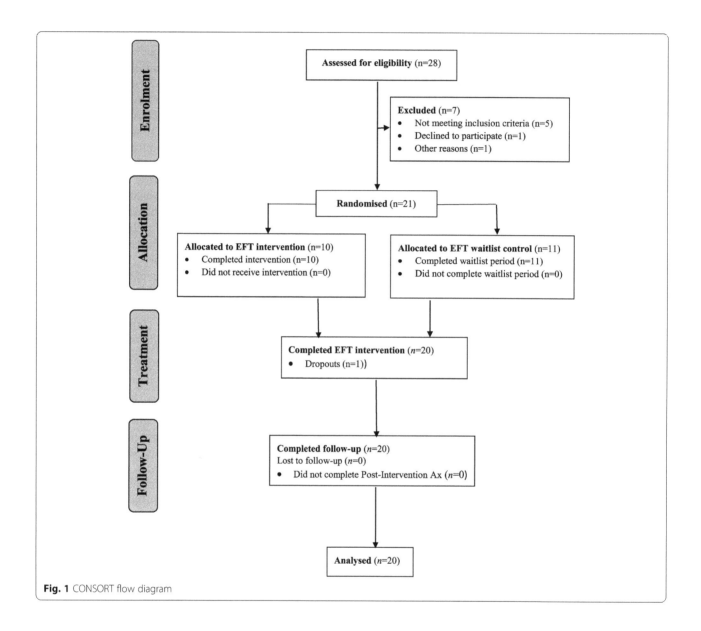

Fig. 1 CONSORT flow diagram

Version - SCID-5-RV [54]. At present, there is limited reliability or validity data available for the SCID-5-RV; however, it has demonstrated internal consistency (.80) and test-retest reliability [55]. Previous versions of Structured Clinical Interview for DSM-IV Axis I Disorders - SCID-I [56], however, have demonstrated a high level of inter-rater reliability (k = .75) for symptoms and 90% accuracy in diagnosis [57].

Feasibility measures
Recruitment
Data were obtained in relation to various aspects of recruitment, including participant willingness to be randomised, and the number of eligible participants during the recruitment process.

Credibility and expectancy
Treatment credibility and participant expectancy for improvement were measured using the Credibility and Expectancy Questionnaire – CEQ [58]. The CEQ is a 6-item self-report measure of treatment expectancy and rationale credibility. Items 1 to 4 are rated based on cognitive appraisal, i.e., asking participants what they think will happen (e.g., "At this point, how logical does the treatment offered to you seem?" and "At this point, how useful do you think the treatment will be in reducing your binge eating disorder symptoms?"), and items 5–6 are rated based on affective aspects of beliefs, i.e., asking participants what they feel will happen (e.g., "At this point, how much do you really feel that therapy will help you reduce your binge eating disorder symptoms?" and "By the end of the therapy period, how much

improvement in your binge eating disorder symptoms do you really feel will occur?"). The original CEQ contains four questions on credibility using a 9-point Likert scale, where 1 = not at all and 9 = very much or very useful, and two questions on expectancy using a scale from 0 to 100% in 10% increments. Given the use of two scales during administration, a composite score is derived for each factor by initially standardising the individual items and then summing those items for each factor. The CEQ has demonstrated adequate test-retest reliability of the expectancy (.82) and credibility factor (.75). The combined overall rating of the treatment rationale resulted in a composite index high test-retest reliability of (.83) and adequate internal consistency [α = .85] [58].

Therapy retention

Participants who completely discontinued attendance were considered dropouts.

Objective binge episodes and days Changes in objective binge episodes and days (occurrence over the previous 7 days) were assessed using items from the Eating Disorder Examination Questionnaire – EDE-Q-6.0 [59]. The EDE-Q-6.0 is a self-report measure of eating disorder psychopathology based on the Eating Disorder Examination Interview [60]. It is a widely used measure of eating disorder attitudes and behaviours in both community and clinical populations [61]. The EDE-Q-6.0 also provides frequency data on the number of episodes of the eating disorder behaviours and the number of days on which the behaviour occurred. The items used to measure objective binge episodes (i.e., a discrete episode of overeating of an objectively large amount of food associated with a feeling of loss of control) in the current study were: "Over the past 7 days how many times have you eaten what other people would regard as an unusually large amount of food (given the circumstances)?" and "On how many of these times did you have a sense of having lost control over your eating (at the time that you were eating)?". The item used to measure the number of days objective binge episodes occurred was "Over the past 7 days, on how many days have such episodes of overeating occurred (i.e., you have eaten an unusually large amount of food and have had a sense of loss of control at the time)?". The EDE-Q-6.0 has received support as a reliable and valid measure of eating-related pathology and specific disordered eating behaviours [62, 63]. Test-retest reliability across studies ranges from 0.66 to 0.94 for scores on the four subscales [64]. The EDEQ-Q-6.0 has demonstrated acceptable levels of internal consistency (α = .90) for the total score in a clinical sample [65]. There are no standardised clinical cut-offs [59].

Binge eating psychopathology Changes in binge-eating psychopathology were assessed using the Binge Eating Scale – BES [66]. The BES is a commonly used self-report screening tool for binge eating in clinical practice and research. A total of 16 items are rated using 3–4 separate responses assigned a numerical value. An example of an item is "(a.) I feel capable to control my eating urges when I want to; (b.) I feel like I have failed to control my eating more than the average person; (c.) I feel utterly helpless when it comes to feeling in control of my eating urges; (d.) Because I feel so helpless about controlling my eating I have become very desperate about trying to get in control". Total scores range from 0 to 46, with higher scores indicating more severe binge-eating symptoms. The BES has demonstrated high test-retest reliability ($r = .71$) and internal consistency ($α = .85$) in an obese population [67], good 2-week test-retest reliability ($r = .87$) in a behavioural weight loss sample [68], high internal consistency ($α = .91$) in a BED sample [69], and good construct reliability and convergent validity [70]. Standardised cut-off scores are as follows: ≤ 17 = no binge eating, 18–26 = mild to moderate binge eating, and ≥ 27 = severe binge eating [66].

Procedures

Participants were initially telephone-screened for BED based on diagnostic criteria, according to DSM-5 [4]. Twenty-eight participants were telephone-screened, of which five did not meet the diagnostic criteria for BED. Twenty-three participants meeting the diagnostic criteria for BED then completed the SCID-5-RV administered by the same research assistant with training in clinical psychology. All met the inclusion criteria, but 1 participant chose not to participate due to being unable to commit fully to weekly treatment sessions, and 1 participant did not respond to contact attempts. Twenty-one participants were randomly allocated to either an immediate EFT intervention or 12-week EFT wait-list using a block randomisation method, by a statistician independent to the research team.

Participants allocated to the immediate EFT intervention completed the BES and EDE-Q-6.0 pretherapy (Week 0). The BES and EDE-Q-6.0 were completed weekly (Weeks 1–12), and CEQ at weeks 1, 3, 5, 7, 9 and 11 during treatment. The BES and EDE-Q-6.0 were completed at follow-up (Weeks 16, 20 and 24). Participants allocated to the EFT wait-list control completed the BES and EDE-Q-6.0at pretherapy (Week 0), and then again 12 weeks later post wait-list period completion. Wait-list control participants then commenced 12 weekly treatment sessions and followed the same protocol as participants initially allocated to the immediate EFT treatment intervention. The therapist was blind to all assessments and randomisation of the participants.

Treatment

Treatment incorporated 12 weekly one-hour sessions of EFT for maladaptive emotions over 3 months. The treatment manual was initially adapted from [45] by [47] in a series of case studies exploring the use of individual EFT to treat BED. Phase 1 of the treatment focused on promoting awareness of emotions, welcoming and accepting emotions, putting emotions into words, and identifying primary emotions. Phase 2 focused on evaluating whether the primary emotion was adaptive or maladaptive, identifying destructive emotions, accessing other adaptive emotions and needs, and transforming maladaptive emotion schemes. Six main marker guided interventions were used in treatment in line with EFT protocol (30, 323). These were: 1. Empathic attunement and validation for vulnerability and establishing the therapeutic alliance 2. Evocative unfolding for problematic reactions 3. Experiential focusing for unclear feelings 4. Two-chair work for self-critical splits 5. Two-chair work for self-interruptive splits and 6. Empty chair work for unfinished business.

Therapist

The therapist was the first author, a Clinical Psychologist with 25 years of practice experience who had undergone Level 1, 2 and 3 training in EFT at the York University Psychology Clinic with the primary developer of this approach, Distinguished ProfessorEmeritus, Leslie Greenberg. The therapist had approximately 4 years of EFT-specific practice experience before the study and was not involved in the initial treatment/wait-list randomisation process, data collection before or during the study, or data analysis until after the study. Supervision was provided by Distinguished Professor Emeritus, Leslie Greenberg, who was also a co-author of the original treatment manual used as a basis for therapy within the current study. Adherence to EFT protocol was reviewed - and rectified where necessary - during supervision based on video recordings of study treatment sessions.

Statistical analyses plan

Initially, a one-way ANOVA was conducted in relation to any significant demographic differences between participants randomly allocated to the immediate EFT and EFT wait-list control group at baseline. Following this, a mixed model approach was utilised with one between effect (group) using a one-way ANOVA to test the hypothesis that participants immediately receiving the EFT treatment would demonstrate a greater degree of improvement on outcome measures relating to objective binge episodes and days, and binge eating psychopathology compared to participants on the EFT wait-list; and one within effect (time) using a repeated-measures ANOVA to test the hypothesis that participation in the EFT intervention would result in significant improvements in outcome measures from pre to post-therapy and then maintained at each follow-up period, for the total sample. Missing data were managed using pairwise deletion.

Results

Demographics

Table 1 outlines the demographics of participants who completed treatment at baseline.

Assessment of feasibility

Recruitment

Participants were recruited over a period of 9 months, and this phase was protracted due to a lower than expected take-up rate. Reports from general practitioners/primary care physicians indicated the one main reason for this was the relatively lower percentage of patients with binge eating disorder within the medical practices. Twenty-eight participants were assessed for eligibility, and 5 five did not meet the diagnostic criteria for BED. All remaining participants met the inclusion criteria, but 1 chose not to participate due to being unable to commit fully to weekly treatment sessions, and 1 did not respond to contact attempts. Twenty-one participants were randomly allocated to either an immediate EFT intervention or 12-week EFT wait-list using a block randomisation method. While 3 participants allocated to an EFT wait-list expressed disappointment about not proceeding to treatment immediately, each expressed a strong willingness to continue involvement in the study.

Credibility and expectancy

The CEQ demonstrated adequate internal consistency ($\alpha = .86$). Mean CEQ credibility scores remained high during early, mid and late therapy: 7.40 (SD = 1.30) at Week 1, 8.01 (SD = .58) at Week 7 and 7.85 (SD = 1.16) at Week 11. Mean CEQ expectancy scores also remained high during early, mid and late therapy: 6.86 (SD = 1.16) at Week 1, 7.13 (SD = 1.30) at Week 7 and 7.06 (SD = 1.32) at Week 11 (See Table 2.) Further, significant differences were not identified in mean treatment credibility and expectancy scores from early to mid-therapy, mid to late therapy or early to late therapy.

Therapy retention

One participant (4.76%) dropped out after Week 4 of the EFT treatment for family health reasons. All completing participants attended all sessions.

Table 1 Participant demographics at baseline for treatment completers ($n = 20$)

Case	Allocation	Gender	Age	Marital Status	Education Status	Employment Status	Age First Binge	Objective Binge Episodes[a]	Binge and Loss Control Days[a]
1	Treatment	Female	36	Separated	2-year college/trade school	School/training	33	7	7
2	Treatment	Female	57	Separated	4-year college	Part-time job	19	4	4
3	Treatment	Female	28	Never married	Part college/trade school	School/training	14	20	6
4	Treatment	Female	23	Married or with someone	High school or equivalent	Keeping house	10	5	5
5	Treatment	Male	58	Separated	High school or equivalent	Disabled	15	1	1
6	Treatment	Female	38	Widowed	4-year college	Keeping house	10	7	5
7	Treatment	Female	32	Married or with someone	4-year college	Full-time job	15	6	6
8	Treatment	Female	45	Divorced or annulled	Part graduate school	Full-time job	24	16	5
9	Treatment	Female	61	Married or with someone	Grades 7–12	Full-time job	8	2	2
10	Treatment	Male	42	Married or with someone	2-year college/ trade school	Full-time job	13	1	1
11	Waitlist	Male	47	Divorced or annulled	4-year college	Full-time job	18	9	7
12	Waitlist	Female	65	Married or with someone	2-year college/trade school	Part-time job	28	5	5
13	Waitlist	Female	42	Married or with someone	4-year college	Full-time job	16	10	7
14	Waitlist	Female	36	Married or with someone	Grades 7–12	Full-time job	15	3	2
15	Waitlist	Female	32	Never married	Part college/trade school	Full-time job	13	2	2
16	Waitlist	Female	50	Married or with someone	Grades 7–12	Part-time job	28	3	2
17	Waitlist	Male	62	Married or with someone	2-year college/trade school	Part-time job	15	5	5
18	Waitlist	Female	45	Never married	2-year college/ trade school	Part-time job	18	1	1
19	Waitlist	Female	41	Separated	High school or equivalent	Full-time job	18	5	6
20	Waitlist	Female	38	Separated	4-year college	Full-time job	13	8	7

[a]In previous 7 days

Table 2 CEQ early, mid and late therapy mean scores for the entire sample ($n = 20$)

	Early therapy[a]	Mid Therapy[b]	Late Therapy[c]	Early therapy to Mid therapy		Mid therapy to Late therapy		Early therapy to Late therapy	
	M (SD)	M (SD)	M (SD)	t-Test	D	t-Test	d	t-Test	d
CEQ credibility	7.40 (1.30)	8.01 (.58)	7.85 (1.16)	−2.04	.45	.93	−.16	−1.53	.32
CEQ expectancy	6.86 (1.16)	7.13 (1.30)	7.06 (1.32)	−1.03	.23	.29	−.07	−.75	.17

CEQ Credibility Expectancy Questionnaire; Week 1[a], Week 7[b], Week 11[c]

Immediate EFT intervention group versus EFT wait-list control group

Demographics No significant demographic differences were found between the immediate EFT intervention and EFT wait-list control groups in relation to mean age (years), mean age at first binge (years), gender, marital status, education, and employment status. See Table 3.

Objective binge episodes Significant differences were found between the immediate EFT intervention group mean scores from Week 0 to Week 12 of treatment, and EFT wait-list control group mean scores from Week 0 to Week 12 of the wait-list period, in relation to objective binge episodes. Compared with the EFT wait-list control group, the immediate EFT intervention group showed significantly greater reductions in objective binge episodes with a large treatment effect ($d = .98$). See Table 4.

Objective binge days Significant differences were also found between the immediate EFT intervention group mean scores from Week 0 to Week 12 of treatment, and EFT wait-list control group mean scores from Week 0 to Week 12 of the wait-list period, in relation to objective binge episodes days. When compared with the EFT wait-list control group, the immediate EFT intervention group experienced significantly greater reductions in objective binge episode days with a very large treatment effect ($d = 1.39$). See Table 4.

Binge eating psychopathology Significant differences were also found between the immediate EFT intervention group mean scores from Week 0 to Week 12 of treatment, and EFT wait-list control group mean scores from Week 0 to Week 12 of the wait-list period, in relation to binge eating psychopathology. Compared with the EFT wait-list control group, the immediate EFT intervention group displayed significantly greater reductions in

Table 3 Participant demographics by treatment group at randomization for treatment completers ($n = 20$)

Demographic	Immediate EFT Group ($n = 10$)	EFT Waitlist Group ($n = 10$)	t (df) or X^2	p-value
	M (SD) or f	M (SD) or f		
Age (years)	42.00 (13.16)	45.80 (10.73)	.67 (18)	.49
Age first binge (years)	16.10 (7.50)	18.20 (5.49)	.73 (18)	.49
Gender				
Male	2	2	.000	1.00
Female	8	8		
Marital Status				
Married or with someone	4	5	1.64	.80
Widowed	1	0		
Divorced or annulled	1	1		
Separated	3	2		
Never married	1	2		
Education				
Grades 7–12	1	2	1.86	.87
High school or equivalent	2	1		
Part college/trade school	1	1		
2-year college/trade school	2	3		
4-year college	3	3		
Part graduate school	1	0		
Employment Status				
Full-time job	4	6	7.20	.13
Part-time job	1	4		
Keeping house	2	0		
School/training	2	0		
Disabled	1	0		

Table 4 Mean Immediate EFT Group (*n* = 10) and EFT Waitlist Group (*n* = 10) EDEQ and BES pretherapy and posttherapy/postwaitlist scores

	Immediate EFT Group	EFT Waitlist Group	Immediate EFT Group	EFT Waitlist Group				
	Pretherapy[a]	Pretherapy	Post Therapy[b]	Post Waitlist[c]				
	M (*SD*)	*M* (*SD*)	*M* (*SD*)	*M* (*SD*)	*F*	*p*-value	η_p^2	Cohen's *d*
Outcome								
EDEQ objective binge episodes	6.90 (6.33)	5.10 (3.03)	2.90 (2.88)	5.10 (2.84)	6.85	.017	.276	.98
EDEQ objective binge episode days	4.20 (2.15)	4.40 (2.41)	1.50 (1.64)	4.70 (2.31)	40.09	.001	.690	1.39
BES binge eating psychopathology	25.60 (9.65)	28.30 (6.93)	20.70 (11.77)	29.20 (7.98)	12.12	.003	.402	.62

EDEQ Eating Disorders Examination Questionnaire *BES* Binge Eating Scale; Week 0[a] Week 12 of treatment[b] Week 12 of wait list[c]

binge eating psychopathology with a moderate treatment effect (d = .62).

Combined immediate EFT intervention group and EFT wait-list control group

Figure 2. and Table 5. outline combined EFT immediate intervention group and EFT wait-list control group within-group changes post the entire sample receiving treatment.

Objective binge episodes There was a significant decrease in objective binge episode frequency scores measured over sixteen-time points including baseline (Week 0), treatment sessions (Week 1, 2, 3, 4, 5, 6, 7, 8, 9, 10, 11 and 12) (Weeks 1 to 12), and follow up at 1 month (Weeks 16), 2 months (Week 20) and 3 months (Week 24) [*F* 1, 2.33) = 4.43, *p* < .014, ηp^2 = .189]. Mauchly's Test of Sphericity indicated that the assumption of sphericity was violated [χ2(119) = 501.42, *p* < .001] and therefore, the Huynh-Feldt correction was used for the ANOVA. The analyses of the changes in objective binge episodes are shown in Table 5.

Pretherapy objective binge episodes significantly decreased from 6.00 (*SD* = 4.92) to 2.05 (*SD* = 2.39) posttherapy with a large effect size (*d* = .99). There was no significant difference between posttherapy and 3 months of follow-up scores, suggesting that treatment gains were maintained.

Objective binge episode days There was a significant decrease in objective binge episode days scores measured over sixteen-time points including baseline (Week 0), treatment sessions (Week 1, 2, 3, 4, 5, 6, 7, 8, 9, 10, 11 and 12) (Weeks 1 to 12), and follow up at 1 month (Weeks 16), 2 months (Week 20) and 3 months (Week 24) [*F* 1, 8.44) = 8.78, *p* < .001, ηp^2 = .316]. Mauchly's Test of Sphericity indicated that the assumption of sphericity was violated [χ2(119) = 245.12, *p* < .001] and therefore, the Huynh-Feldt correction was used for the ANOVA. The analyses of the changes in objective binge episode days are shown in Table 5. Mean objective binge

episode days decreased from 4.30 (*SD* = 2.23) pretherapy to 1.25 (*SD* = 1.33) posttherapy with a very large effect size (*d* = 1.51). There was no significant difference between posttherapy and 3 months of follow-up scores, suggesting that treatment gains were maintained.

Binge eating psychopathology The BES demonstrated adequate internal consistency (α = .90). There was a significant decrease in binge eating psychopathology within-group scores measured over sixteen-time points including baseline (Week 0), treatment sessions (Week 1, 2, 3, 4, 5, 6, 7, 8, 9, 10, 11 and 12) (Weeks 1 to 12), and follow up at 1 month (Weeks 16), 2 months (Week 20) and 3 months (Week 24) [*F* 1, 4.04) = 9.84, *p* < .001, ηp^2 = .341]. Mauchly's Test of Sphericity indicated that the assumption of sphericity was violated [χ2(119) = 314.28, *p* < .001] and therefore, the Huynh-Feldt correction was used. Pretherapy mean BES scores significantly decreased from 26.95 (*SD* = 8.29) to 18.65 (*SD* = 10.45) posttherapy with a large effect size (*d* = 1.10) (see Table 5). Pre to posttherapy, the number of participants with severe binge eating range decreased from 14 to 6, and the number of non-binge eating participants increased from 3 to 11. There were 3 participants with mild to moderate binge eating at pre and posttherapy. At 3-month follow-up, there were 12 participants in the non-binge eating range, 1 mild to moderate and 7 in the severe range. There was no significant difference between posttherapy and 3-month follow-up scores, indicating that treatment gains were maintained.

Discussion

To our knowledge, this is one of the first pilot randomised controlled trials to test the feasibility of individual EFT for BED. It builds upon more extensive previous research exploring the efficacy and feasibility of group therapy based EFT for BED [46] which used a non-randomised observational study, and a less extensive feasibility trial of individual therapy based EFT for BED which used a case study approach [47]. It was initially hypothesised that participants would be willing to be

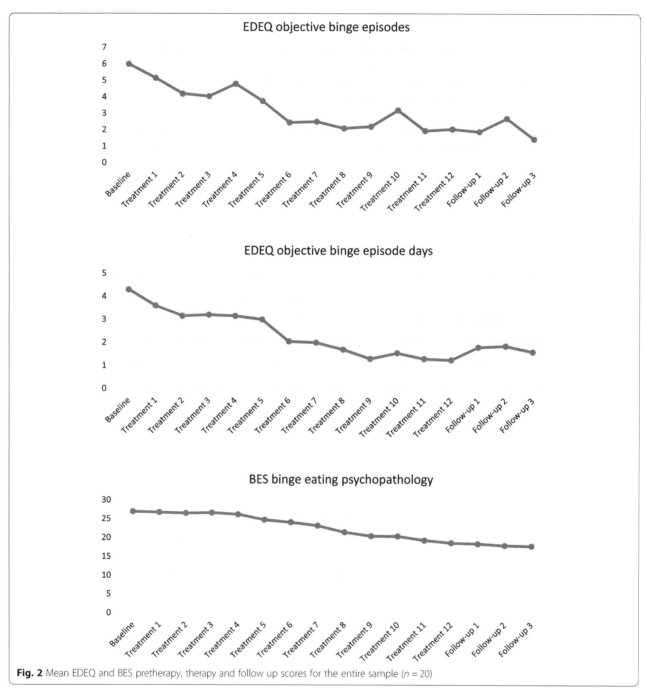

Fig. 2 Mean EDEQ and BES pretherapy, therapy and follow up scores for the entire sample (*n* = 20)

randomised; and an appropriate number of participants would be deemed eligible for the research. While a relatively small number of participants allocated to the EFT wait-list group expressed disappointment about not proceeding to treatment immediately, each expressed a strong willingness to continue involvement in the study. Further, while the recruitment phase was protracted due to a lower than expected take-up rate, this was mainly due to the relatively lower percentage of patients with binge eating disorder within the medical practices of referring general practitioner/primary care physicians.

Future research could improve recruitment through liaison with relevant specialised eating disorder treatment and support services.

The second hypothesis was that that participation in EFT would result in higher participant treatment credibility and expectancy for improvement scores. Mean CEQ credibility scores remained high during early, mid and late therapy, and significant differences were not identified in scores from early to mid-therapy, mid to late therapy or early to late therapy. This finding suggests that EFT is a feasible treatment approach for BED.

Table 5 Mean EDEQ and BES pretherapy, posttherapy and follow up scores for the entire sample ($n = 20$)

	Pretherapy[a] M (SD)	Posttherapy[b] M (SD)	F	p-value	η_p^2	Cohen's d
Outcome						
EDEQ objective binge episodes	6.0 (4.92)	2.05 (2.39)	19.70	.001	.509	.99
EDEQ objective binge episode days	4.30 (2.23)	1.25 (1.33)	45.93	.001	.707	1.51
BES binge eating psychopathology	26.95 (8.30)	18.65 (10.45)	24.50	.001	.563	1.10
	Posttherapy[b] M (SD)	Follow-up[c] M (SD)	F	p-value	η_p^2	Cohen's d
EDEQ objective binge episodes	2.05 (2.39)	1.45 (1.90)	1.21	.285	.060	.25
EDEQ objective binge episode days	1.25 (1.33)	1.60 (1.82)	.721	.406	.037	.19
BES binge eating psychopathology	18.65 (10.45)	17.80 (14.69)	.172	.683	.009	.09

EDEQ Eating Disorders Examination Questionnaire BES Binge Eating Scale; Week 0[a]. Week 12[b]. Week 24[c]

Our third hypothesis was that there would be a lower dropout rate using EFT for BED compared to more commonly used psychological treatment approaches. The 4.76% EFT for BED dropout rate in the current study compares favourably with dropout rates for other psychological treatment approaches for this condition including CBT - 11.1% [71] and 21.3% [72]; guided self-help cognitive behaviour therapy (CBTgsh) - 30% [73]; IPT - 8.6% [74] and 7% [75]; DBT - 4% [76]; and group psychodynamic interpersonal psychotherapy (GPIP) - 22.9% [72].

Our fourth hypothesis was that the immediate EFT treatment group participants would demonstrate a significantly greater degree of improvement in objective binge episodes, the number of days on which objective binge episodes occurred, and binge eating psychopathology, compared to participants in an EFT wait-list control group who had not received the treatment. Compared with the EFT wait-list control group, the immediate EFT intervention group showed significantly greater reductions in objective binge episodes with a large treatment effect (d = .98), objective binge days with a very large treatment effect (d = 1.39), and binge eating psychopathology with moderate treatment effect (d = .62). These findings provide support for the feasibility of EFT as a treatment approach for BED.

Our final and fifth hypothesis was that all participants receiving EFT (i.e. the EFT treatment group who initially received treatment, and also EFT wait-list group post receiving treatment), would experience significant improvements in objective binge episodes, the number of days on which objective binge episodes occurred, and binge eating psychopathology. There was a significant decrease from pretherapy to post-therapy in objective binge episodes with a large effect size (d = .99), objective binge episode days with a very large effect size (d = 1.51), and binge eating psychopathology with a large effect size (d = 1.10). The current findings compare favourably with posttherapy effect sizes for pooled primary outcome measures using bona fide vs non-bona fide therapies

(d = .36) and CBT versus non-bona fide CBT (d = .30) for BED [77].

There was no significant difference between posttherapy and 3-month follow-up scores, indicating that objective binge episodes, objective binge episode days and binge eating psychopathology treatment gains were maintained. The number of participants classified as non-binge eating according to the BES in the current study was 11/20 (55%) at the end of treatment and 12/20 (60%) at 3 months follow up; and weekly mean objective binge episodes (in the previous 7 days) scores were 2.05 at the end of treatment and 1.45 at 3 months follow up. These findings compare favourably with results from a systematic review and network meta-analysis of the comparative effectiveness of treatments for BED [74] where abstinence rates for therapist-led, partially therapist-led and structured self-help variants of CBT ranged from 17.9 to 86.7% at the end of treatment, and 20.8 to 84.6% at twelve-month follow-up; and binge episodes (in the previous 28 days) ranged from an average of 11.9 to .04 at the end of treatment, and 16.2 and .5 at twelve-month follow up [73, 78, 79].

The following future sample size calculations were made using GPower 3.1.9.2 with alpha = .05, power = 0.95, 2 groups and 4-time points. Using our between-group effect size for objective binge eating frequency (d = .98), future studies comparing EFT to a wait-list control group will need a minimum sample size of 12. However, if comparing individual EFT with an active psychotherapy (d = 0.82) [79], future studies would require a minimum sample size of 320 participants to find an effect. Using our between-group effect size for days without bingeing and loss of control (d = 1.39), future studies comparing EFT to a wait-list control group will need a minimum sample size of 8 participants. If comparing EFT with an active psychotherapy (d = 1.04) [80], future studies will need a minimum of 70 participants to find an effect.

The main limitation of the current research is the relatively small sample size which may limit the extent to which the sample is representative of people with binge eating disorder. Additionally, the majority of the sample was female, and outcome measures were confined to self-report measures which limited a participant's descriptions of attitudes and behaviours to those within their awareness. Posttreatment follow-up at 4, 8 and 12 weeks was also relatively short, which limited the analysis of participant trajectory and capacity to maintain gains. Finally, therapist effects cannot be ruled out given that the same therapist delivered the treatment; however, a recent investigation indicated that therapist effects account for only 5.8% of the variance in patient outcomes (e.g., [81]).

The present study has several implications. Firstly, it provides further preliminary evidence for the feasibility of EFT for BED and builds upon previous findings (e.g., [46, 47]). It also identified changes in objective binge episodes and days, and binge eating psychopathology that are theoretically important to EFT, including emotion and emotion regulation. The dropout rate was also relatively low compared to other psychological therapy interventions for BED, which indicates the acceptability of the EFT intervention.

Conclusion

In conclusion, the evidence is emerging for the benefits of EFT for BED which has a focus on assisting clients in experiencing and processing unpleasant emotions and decreasing the reliance on an eating disorder as an emotional coping mechanism. Future research assessing EFT for BED needs to include a more extensive randomised control trial to assess efficacy with a larger sample size to establish causal conclusions and equal gender representation to improve the generalisability of findings. Consideration could also be given to a more extended follow-up period to improve the analysis of participant trajectory and capacity to maintain gains, and the use of more than one therapist to rule out therapist effects.

Abbreviations
ANOVA: Analyses of variance; BED: Binge-eating disorder; BES: Binge Eating Scale; BN: Bulimia nervosa; CBT: Cognitive behaviour therapy; CBTgsh: Guided self-help cognitive behaviour therapy; CEQ: Credibility Expectancy Questionnaire; CONSORT: Consolidated Standards of Reporting Trials; CT: Combined therapy; DBT: Dialectical behaviour therapy; DSM-5: Diagnostic and Statistical Manual of Mental Disorders: DSM-V; EDE-Q-6.0: Eating Disorder Examination Questionnaire 6.0; EFGT: Emotionally focused group therapy; EFT: Emotion-focused therapy; GPIP: Group psychodynamic interpersonal psychotherapy; IPT: Interpersonal therapy; NICE: National Institute of Clinical Excellence; QUT: Queensland University of Technology; RCT: Randomised control trial; SCID-5-RV: Structured Clinical Interview for DSM-5-Research Version; SCID-I: Structured Clinical Interview for DSM-IV Axis I Disorders; SD: Standard deviation; UHREC: University Human Research Ethics Committee

Acknowledgements
We gratefully acknowledge the clients who participated in the study, and Kathleen Edwards – Research Assistant for the administration of the SCID-5-RV and data entry.

Authors' contributions
KG, ES and RK designed the study; KG performed the treatment, and LG provided clinical supervision. KG and ES analysed the data; and KG, ES, RK and LG drafted the manuscript. All author(s) read and approved the final manuscript.

Competing interests
The authors declare that they have no competing interests.

Author details
School of Psychology and Counselling, Queensland University of Technology, Faculty of Health, Brisbane, Queensland, Australia. ²Department of Psychology, York University, Faculty of Health, Toronto, Canada.

References
1.   Kornstein S. Epidemiology and recognition of binge-eating disorder in psychiatry and primary care. J Clin Psychiat. 2017;78(1):3–8.
2.   The National Eating Disorders Collaboration. Eating disorders prevention, treatment and management: an evidence review. Sydney: NEDC; 2010.
3.   Hay P, Girosi F, Mond J. Prevalence and sociodemographic correlates of DSM-5 eating disorders in the Australian population. J Eat Disord. 2015;3(1): 19–25.
4.   American Psychiatric Association. Diagnostic and statistical manual of mental disorders. 5th ed. Arlington, VA: American Psychiatric Association; 2013.
5.   Dingemans A, Danner U, Parks M. Emotion regulation in binge eating disorder: a review. Nutri. 2017;9(11):1274.
6.   Becker D, Jostmann N, Holland R. Does approach bias modification really work in the eating domain? A commentary on Kakoschke et al. (2017). Add Behav. 2018;77:293–4.
7.   Blomquist KK, Grilo CM. Family histories of anxiety in overweight men and women with binge eating disorder: a preliminary investigation. Compr Psychiatry. 2015;62:161–9.
8.   Araujo DMR, Santos GFDS, Nardi AE. Binge eating disorder and depression: a systematic review. World J Biol Psychiatry. 2010;11(2–2):199–207.
9.   Udo T, McKee SA, Grilo CM. Factor structure and clinical utility of the Beck depression inventory in patients with binge eating disorder and obesity. Gen Hosp Psychiat. 2014;37(2):120–5.
10. American Psychiatric Association. Treatment of patients with eating disorders. Third edition. Am J Psychiat. 2006;163(7):4–54.
11. National Collaborating Centre for Mental Health. Eating disorders core interventions in the treatment and management of anorexia nervosa, bulimia nervosa, and related eating disorders. 2004. Place of publication not identified: British Psychological Society.
12. Hilbert A, Petroff D, Herpertz S, Pietrowsky R, Tuschen-Caffier B, Vocks S, et al. Meta-analysis of the efficacy of psychological and medical treatments for binge-eating disorder. J Consult Clin Psychol. 2019;87(1):91–105.
13. Linardon J. Review of rates of abstinence following psychological or behavioural treatments for binge-eating disorder: meta-analysis. Int J Eat Disord. 2018;51(8):785–97.
14. Gross J. The emerging field of emotion regulation: an integrative review. Rev Gen Psychol. 1998;2(3):271–99.
15. Bennett J, Greene G, Schwartz-Barcott D. Perceptions of emotional eating behaviour. A qualitative study of college students. App. 2013 Jan 1;60:187–92.
16. Bruch H. Eating disorders. Obesity, anorexia nervosa, and the person within: Routledge & Kegan Paul; 1974.
17. Heatherton TF, Baumeister RF. Binge eating as escape from self-awareness. Psychol Bull. 1991 Jul;110(1):86.
18. Polivy J, Herman CP. Aetiology of binge eating: psychological mechanisms (1993). In C. G. Fairburn & G. T. Wilson (Eds.), binge eating: nature, assessment, and treatment (p. 173–205). Guilford Press.
19. Pine CJ. Anxiety and eating behaviour in obese and nonobese American Indians and white Americans. J Pers Soc Psychol. 1985 Sep;49(3):774.
20. Leehr EJ, Krohmer K, Schag K, Dresler T, Zipfel S, Giel KE. Emotion regulation model in binge eating disorder and obesity - a systematic review. Neurosci Biobehav Rev. 2015;49:125–34.

21. Iacovino J, Gredysa D, Altman M, Wilfley D. Psychological treatments for binge eating disorder. Curr Psychiatry Rep. 2012;14(4):432–46.

22. Blocher-McCabe E, La Via M, Marcus MD. Dialectical behaviour therapy for eating disorders. In: Thompson K, editor. Handbook of eating disorders and obesity. Hoboken, NJ: Wiley; 2004. p. 232–45.

23. Brockmeyer T, Skunde M, Wu M, Bresslein E, Rudofsky G, Herzog W, Friederich HC. Difficulties in emotion regulation across the spectrum of eating disorders. Compr Psychiatry. 2014;55(3):565–71.

24. Kenny T, Singleton C, Carter J. Testing predictions of the emotion regulation model of binge-eating disorder. Int J Eat Disord. 2017;50(11):1297–305.

25. Svaldi J, Tuschen-Caffier B, Trentowska M, Caffier D, Naumann E. Differential caloric intake in overweight females with and without binge eating: effects of a laboratory-based emotion-regulation training. Behav Res Ther. 2014; 56(1):39–46.

26. Peterson CB, Engel SG, Crosby RD, et al. Comparing integrative cognitive-affective therapy and guided self-help cognitive-behavioural therapy to treat binge-eating disorder using standard and naturalistic momentary outcome measures: a randomised controlled trial. Int J Eat Disord. 2020:1–10.

27. Torres S, Sales C, Guerra M, Simões M, Pinto M, Vieira F. Emotion-focused cognitive behavioural therapy in comorbid obesity with binge eating disorder: a pilot study of feasibility and long-term outcomes. Front Psychol. 2020;11:343.

28. Dolhanty J, Greenberg LS. Emotion-focused therapy in the treatment of eating disorders. Eur Psychother. 2007;7:97–116.

29. Ivanova I, Watson J. Emotion-focused therapy for eating disorders: enhancing emotional processing. Pers-Cent Exp Psychoth. 2014;13(4):278–93.

30. Greenberg LS. Emotion-focused therapy. Washington, DC: American Psychological Association; 2010.

31. Greenberg LS. Emotion-focused therapy: coaching clients to work through their feelings. Washington, DC: American Psychological Association; 2002.

32. Elliott R, Watson JC, Goldman RN, Greenberg LS. Learning emotion-focused therapy: the process experiential approach to change. Washington, DC: American Psychological Association; 2004.

33. Goldman R, Greenberg L, Angus L. The effects of adding emotion-focused interventions to the client-centred relationship conditions in the treatment of depression. Psychother Res. 2006;16(5):537–49.

34. Greenberg L, Watson J. Emotion-focused therapy for depression. Washington, DC: American Psychological Association; 2005.

35. Robinson A, McCague E, Whissell C. That chair work thing was great: a pilot study of group-based emotion-focused therapy for anxiety and depression. Pers-Cent Exp Psychot. 2014;13(4):263–77.

36. Holowaty K, Paivio S. Characteristics of client-identified helpful events in emotion-focused therapy for child abuse trauma. Psychother Res. 2012; 22(1):56–66.

37. Paivio S, Nieuwenhuis J. Efficacy of emotion-focused therapy for adult survivors of child abuse: a preliminary study. J Trau Str. 2001;14(1):115–33.

38. Paivio S, Pascual-Leone A. Emotion-focused therapy for complex trauma. Washington, D.C: American Psychological Association; 2010.

39. Shahar B, Bar-Kalifa E, Alon E. Emotion-focused therapy for social anxiety disorder: results from a multiple-baseline study. J Con Clin Psychol. 2017; 85(3):238–49.

40. Timulak L, McElvaney J, Keogh D, Martin E, Clare P, Chepukova E, et al. Emotion-focused therapy for generalised anxiety disorder: an exploratory study. Psychot. 2017;54(4):361–14.

41. Watson J, Greenberg L. Emotion-focused therapy for generalised anxiety. Washington, DC: American Psychological Association; 2017.

42. Dolhanty J, Greenberg L. Emotion-focused therapy in the treatment of eating disorders. Eur Psychot. 2009;7:97–116.

43. Robinson AL, Dolhanty J, Greenberg L. Emotion-focused family therapy for eating disorders in children and adolescents. Clin Psychol Psychother. 2013; 22(1):75–82.

44. Brennan MA, Emmerling ME, Whelton WJ. Emotion-focused group therapy: addressing self-criticism in the treatment of eating disorders. Couns Psychother Res. 2015;15(1):67–75.

45. Wnuk SM, Greenberg L, Dolhanty J. Emotion-focused group therapy for women with symptoms of bulimia nervosa. Eat Disord. 2015;23(3):253–61.

46. Compare A, Tasca GA. The rate and shape of change in binge-eating episodes and weight: an effectiveness trial of emotionally focused group therapy for binge-eating disorder. Clin Psychol Psychother. 2016;23(1):24–34.

47. Glisenti K, Strodl E, King R. Emotion-focused therapy for binge-eating disorder: a review of six cases. Clini Psychol and Psychoth. 2018;25(6): 842–55.

48. Arain M, Campbell MJ, Cooper CL, Lancaster GA. (2010). What is a pilot or feasibility study? A review of current practice and editorial policy. BMC Med Res Meth. 2010;10:1–10.

49. Leon A, Davis L, Kraemer H. The role and interpretation of pilot studies in clinical research. J Psychiatr Res. 2011;45(5):626–9.

50. Fischer S, Peterson C. Dialectical behaviour therapy for adolescent binge eating, purging, suicidal behaviour, and non-suicidal self-injury: a pilot study. Psychoth. 2015;52(1):78–92.

51. Lewer M, Kosfelder J, Michalak J, Schroeder D, Nasrawi N, Vocks S. Effects of a cognitive-behavioural exposure-based body image therapy for overweight females with binge eating disorder: a pilot study. J Eat Dis. 2017;5(1):36.

52. Kelly A, Carter J. Self-compassion training for binge eating disorder: a pilot randomised controlled trial. Psychol and Psychothy: Theo, Res and Prac. 2014;88(3):285–303.

53. Efird J. Blocked randomisation with randomly selected block sizes. Int J Environ Res Public Health. 2011;8(1):15–20.

54. First MB, Williams JBW, Karg RS, Spitzer RL. Structured clinical interview for DSM-5-research version (SCID-5 for DSM-5, research version; SCID-5-RV). Arlington: American Psychiatric Association; 2015.

55. Shankman S, Funkhouser C, Klein D, Davila J, Lerner D, Hee D. Reliability and validity of severity dimensions of psychopathology assessed using the Structured Clinical Interview for DSM-5. Int J Meth Psychiatr Res. 2018;27:1.

56. First M, Spitzer R, Gibbon M, Williams J. Structured clinical interview for DSM-IV-TR Axis I disorders, research version, patient edition. (SCID-I/P). New York: biometrics research, New York state psychiatric institute; 1996.

57. Ventura J, Liberman RP, Green MF, Shaner A, Mintz J. Training and quality assurance with the structured clinical interview for DSM-IV (SCID-I/P). Psychiatry Res. 1998;79(2):163–73.

58. Devilly G, Borkovec T. Psychometric properties of the credibility/expectancy questionnaire. J Behav Ther Exp Psychiat. 2000;31(2):73–86.

59. Fairburn CG, Beglin SJ. Assessment of eating disorders: interview or self-report questionnaire? Int J Eat Disord. 1994;16(4):363–70.

60. Fairburn CG, Cooper Z. The eating disorder examination. In: Fairburn CG, Wilson GT, editors. Binge eating: nature, assessment and treatment. New York, NY: Guilford Press; 1993. p. 317–60.

61. Rose JS, Vaewsorn A, Rosselli-Navarra F, Wilson G, Weissman R. Test-retest reliability of the eating disorder examination-questionnaire (EDE-Q) in a college sample. J Eat Disord. 2013;1(1):43–52.

62. Mond J, Hay P, Rodgers B, Owen C, Beumont P. Validity of the eating disorder examination questionnaire (EDE-Q) in screening for eating disorders in community samples. Behav Res Ther. 2004;42(5):551–67.

63. Reas DL, Grilo CM, Masheb RM. Reliability of the eating disorder examination-questionnaire in patients with binge eating disorder. Behav Res Ther. 2006;44(1):43–51.

64. Berg KC, Peterson CB, Frazier P, Crow SJ. Psychometric evaluation of the eating disorder examination and eating disorder examination-questionnaire: a systematic review of the literature. Int J Eat Disord. 2012;45(3):428–38.

65. Peterson C, Crosby R, Wonderlich S, Joiner T, Crow S, Mitchell J, et al. Psychometric properties of the eating disorder examination-questionnaire: factor structure and internal consistency. Int J Eat Disord. 2007;40(4):386–9.

66. Gormally J, Black S, Daston S, Rardin D. The assessment of binge eating severity among obese persons. Add Behav. 1982;7(1):47–55.

67. Dezhkam M, Moloodi R, Mootabi F, Omidvar N. Standardisation of the binge eating scale among an Iranian obese population. Iran J Psychiatry. 2009;4(4): 143–6.

68. Timmerman GM. Binge eating scale: further assessment of validity and reliability. J Appl Biobehav Res. 1999;4(1):1–12.

69. Carano A, De Berardis D, Gambi F, Di Paolo C, Campanella D, Pelusi L, et al. Alexithymia and body image in adult outpatients with binge eating disorder. Int J Eat Disord. 2006;39(4):332–40.

70. Duarte C, Pinto-Gouveia J, Ferreira C. Expanding binge eating assessment: validity and screening value of the binge eating scale in women from the general population. Eat Behav. 2015;18:41–7.

71. Wilfley DE, Welch RR, Stein RI, Spurrell EB, Cohen LR, Saelens BE, et al. A randomised comparison of group cognitive-behavioural therapy and group interpersonal psychotherapy for the treatment of overweight individuals with binge-eating disorder. Arch Gen Psychiatry. 2002;59(8):713–21.

72. Tasca GA, Ritchie K, Conrad G, Balfour L, Gayton J, Lybanon V, Bissada H. Attachment scales predict outcome in a randomised controlled trial of two group therapies for binge eating disorder: an aptitude by treatment interaction. Psychother Res. 2006;16(1):106–21.

73. Peterson C, Mitchell J, Engbloom S, Nugent S, Mussell M, Miller J. Group

cognitive-behavioural treatment of binge eating disorder: a comparison of therapist-led versus self-help formats. Int J Eat Disord. 1998;24(2):125–36.

74. Peat C, Berkman N, Lohr K, Brownley K, Bann C, Cullen K, et al. Review of comparative effectiveness of treatments for binge-eating disorder: systematic review and network meta-analysis. Eur Eat Disord Rev. 2017;25(5): 317–28.

75. Wilson GT, Wilfley DE, Agras WS, Bryson SW. Psychological treatments of binge eating disorder. Arch Gen Psychiatry. 2010;67(1):94–101.

76. Safer DL, Robinson AH, Jo B. Outcomes from a randomised controlled trial of group therapy for binge eating disorder: comparing dialectical behaviour therapy adapted for binge eating to an active comparison group therapy. Behav Ther. 2010;41(1):106–20.

77. Spielmans G, Benish S, Marin C, Bowman W, Menster M, Wheeler A. Specificity of psychological treatments for bulimia nervosa and binge eating disorder? A meta-analysis of direct comparisons. Clin Psychol Rev. 2013; 33(3):460–9.

78. Peterson C, Mitchell J, Engbloom S, Nugent S, Mussell M, Crow S, Thuras P. Self-help versus therapist-led group cognitive-behavioural treatment of binge eating disorder at follow-up. Int J Eat Disord. 2001;30(4):363–74.

79. Peterson C, Mitchell J, Crow S, Crosby R, Wonderlich S. The efficacy of self-help group treatment and therapist-led group treatment for binge eating disorder. Am J Psychiatry. 2009;12:1347–54.

80. Vocks S, Tuschen-Caffier B, Pietrowsky R, Rustenbach SJ, Kersting A, Herpertz S. Meta-analysis of the effectiveness of psychological and pharmacological treatments for binge eating disorder. Int J Eat Disord. 2010;43(3):205–17.

81. Saxon D, Firth N, Barkham M. The relationship between therapist effects and therapy delivery factors: therapy modality, dosage, and non-completion. Admin Pol Ment Health. 2017;44(5):705–15.

5

Metacognition and emotion regulation as treatment targets in binge eating disorder: a network analysis study

Matteo Aloi[1,2], Marianna Rania[1,2], Elvira Anna Carbone[1,2], Mariarita Caroleo[1,2], Giuseppina Calabrò[1,2], Paolo Zaffino[3], Giuseppe Nicolò[4], Antonino Carcione[4], Gianluca Lo Coco[5], Carlo Cosentino[3] and Cristina Segura-Garcia[1,6]*

Abstract

Background: This study aims to examine the underlying associations between eating, affective and metacognitive symptoms in patients with binge eating disorder (BED) through network analysis (NA) in order to identify key variables that may be considered the target for psychotherapeutic interventions.

Methods: A total of 155 patients with BED completed measures of eating psychopathology, affective symptoms, emotion regulation and metacognition. A cross-sectional network was inferred by means of Gaussian Markov random field estimation using graphical LASSO and the extended Bayesian information criterion (EBIC-LASSO), and central symptoms of BED were identified by means of the strength centrality index.

Results: Impaired self-monitoring metacognition and difficulties in impulse control emerged as the symptoms with the highest centrality. Conversely, eating and affective features were less central. The centrality stability coefficient of strength was above the recommended cut-off, thus indicating the stability of the network.

Conclusions: According to the present NA findings, impaired self-monitoring metacognition and difficulties in impulse control are the central nodes in the psychopathological network of BED whereas eating symptoms appear marginal. If further studies with larger samples replicate these results, metacognition and impulse control could represent new targets of psychotherapeutic interventions in the treatment of BED. In light of this, metacognitive interpersonal therapy could be a promising aid in clinical practice to develop an effective treatment for BED.

Keywords: Binge eating disorder, Network analysis, Metacognition, Emotion dysregulation, Binge severity, Psychotherapy

Plain English summary

This study sought to examine the key symptoms for the psychotherapy of patients with binge eating disorder (BED). For this purpose, we applied a network analysis approach to examine the reciprocal association between clinical variables and how eating symptoms, metacognition, emotion regulation, depression and anxiety mutually interact. A total of 155 outpatients with BED completed measures related to their eating behaviour, affectivity, emotion regulation and metacognition. The central elements of BED were found to be impaired metacognition and difficulty in impulse control, whereas affective and eating symptoms appeared to be marginal. Therefore, metacognitive alterations and emotion dysregulation should be considered important targets for the psychotherapy of patients with BED.

* Correspondence: segura@unicz.it
[1]Outpatient Unit for Clinical Research and Treatment of Eating Disorders, University Hospital "Mater Domini", Catanzaro, Italy
[6]Department of Medical and Surgical Sciences, University "Magna Graecia" of Catanzaro, Catanzaro, Italy
Full list of author information is available at the end of the article

Background

Binge eating disorder (BED) is characterized by recurrent episodes of binge eating with a sense of loss of control over eating, accompanied by negative feelings [1]. To date, the guidelines recommend cognitive behavioural therapy (CBT) as the first-line treatment option for BED [2, 3]. Although CBT is quite effective in patients with BED, about 50% do not fully respond to treatment [4–6]. A possible explanation could be that only a small portion of patients with BED report the overvaluation of body shape and weight that forms the core of the CBT protocol [7]. Other treatments such as dialectical behaviour therapy [8, 9] and interpersonal psychotherapy [10, 11] have shown promising results but failed to bridge the efficacy gap in treating BED. In other words, the available data do not favour one treatment over the other.

New therapeutic approaches able to target the key elements of the complex psychopathology of BED are therefore a priority. Investigating the specific weight of each psychopathological dimension could help in developing more tailored psychological interventions for BED.

Network analysis (NA) emerged as a novel approach to conceptualize mental disorders [12]. According to this approach, symptoms of psychiatric disorders are distinct entities that can influence, maintain and/or interact with other symptoms [13]. Mental disorders can be characterized as complex systems in which symptoms are represented as distinct nodes, connected by edges that represent the strength (e.g. strong/weak correlations) and direction (e.g. positive/negative correlations) between pairs of symptoms. NA allows the identification of the central symptoms (i.e. when a node has many strong associations with other nodes and strong correlations with other nodes within the network) [14].

Development of the NA approach over the past decade has provided a theoretical framework that was adopted to identify the central symptoms of different psychiatric disorders, such as bipolar disorder [15], depression [16], obsessive compulsive disorder [17] and schizophrenia [18]. More recently, researchers in the field of eating disorders have applied NA to examine the symptoms of anorexia nervosa [19–22] and bulimia nervosa [23–25].

To date, only three studies [26–28] dealing with BED have used the NA approach. In the first investigation, overvaluation of shape and weight emerged as central symptoms of BED whereas behavioural symptoms (i.e. binge eating, restriction, secret eating) were less central [26]. The study by Solmi et al. revealed affective symptoms, interoceptive awareness, ineffectiveness, interpersonal functioning and drive for thinness as the central variables among patients with BED [27]. Finally, the third study showed that CBT provides high integration and connectivity of the psychopathology network in BED,

suggesting an improved patient understanding of associations between binge eating and other symptoms [28].

However, no research has used NA to investigate the complex connections between the eating (i.e. binge eating and eating psychopathology), affective (i.e. anxiety and mood) and psychological (i.e. metacognition and emotion regulation) features of patients with BED.

Prior research evidenced a significant relationship among negative affect, difficulties with emotion regulation and binge eating symptoms [29–33]. For example, binge eating can be the result of a dysfunctional strategy to avoid interpersonal difficulties and negative emotions [34], especially in individuals who experience difficulties with regulating their emotional state [32]. However, the role of metacognition in BED has received less research attention. In the current study, we refer to metacognition as a psychological function that plays a key role in identifying mental states and ascribing them to oneself and others, reflecting and reasoning on mental states and, finally, using this information to manage interpersonal conflicts [35]. According to this model, metacognition is made up of different sub-functions that interact with each other and can be singularly impaired [35]. A previous study suggested that the severity of BED can worsen in relation to the impaired self-monitoring metacognition through the mediation of emotion dysregulation [36].

In the present study, we sought to extend the research on the clinical characteristics of BED by applying an NA model to provide an examination of the pathways that underlie eating symptoms and their relations to metacognition, emotion regulation and distress. These NA results may lead to more nuanced insights regarding the core targets for psychotherapeutic interventions. Given the explorative nature of our study, no a priori hypotheses were formulated.

Methods
Procedure

We performed a consecutive sampling of male and female patients attending the Outpatient Unit for Clinical Research and Treatment of Eating Disorders in Catanzaro (Italy). Patients were invited to participate in the present study if they met the following criteria: age 18–65 years; current diagnosis of BED according to the fifth edition of the *Diagnostic and Statistical Manual of Mental Disorders* (DSM-5) criteria; absence of current Axis I comorbid psychiatric disorders; and capable of answering self-report questionnaires and expressing valid consent.

Participants were deemed ineligible if they had: IQ < 70 [37]; drug dependence and/or abuse; severe mental illness that could interfere with clinical assessment (i.e. psychosis); history of chronic medical illness (i.e. chronic cardiovascular diseases) or neurological conditions (i.e. dementia) affecting cognitive functioning; other severe medical comorbidities (i.e. epilepsy); medical conditions that influenced eating/weight (i.e. diagnosis of diabetes mellitus); or a history of malignant disease.

Trained psychiatrists interviewed all participants using the Structured Clinical Interview for DSM-5 Disorders – Research Version [38] for diagnostic purposes and collected sociodemographic and clinical data. Researchers informed participants about the aims, procedures, anonymity and voluntary participation in this research. Participants gave their written informed consent to participate in accordance with the latest version of the Declaration of Helsinki [39] and the local ethical committee.

Measures

The Eating Disorders Inventory-2 (EDI-2) [40, 41] is a self-report questionnaire made up of 91 items that evaluates the psychopathology and symptomatology of eating disorders. The EDI-2 provides 11 subscale scores and a global measure of eating disorder severity obtained from the sum of all the items (ranging from 0 to 273). Higher scores indicate more severe symptoms. Cronbach's alpha for the total score in this study was good (.840).

The Binge Eating Scale (BES) [42] measures the severity of BED. It consists of 16 items that describe the behaviours, feelings and cognitions associated with binge eating. Total BES scores of < 17, 17–27 and > 27 indicate improbable, possible and probable BED, respectively. The internal consistency in this study was .880.

The Metacognition Self-Assessment Scale (MSAS) [43] is an 18-item five-point Likert-type (1 = never, 5 = almost always) self-report questionnaire that evaluates metacognitive functioning. The raw score ranges from 18 to 90 and lower scores indicate impaired self-evaluation of metacognitive function. Specifically, the MSAS measures four abilities of metacognition: monitoring, differentiation/decentration, integration and mastery. In this study, Cronbach's alpha ranges from .820 to .840.

The Difficulties in Emotion Regulation Scale (DERS) [44] is a 36-item five-point Likert-type scale that assesses emotion dysregulation across six subscales: non-acceptance of emotions; difficulties in pursuing goals when having strong emotions; difficulties in controlling impulsive behaviours when experiencing negative emotions; lack of emotional awareness; limited access to emotion regulation strategies; and lack of emotional clarity. Higher scores indicate more problems in emotion regulation. In the current study, the internal consistency ranges from .870 to .895.

The Beck Depression Inventory II (BDI-II) [45] assesses depressive symptoms through 21 items on a Likert scale (0–3); scores of 0–9, 10–16, 17–29 and ≥ 30 indicate minimal, mild, moderate and severe depression, respectively. Cronbach's alpha in the present research was .820.

The State-Trait Anxiety Inventory (STAI) consists of 20 items that assess state anxiety (STAI-St) and 20 items that measure trait anxiety (STAI-Tr) [46]. The present study only included the STAI-Tr for statistical purposes. Cronbach's alpha was .795.

Network estimation and accuracy

NA was performed using the R (version 3.6.2) *qgraph* and *bootnet* packages in accordance with Epskamp and colleagues [47].

The network has been inferred by means of Gaussian Markov random field estimation, applying 'Least Absolute Shrinkage and Selection Operator'(LASSO) regularization to limit the number of spurious associations [48]. Moreover, the extended Bayesian information criterion (EBIC) [49], a tuning parameter that sets the degree of regularization/penalty applied to sparse correlations, was set to 0.20 in the current study (values between 0 and 0.5 are typically chosen). Network estimation was performed using the *estimateNetwork* routine of the *bootnet* package [50].

The centrality of a node is used to infer its influence, or structural importance, in the network. Three main indices estimate the centrality: *betweenness* (how a node influences the average path between other pairs of nodes); *closeness* (how a node is indirectly connected to the other nodes); and *strength* (how a node is directly connected to the other nodes). The centrality Plot function in *qgraph* was used to calculate indices of centrality.

According to the recommendations of Epskamp et al. [51], in order to assess the internal reliability of the network we calculated the correlation stability (CS) coefficient, which is the maximum proportion of the population that can be dropped so that the correlation between the re-calculated indices of the obtained networks and those of the original network is at least 0.7. It is recommended that the minimum cut-off to consider a network stable is 0.25 for *betweenness, closeness* and *strength* [51]. The CS coefficient was computed using case-drop bootstrapping (nboots = 2000). Then we estimated the accuracy of edge-weights by drawing bootstrapped confidence intervals calculated using nonparametric bootstrapping (nboots = 2000). Both for case-drop and non-parametric bootstrapping, network stability analyses were performed using the *bootnet* function in the *bootnet* package.

Visual inspection of the network reveals that thicker edges indicate stronger associations between symptoms, with positive associations typically illustrated in blue and negative associations typically represented in red.

Results

Sample characteristics

In total, 155 BED patients (86.5% females) aged 41.2 ± 13.2 years and with body mass index 37.9 ± 10.4 kg/m², took part in the current study. Table 1 displays the clinical characteristics of the sample.

Network analysis

Figure 1 illustrates the network of BED symptoms. Nodes belonging to each domain (i.e. eating symptoms, emotion dysregulation and metacognition) are generally associated and close to each other. There is a strong negative connection between self-monitoring and DERS-Clarity, and a strong positive connection among self-monitoring, differentiation and mastery. The associations between BED symptoms and depression, and between EDI-2 total score, depression and anxiety, are moderately strong. The psychopathological variables (BES, EDI-2 total score, STAI-Tr and BDI) and emotion regulation (DERS) are moderately connected. The BED symptom node (BES) has a direct connection with non-acceptance of emotions, whereas the depression node (BDI) connects both with difficulties in controlling impulsive behaviour and lack of emotional clarity. Figure 2 displays the strength centrality index of the variables included in the network. The CS coefficient is 0.301 for *strength*, which is above the recommended cut-off value (i.e. 0.25); however, the CS coefficients for *betweenness* and *closeness* are below 0.25. Therefore, we decided to

Table 1 Clinical characteristics of the sample

	Mean	SD
EDI-2 Total	83.9	60.2
BES	23.4	9.3
STAI Trait	52.8	12.1
BDI	23.2	11.3
DERS		
Non acceptance	16.3	6.2
Goals	15.6	5.4
Impulse	15.8	6.2
Awareness	17.4	5.3
Strategies	22.1	8.8
Clarity	11.8	4.8
MSAS		
Self monitoring	18.4	5.0
Differentiation/Decentration	18.9	4.3
Mastery	16.5	4.2
Others monitoring	10.3	2.8

EDI-2 Eating Disorder Inventory-2, *BES* Binge Eating Scale, *STAI* State and Trait Anxiety Inventory, *BDI* Beck Depression Inventory, *DERS* Difficulties in Emotion Regulation Scale, *MSAS* Metacognition Self-Assessment Scale, *SD* Standard Deviation

choose the strength index as the main CS coefficient. This choice is not surprising because the interpretation of betweenness and closeness in networks is somewhat unclear [52] and the strength index is considered a more stable centrality index than betweenness and closeness [53]. Furthermore, because we aimed to understand the core symptoms to target using psychological treatment, we relied on the strength index because it exactly performs this function. Additional file 1 (Fig. S1) shows the accuracy of the CS indices.

The nodes with the highest strength centrality are MSAS-Self-monitoring (M = 1.98) and DERS-Impulse (M = 1.27) (Fig. 2). The strongest connections of MSAS-Self-monitoring are with MSAS-Mastery (0.352) and DERS-Clarity (− 0.350). The strongest connections of DERS-Impulse are with DERS-Goals (0.38) and DERS-Strategies (0.318). Additional file 2 (Fig. S2) reports the bootstrapped confidence intervals of the estimated edge-weights.

Discussion

This is the first study to investigate the associations between eating (i.e. binge eating and eating psychopathology), affective (i.e. anxiety and depression) and psychological features (i.e. metacognition and emotion regulation) through the NA method among patients with BED.

Our results showed that impaired self-monitoring metacognition and difficulties in impulse control were the nodes with the highest centrality strength and thus the nodes most directly connected to the other nodes in the network [53]. According to the NA approach, activation of a node may cause the development of the connected symptoms; therefore, the most central nodes have been conceptualized as core symptoms [54]. Our findings suggest that impaired self-monitoring metacognition and difficulties in impulse control may be important clinical characteristics among patients with BED. Although the high centrality of a node may be the effect of connections with other symptoms [55] and a cross-sectional study cannot show causal associations, the metacognitive and emotion regulation dysfunctions may represent potential targets for treatment, therefore these outcome variables of BED warrant further research.

This finding is in line with our previous study where low self-monitoring led BED-obese patients to express the worsening of binge severity through emotion dysregulation [36]. Consistent with this hypothesis, other researchers found that difficulties in emotion recognition could play a key role in the development and maintenance of BED [56, 57].

Another important finding of the current NA was the strong correlation of the self-monitoring node with mastery strategies. According to metacognitive

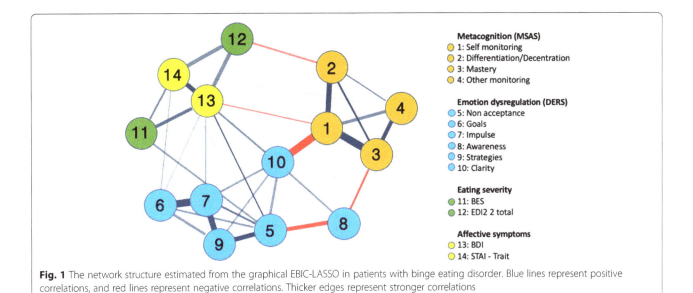

Fig. 1 The network structure estimated from the graphical EBIC-LASSO in patients with binge eating disorder. Blue lines represent positive correlations, and red lines represent negative correlations. Thicker edges represent stronger correlations

theory, a high level of self-monitoring allows the use of functional mastery strategies. In more detail, mastery is '*the ability to work through one's representations and mental states, with a view to implementing effective action strategies, in order to accomplish cognitive tasks or cope with problematic mental states*' [35, 58]. Thus, it could be inferred that enhancing metacognitive abilities leads to reduced dysfunctional strategies among patients with BED, who usually manage intense emotions with binges [8, 59].

It is worth noting that both dysfunctional eating (i.e. BES and EDI-2 total scores) and affective symptoms (i.e. BDI and STAI-Tr) were peripheral to the network structure of patients with BED, indicating that they had weaker connections to the rest of the network compared with other nodes. Regarding eating psychopathology, in the current study the lowest strength was found for the BES (M = – 1.39) and the EDI-2 total score (M = – 1.22). Notwithstanding the weak centrality of eating symptoms in the network structure, our findings suggest that the BES score is connected to non-acceptance of emotions, whereas the EDI-2 total score is connected to poor metacognitive ability to distance from one's own thoughts and evaluate them critically. Overall, our results confirm recent literature data on NA in BED (that binge eating was not central to the psychopathology) [26, 28] but contrast with the typical approach to diagnosing BED (relying upon the presence of binge eating behaviours).

Consistent with the present findings, we could argue that the clinical constructs such as impaired self-monitoring, difficulties in impulse control and lack of emotional clarity could be the vulnerability factors of BED whereas the pathological eating behaviour (i.e. binge eating) itself seems to be the consequent

behaviour. This observation is in line with recent literature that investigated predisposing and precipitating factors in BED [32, 60, 61].

Furthermore, depressive and anxious symptoms were not central nodes in our network model whereas they had high centrality in Solmi and colleagues' model [27]. This discrepancy could be due to the use of different psychometric instruments. Solmi and colleagues used the Symptom Checklist-90 (SCL-90), which is not so specific and only takes into consideration the prior week; instead, the BDI-II and the STAI-Tr are more specific for diagnostic purposes and consider a longer temporal range of assessment (i.e. 2 weeks for BDI following the DSM-5 temporal criterion for major depressive episode; 'usually feeling' for STAI-Tr). Therefore, their study could have overestimated the weight of anxious and depressive symptoms in BED.

The present results should be read in light of some limitations. First, the sample size is smaller than in other studies that used NA in BED. Nevertheless, according to the recommendations of Levinson and colleagues [62] on the use of NA in the field of eating disorder ('*to date, the best recommendation is to use the largest sample size possible and make sure that your network is stable*'), our model was demonstrated to be stable. Second, it was not possible to evaluate the differences in NA according to gender; however, a recent NA study among patients with eating disorders showed more similarities than differences between men and women [63]. Finally, the cross-sectional design does not allow the investigation of causality in the associations between dimensions, therefore future longitudinal research could explore whether psychotherapeutic interventions that target metacognitive and impulsive dimensions may be more effective in treating BED.

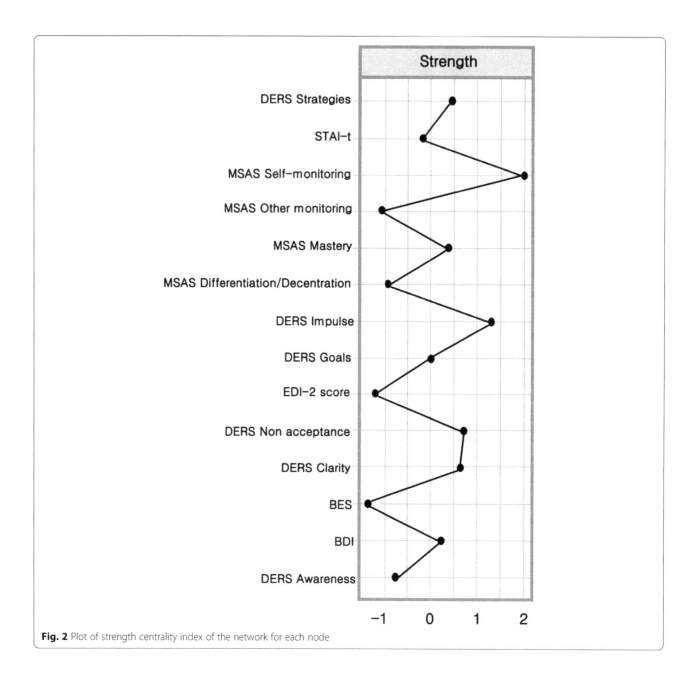

Fig. 2 Plot of strength centrality index of the network for each node

Conclusions

The current study suggests a link between reduced ability to identify and describe mental states and the lack of emotion awareness and clarity among patients with BED. Moreover, according to the present NA findings, impaired self-monitoring metacognition and difficulties in impulse control are the central nodes in the psychopathological network of BED, whereas eating symptoms seem to be marginal.

These results could lead to a change in the current conceptualization of BED and the consideration of new targets of psychotherapeutic interventions, if confirmed in larger samples. Also, approaches focused on the

improvement of metacognitive dysfunctions could be considered. With this aim, metacognitive interpersonal therapy [64] could be a promising aid in clinical practice to develop an effective treatment for BED.

Abbreviations
BED: Binge eating disorder; BES: Binge eating scale; BDI-II: Beck Depression Inventory II; CBT: Cognitive behavioral therapy; CS: Correlation stability; DBT: Dialectical behavioral therapy; DERS: Difficulties in Emotion Regulation Scale; DSM-5: Diagnostic and Statistical Manual of Mental Disorders – 5; EBIC: Extended Bayesian Information Criterion; ED: Eating disorder; EDI-2: Eating Disorders Inventory-2; IPT: Interpersonal psychotherapy; LASSO: Least Absolute Shrinkage and Selection Operator; MIT: Metacognitive Interpersonal Therapy; MSAS: Metacognition Self-Assessment Scale; NA: Network analysis; SCL-90: Symptom checklist – 90; STAI-Tr: State-Trait Anxiety Inventory-Trait

Acknowledgements
The authors would like to thank all the participants for the time they spent for this study.

Authors' contributions
MA and CSG designed the study; MA, MR, EAC, GC, MC collected the data; PZ and CC analysed the data; MA wrote the first draft of the manuscript; CSG, GLC, GN, AC made the first critical review and participated to write the final manuscript. All authors approved the final manuscript.

Competing interests
All the authors declare that they have no conflict of interest.

Author details
[1]Outpatient Unit for Clinical Research and Treatment of Eating Disorders, University Hospital "Mater Domini", Catanzaro, Italy. [2]Department of Health Sciences, University "Magna Graecia" of Catanzaro, Catanzaro, Italy. [3]Department of Experimental and Clinical Medicine, School of Computer and Biomedical Engineering, University "Magna Graecia" of Catanzaro, Catanzaro, Italy. [4]Third Centre of Cognitive Psychotherapy – Italian School of Cognitive Psychotherapy (SICC), Rome, Italy. [5]Department of Psychology, Educational Science and Human Movement, University of Palermo, Palermo, Italy. [6]Department of Medical and Surgical Sciences, University "Magna Graecia" of Catanzaro, Catanzaro, Italy.

References
1. APA AAP. Diagnostic and statistical manual of mental disorders (DSM-5®). 5th ed. Arlington: American Psychiatric Association; 2013. Available from: https://books.google.com.mx/books?id=-JivBAAAQBAJ

2. Hay P, Chinn D, Forbes D, Madden S, Newton R, Sugenor L, et al. Royal Australian and new Zealand College of Psychiatrists clinical practice guidelines for the treatment of eating disorders. Aust New Zeal J Psychiatry. 2014;48:977–1008 Available from: http://journals.sagepub.com/doi/10.1177/0004867414555814.

3. National Institute for Health and Care Excellence. Eating disorders: Recognition and treatment. 2017. Available from: https://www.nice.org.uk/guidance/ng69/%0Achapter/Recommendations#treating-binge-eating-disorder

4. Grilo CM. Psychological and behavioral treatments for binge-eating disorder. J Clin Psychiatry. 2017;78:20–4 Available from: http://www.psychiatrist.com/jcp/article/pages/2017/v78n01/v78s0104.aspx.

5. Hay P. A systematic review of evidence for psychological treatments in eating disorders: 2005-2012. Int J Eat Disord. 2013;46:462–9 Available from: http://doi.wiley.com/10.1002/eat.22103.

6. Brownley KA, Berkman ND, Peat CM, Lohr KN, Cullen KE, Bann CM, et al. Binge-Eating Disorder in Adults. Ann Intern Med. 2016;165:409 Available from: http://annals.org/article.aspx?doi=10.7326/M15-2455.

7. Grilo CM. Why no cognitive body image feature such as overvaluation of shape/weight in the binge eating disorder diagnosis? Int J Eat Disord. 2013;46:208–11 Available from: https://onlinelibrary.wiley.com/doi/abs/10.1002/eat.22082.

8. Chen EY, Cacioppo J, Fettich K, Gallop R, McCloskey MS, Olino T, et al. An adaptive randomized trial of dialectical behavior therapy and cognitive behavior therapy for binge-eating. Psychol Med. 2017;47:703–17 Available from: https://www.cambridge.org/core/product/identifier/S0033291716002543/type/journal_article.

9. Lammers MW, Vroling MS, Crosby RD, van Strien T. Dialectical behavior therapy adapted for binge eating compared to cognitive behavior therapy in obese adults with binge eating disorder: a controlled study. J Eat Disord. 2020;8:27 Available from: https://jeatdisord.biomedcentral.com/articles/10.1186/s40337-020-00299-z.

10. Linardon J. Rates of abstinence following psychological or behavioral treatments for binge-eating disorder: meta-analysis. Int J Eat Disord. 2018;51:785–97.

11. Hilbert A, Hildebrandt T, Agras WS, Wilfley DE, Wilson GT. Rapid response in psychological treatments for binge eating disorder. J Consult Clin Psychol. 2015;83:649–54 Available from: http://doi.apa.org/getdoi.cfm?doi=10.1037/ccp0000018.

12. Robinaugh DJ, Hoekstra RHA, Toner ER, Borsboom D. The network approach to psychopathology: a review of the literature 2008–2018 and an agenda for future research. Psychol Med. 2020;50:353–66 Available from: https://www.cambridge.org/core/product/identifier/S0033291719003404/type/journal_article.

13. McNally RJ. Can network analysis transform psychopathology? Behav Res Ther. 2016;86:95–104 Available from: https://linkinghub.elsevier.com/retrieve/pii/S0005796716301103.

14. Freeman LC. Centrality in social networks conceptual clarification. Soc Networks. 1978;1:215–39 Available from: https://linkinghub.elsevier.com/retrieve/pii/0378873378900217.

15. Scott J, Bellivier F, Manchia M, Schulze T, Alda M, Etain B, et al. Can network analysis shed light on predictors of lithium response in bipolar I disorder? Acta Psychiatr Scand. 2020;141:522–33 Available from: https://onlinelibrary.wiley.com/doi/abs/10.1111/acps.13163.

16. Corponi F, Anmella G, Verdolini N, Pacchiarotti I, Samalin L, Popovic D, et al. Symptom networks in acute depression across bipolar and major depressive disorders: A network analysis on a large, international, observational study. Eur Neuropsychopharmacol. 2020;35:49–60 Available from: https://linkinghub.elsevier.com/retrieve/pii/S0924977X20300924.

17. Olatunji BO, Christian C, Brosof L, Tolin DF, Levinson CA. What is at the core of OCD? A network analysis of selected obsessive-compulsive symptoms and beliefs. J Affect Disord. 2019;257:45–54 Available from: https://linkinghub.elsevier.com/retrieve/pii/S0165032719305774.

18. Galderisi S, Rucci P, Mucci A, Rossi A, Rocca P, Bertolino A, et al. The interplay among psychopathology, personal resources, context-related factors and real-life functioning in schizophrenia: stability in relationships after 4 years and differences in network structure between recovered and non-recovered patients. World Psychiatry. 2020;19:81–91 Available from: https://onlinelibrary.wiley.com/doi/abs/10.1002/wps.20700.

19. Calugi S, Sartirana M, Misconel A, Boglioli C, Dalle GR. Eating disorder psychopathology in adults and adolescents with anorexia nervosa: a network approach. Int J Eat Disord. 2020;53:690–701 Available from: https://onlinelibrary.wiley.com/doi/abs/10.1002/eat.23270.

20. Cascino G, Castellini G, Stanghellini G, Ricca V, Cassioli E, Ruzzi V, et al. The Role of the Embodiment Disturbance in the Anorexia Nervosa Psychopathology: A Network Analysis Study. Brain Sci. 2019;9:276 Available from: https://www.mdpi.com/2076-3425/9/10/276.

21. Monteleone AM, Cascino G, Pellegrino F, Ruzzi V, Patriciello G, Marone L, et al. The association between childhood maltreatment and eating disorder psychopathology: a mixed-model investigation. Eur Psychiatry. 2019;61:111–8 Available from: https://linkinghub.elsevier.com/retrieve/pii/S092493381930 1257.

22. Kerr-Gaffney J, Halls D, Harrison A, Tchanturia K. Exploring Relationships Between Autism Spectrum Disorder Symptoms and Eating Disorder Symptoms in Adults With Anorexia Nervosa: A Network Approach. Front Psychiatry. 2020;11 Available from: https://www.frontiersin.org/article/10.3389/fpsyt.2020.00401/full.

23. Levinson CA, Zerwas S, Calebs B, Forbush K, Kordy H, Watson H, et al. The core symptoms of bulimia nervosa, anxiety, and depression: a network analysis. J Abnorm Psychol. 2017;126:340–54 Available from: http://doi.apa.org/getdoi.cfm?doi=10.1037/abn0000254.

24. Monteleone AM, Corsi E, Cascino G, Ruzzi V, Ricca V, Ashworth R, et al. The Interaction Between Mentalizing, Empathy and Symptoms in People with Eating Disorders: A Network Analysis Integrating Experimentally Induced and Self-report Measures. Cognit Ther Res. 2020; Available from: http://link.springer.com/10.1007/s10608-020-10126-z.

25. Brown TA, Vanzhula IA, Reilly EE, Levinson CA, Berner LA, Krueger A, et al. Body mistrust bridges interoceptive awareness and eating disorder symptoms. J Abnorm Psychol. 2020;129:445–56 Available from: http://doi.apa.org/getdoi.cfm?doi=10.1037/abn0000516.

26. Wang SB, Jones PJ, Dreier M, Elliott H, Grilo CM. Core psychopathology of treatment-seeking patients with binge-eating disorder: a network analysis investigation. Psychol Med. 2019;49:1923–8 Available from: https://www.cambridge.org/core/product/identifier/S0033291718002702/type/journal_article.

27. Solmi M, Collantoni E, Meneguzzo P, Degortes D, Tenconi E, Favaro A. Network analysis of specific psychopathology and psychiatric symptoms in patients with eating disorders. Int J Eat Disord. 2018;51:680–92 Available from: http://doi.wiley.com/10.1002/eat.22884.

28. Hilbert A, Herpertz S, Zipfel S, Tuschen-Caffier B, Friederich H-C, Mayr A, et al. Psychopathological Networks in Cognitive-Behavioral Treatments for Binge-Eating Disorder. Psychother Psychosom. 2020:1–7 Available from: https://www.karger.com/Article/FullText/509458.

29. Aloi M, Rania M, Caroleo M, Carbone EA, Fazia G, Calabrò G, et al. How are early maladaptive schemas and DSM-5 personality traits associated with the severity of binge eating? J Clin Psychol. 2020;76:539–48 Available from: https://onlinelibrary.wiley.com/doi/abs/10.1002/jclp.22900.

30. Araujo DMR, da Silva Santos GF, Nardi AE. Binge eating disorder and depression: a systematic review. World J Biol Psychiatry. 2010;11:199–207 Available from: http://www.tandfonline.com/doi/full/10.3109/15622970802563171.

31. Caroleo M, Primerano A, Rania M, Aloi M, Pugliese V, Magliocco F, et al. A real world study on the genetic, cognitive and psychopathological differences of obese patients clustered according to eating behaviours. Eur Psychiatry. 2018;48:58–64. https://doi.org/10.1016/j.eurpsy.2017.11.009. Epub 2018 Jan 10. PMID: 29331600.

32. Burton AL, Abbott MJ. Processes and pathways to binge eating: development of an integrated cognitive and behavioural model of binge eating. J Eat Disord. 2019;7:–18 Available from: https://jeatdisord.biomedcentral.com/articles/10.1186/s40337-019-0248-0.

33. Leehr EJ, Krohmer K, Schag K, Dresler T, Zipfel S, Giel KE. Emotion regulation model in binge eating disorder and obesity - a systematic review. Neurosci Biobehav Rev. 2015;49:125–34 Available from: https://linkinghub.elsevier.com/retrieve/pii/S0149763414003455.

34. Lo Coco G, Sutton R, Tasca GA, Salerno L, Oieni V, Compare A. Does the interpersonal model generalize to obesity without binge eating? Eur Eat Disord Rev. 2016;24:391–8 Available from: http://doi.wiley.com/10.1002/erv.2459.

35. Semerari A, Carcione A, Dimaggio G, Falcone M, Nicolò G, Procacci M, et al. How to evaluate metacognitive functioning in psychotherapy? The metacognition assessment scale and its applications. Clin Psychol Psychother. 2003;10:238–61.

36. Aloi M, Rania M, Carbone EA, Calabrò G, Caroleo M, Carcione A, et al. The role of self-monitoring metacognition sub-function and negative urgency related to binge severity. Eur Eat Disord Rev. 2020;28:580–6 Available from: https://onlinelibrary.wiley.com/doi/abs/10.1002/erv.2742.

37. Wechsler D. WAIS-iv. Wechsler Adult Intelligence Scale. 4th ed. Firenze: Organizzazioni Speciali; 2013.

38. First MB, Williams JBW, Karg RS, Spitzer RL. User's guide for the structured clinical interview for DSM-5 disorders, research version (SCID-5-RV). Arlington: American Psychiatric Association; 2015.

39. World Medical Association. Declaration of Helsinki. JAMA. 2013;310:2191 Available from: http://jama.jamanetwork.com/article.aspx?doi=10.1001/jama.2013.281053.

40. Garner DM. Eating disorder Inventory-2. Professional manual. Odessa: Psychological Assessment Resources Inc; 1991.

41. Segura-García C, Aloi M, Rania M, Ciambrone P, Palmieri A, Pugliese V, et al. Ability of EDI-2 and EDI-3 to correctly identify patients and subjects at risk for eating disorders. Eat Behav. 2015;19:20–3 Available from: https://linkinghub.elsevier.com/retrieve/pii/S1471015315000793.

42. Ricca V, Mannucci E, Moretti S, Di Bernardo M, Zucchi T, Cabras PL, et al. Screening for binge eating disorder in obese outpatients. Compr Psychiatry. 2000;41:111–5.

43. Pedone R, Semerari A, Riccardi I, Procacci M, Nicolò G, Carcione A. Development of a self-report measure of metacognition: the metacognition self-assessment scale (MSAS). Instrument description and factor structure. Clin Neuropsychiatry J Treat Eval. 2017;14:185–94.

44. Giromini L, Velotti P, de Campora G, Bonalume L, Cesare ZG. Cultural adaptation of the difficulties in emotion regulation scale: reliability and validity of an Italian version. J Clin Psychol. 2012;68:989–1007 Available from: http://doi.wiley.com/10.1002/jclp.21876.

45. Ghisi M, Flebus GB, Montano A, Sanavio E, Sica C. Beck depression inventory-II. Manuale italiano. Firenze: Organizzazioni Speciali; 2006.

46. Pedrabissi L, Santinello M. Inventario per l Ansia di Stato e di Tratto: Nuova Versione Italiana dello STAI —Forma Y: Manuale. Firenze: Organizzazioni Speciali; 1989.

47. Epskamp S, Cramer AOJ, Waldorp LJ, Schmittmann VD, Borsboom D. qgraph: Network Visualizations of Relationships in Psychometric Data. J Stat Softw. 2012;48 Available from: http://www.jstatsoft.org/v48/i04/.

48. Friedman J, Hastie T, Tibshirani R. Glasso: graphical Lasso-estimation of Gaussian graphical models; R package version 1. Vienna: R Core Team; 2014.

49. Chen J, Chen Z. Extended Bayesian information criteria for model selection with large model spaces. Biometrika. 2008;95:759–71 Available from: https://academic.oup.com/biomet/article-lookup/doi/10.1093/biomet/asn034.

50. Epskamp S, Maris G, Waldorp L, Borsboom D. Network psychometrics. In: Irwing P, Hughes D, Booth T, editors. Handb Psychom. New York: Wiley; 2016.

51. Epskamp S, Borsboom D, Fried EI. Estimating psychological networks and their accuracy: a tutorial paper. Behav Res Methods. 2018;50:195–212.

52. Forbes MK, Wright AGC, Markon KE, Krueger RF. Evidence that psychopathology symptom networks have limited replicability. J Abnorm Psychol. 2017;126:969–88 Available from: http://doi.apa.org/getdoi.cfm?doi=10.1037/abn0000276.

53. Epskamp S, Fried EI. A tutorial on regularized partial correlation networks. Psychol Methods. 2018;23:617–34 Available from: http://doi.apa.org/getdoi.cfm?doi=10.1037/met0000167.

54. Fried EI, Cramer AOJ. Moving forward: challenges and directions for psychopathological network theory and methodology. Perspect Psychol Sci. 2017;12:999–1020 Available from: http://journals.sagepub.com/doi/10.1177/1745691617705892.

55. Forbes MK, Wright AGC, Markon KE, Krueger RF. The network approach to psychopathology: promise versus reality. World Psychiatry. 2019;18:272–3 Available from: https://onlinelibrary.wiley.com/doi/abs/10.1002/wps.20659.

56. Prefit A-B, Cândea DM, Szentagotai-Tătar A. Emotion regulation across eating pathology: A meta-analysis. Appetite. 2019;143:104438 Available from: https://linkinghub.elsevier.com/retrieve/pii/S0195666319304623.

57. Westwood H, Kerr-Gaffney J, Stahl D, Tchanturia K. Alexithymia in eating disorders: systematic review and meta-analyses of studies using the Toronto alexithymia scale. J Psychosom Res. 2017;99:66–81 Available from: https://linkinghub.elsevier.com/retrieve/pii/S0022399917302295.

58. Carcione A, Nicolò G, Pedone R, Popolo R, Conti L, Fiore D, et al. Metacognitive mastery dysfunctions in personality disorder psychotherapy. Psychiatry Res. 2011;190:60–71 Available from: https://linkinghub.elsevier.com/retrieve/pii/S0165178111000035.

59. Safer DL, Telch CF, Chen EY. Dialectical behavior therapy for binge eating and bulimia. New York: The Guilford Press; 2009.

60. Dingemans A, Danner U, Parks M. Emotion Regulation in Binge Eating Disorder: A Review. Nutrients. 2017;9:1274 Available from: http://www.mdpi.com/2072-6643/9/11/1274.

61. Treasure J, Duarte TA, Schmidt U. Eating disorders. Lancet. 2020;395:899 91-1 Available from: https://linkinghub.elsevier.com/retrieve/pii/S0140673620300593.

62. Levinson CA, Vanzhula IA, Brosof LC, Forbush K. Network Analysis as an Alternative Approach to Conceptualizing Eating Disorders: Implications for Research and Treatment. Curr Psychiatry Rep [Internet]. 2018;20:67. Available from: http://link.springer.com/10.1007/s11920-018-0930-y

63. Perko VL, Forbush KT, Siew CSQ, Tregarthen JP. Application of network analysis to investigate sex differences in interactive systems of eating-disorder psychopathology. Int J Eat Disord. 2019;52:1343–52 Available from: https://onlinelibrary.wiley.com/doi/abs/10.1002/eat.23170.

64. Carcione A, Riccardi I, Bilotta E, Leone L, Pedone R, Conti L, et al. Metacognition as a Predictor of Improvements in Personality Disorders. Front Psychol. 2019;10 Available from: https://www.frontiersin.org/article/10.3389/fpsyg.2019.00170/full.

6

Binge eating among older women: prevalence rates and health correlates across three independent samples

Salomé Adelia Wilfred[1], Carolyn Black Becker[2], Kathryn E. Kanzler[3], Nicolas Musi[4,5], Sara E. Espinoza[4,5] and Lisa Smith Kilpela[3,4*] (iD)

Abstract

Background: Emerging research indicates that binge eating (BE; consuming unusually large amounts of food in one siting while feeling a loss of control) is prevalent among older women. Yet, health correlates of BE in older adult populations are poorly understood. The original study aimed to investigate BE prevalence, frequency, and health correlates in a sample of older adult women. Based on results from this first study, we then sought to replicate findings in two additional samples of older adult women from separate studies.

Method: Using self-reported frequencies of BE from three separate samples of older women with very different demographics, we compared BE prevalence, frequency, and health correlates among older women. Study 1 ($N = 185$) includes data collected online (86% White; 59% overweight/obese status). Study 2 ($N = 64$) was conducted in person at a local food pantry (65% Hispanic; 47% household income < $10,000/year). Study 3 ($N = 100$) comprises data collected online (72% White; 50% Masters/Doctoral Degree).

Results: Per DSM-5 frequency criterion of BE at least weekly, we found prevalence rates ranging from 19 to 26% across the three samples. Correlates of BE frequency included elevated negative mood, worry, BMI, and less nutritious food consumption.

Conclusions: Across three very different samples in terms of race/ethnicity, education, food security status, measurements, and sampling methodology, we found fairly consistent rates of self-reported BE at least weekly (19–26%). Results suggest that BE is related to negative health indices among older women and support the need for more research in this population.

Keywords: Aging, Binge eating, Women's health

Plain English summary

Historically viewed as problems of youth, eating disorders are understudied in older women. Yet, disordered eating, especially binge eating (BE; eating an unusually large amount of food with loss of control), appears to be more prevalent among older women than previously thought.

Importantly, BE is associated with various health problems in the general population, but less is known about health outcomes related to BE in older populations. We compared prevalence rates of weekly BE measured in three separate samples of older women, as well as various health and wellness indices. We found fairly consistent rates of BE at least weekly (19–26%) across the three samples, and that BE frequency was related to negative health outcomes among older adult women. There is still much to be learned about BE among older adult populations.

*Correspondence: kilpela@uthscsa.edu
[3] ReACH Center, UT Health San Antonio, San Antonio, TX, USA
Full list of author information is available at the end of the article

Future research is needed to better understand how specific age-related experiences may comprise risk factors for disordered eating among older women.

Background

Nutrition pathology can significantly interfere with healthy aging. One form of nutrition pathology is disordered eating. Although clinical eating disorders and subclinical disordered eating are commonly viewed as problems of youth, emerging research indicates that older women indeed struggle with the spectrum of disordered eating [1, 2]. One of the most common forms of disordered eating among midlife and older women appears to be binge eating (BE) [3], which refers to recurrently consuming unusually large amounts of food in one siting while simultaneously feeling a loss of control, often resulting in significant distress [4]. BE is one of the core symptoms of binge eating disorder [4].

In the general population, binge eating disorder is associated with significant medical morbidity, including sleep problems, chronic pain, dyslipidemias, and metabolic and cardiac dysfunction [5, 6]. BE also increases risk for poorer micronutrient intake, as binge episodes typically involve consumption of foods high in sugar, fat, and salt [7, 8]. Frequent consumption of such foods and in large quantities can cause spikes in blood glucose [9] and research indicates that BE is linked prospectively with both type 2 diabetes and metabolic syndrome [10, 11]. Additionally, binge eating disorder is associated with higher levels of disability, psychosocial stress, and poorer quality of life [5, 6]. Importantly, BE also is closely associated with obesity and depression [12], which can amplify existing medical morbidities common among older adults. In older women, the health consequences of any form of disordered eating may be even more severe than seen in the general population, as older women have pre-existing risk for nutritional disorders (both over- and under-nutrition), sarcopenia, and frailty [13]. Despite this, older women historically have been excluded from BE research, leaving a major gap in understanding the risk, maintenance, and health consequences of BE among older women.

Eating disorder researchers have historically paid scant attention to older women. Despite this lack of research, numerous aging-related factors may contribute to elevating risk for BE in this population. Specifically, experiences related to the menopausal transition comprise risk for BE [3, 14]. For instance, a recent pilot study found that elevated daily estradiol, when progesterone was also elevated, was associated with BE episodes in perimenopausal women [14]. Sleep disturbances and negative affect, both of which are common experiences of women during the menopausal transition [15], also are well-established

risk factors for BE [16, 17]. Additionally, psychosocial stressors, such as caregiving demands and interpersonal strain, may increase further risk for dysregulated eating behaviors, especially for women [18]. Indeed, preliminary research suggests that older women who experience life stressors such as divorce, marital conflicts, traumatic illness, empty nest syndrome, and loss of parents, siblings or children are at increased risk for onset of disordered eating [19].

Additionally, aging-related changes in body shape/appearance (e.g., increased adipose tissue, decreased muscle mass, increased body fat distribution towards the torso, and changes in skin coloration, firmness, and elasticity; [20–22] may also increase risk for disordered eating [3, 23]. These changes shift women's bodies further away from the thin-young-ideal standard of female beauty in Western societies. This increased deviation from societal standards of female beauty, in turn, further increases risk for harmful comparisons of self to media representations and/or one's younger body weight or shape [24]. Such upward body comparisons often lead to or exacerbate negative body image (also referred to as body dissatisfaction), which is a well-established and robust risk factor for BE [25].

Notably, recent research indicates that older women experience high levels of body dissatisfaction. For instance, Mangweth-Matzek et al. [2] found that over 60% of women age 60–70 years endorsed body dissatisfaction. Kilpela et al. [26] found that negative body image mediated the relation between BMI and both health/wellness behaviors as well as quality of life among women aged 50 and over. Thus, negative body image appears to be prevalent among older women and increase risk for both disordered eating and poorer health outcomes. In sum, early research investigating prevalence rates of BE among older women indicate that this pathology is more pervasive than previously thought. Yet, given that the aging process poses unique risk for women with regards to BE, there is still much to learn about both prevalence and health correlates of BE among older women.

As noted above, the intersection of aging and eating disorders is an emerging field of research. When broaching a new area of science, it is important that researchers are accountable and present well-informed findings, specifically when researching populations not often represented in research. The replication of research findings is one way to increase accountability, especially when presenting research findings in emerging domains.

Indeed, recent literature has documented a "replication crisis" in psychological science highlighting the importance of replicating findings in independent studies [27]. In their seminal paper, Open Science Collaboration set out to replicate 100 experiments; only 36% yielded a statistically significant effect in the replication effort. This outcome signaled a concerning lack of replication and raised significant questions regarding the validity of the original findings. In response to rising concerns about replication in psychological science and the paper by the Open Science Collaboration, Lindsay and editors at Psychological Science [28] identified three factors (referred to as the "troubling trio") that appeared to contribute to lack of replication. These factors are, in terms coined by Lindsay: (1) "low statistical power," (2) "a surprising finding," and (3) "a p value of only slightly less than $p = 0.05$" [28]. According to Lindsay [28], any research findings that meet one or more of these criteria warrant efforts for replication.

The present research

The original purpose of this research was to examine the prevalence of BE and health correlates in older women in a single study. However, the primary finding of this original study (hereafter referred to as the index study) met Lindsay's criterion of a "surprising finding," which is one of the "troubling trio" [28]. Specifically, the prevalence rate of weekly BE in the index study was higher than those seen in the limited existing research (e.g., [1–3]). This raised the specter of a spurious finding which led to the development of three specific aims for a series of studies presented in this paper. First, we sought to describe the frequency of binge eating in older women. Per DSM-5 diagnostic criteria for bulimia nervosa and binge eating disorder [4], which require binge eating once per week on average, we used the frequency criterion of weekly or more BE in our descriptions of prevalence rates within each sample. Second, we sought to identify the health behaviors correlated with binge eating in older women. Finally, we sought to determine if findings from the index study would replicate by comparing the findings of two additional samples of older women.

Method

Index study: general online sample of women
Participants

Participants were 185 women recruited online. Participants ranged from 60 to 83 years of age ($M = 65.91$, $SD = 5.09$); 86.4% identified as White and 2.2% endorsed Hispanic/Latina ethnicity (Table 1). Over one-third of participants (36.4%) reported a body mass index (BMI) greater than 30 (i.e., obese status), while 23.2% reported a BMI in the overweight range (25–29.9).

Procedure

The Institutional Review Board (IRB) of the senior author's institution deemed this study as IRB-exempt (i.e., no more than minimal risk to study participants).

Participants were recruited via email using personal and professional networks (i.e., non-randomized snowball sampling) and Amazon Mechanical Turk within the United States. We recruited women, aged 60 and over, to complete an online survey on health and wellness among older women. After providing informed consent, participants completed self-report questionnaires online.

Measures
Demographic information

Participants reported age, height, weight, race and ethnicity. Although self-report is not optimal for assessing height and weight, research indicates that self-report weights are reasonably accurate [29] and we were limited to self-report due to the online nature of the study.

Binge eating

As our primary measure of BE, we used the VA-Binge Eating Screener (VA-BES; [30]), which asks: "On average, how often have you eaten extremely large amounts of food at one time and felt that your eating was out of control at that time?" Response options include: Never, < 1 time/week, 1 time/week, 2–4 times/week, and 5+ times/week. This measure demonstrated good psychometric properties [30].

Eating disorder (ED) symptoms

We assessed ED symptoms using the Eating Disorder Examination Questionnaire (EDE-Q Short; [31]), which is a 12-item version of the full EDE-Q [32]. The EDE-Q Short measures ED symptoms over the past week, using a 0–3 scale ranging from 0 to 7 days in the past week. Within this measure, one item asks about number of BE episodes in the past week. We did not isolate this item for any inferential statistics; however, we used self-reported BE frequency on this measure as an indicator of convergent validity participant responses to the primary measure of BE frequency (i.e., the VA-BES) to evaluate consistency of reporting. Past research demonstrated good internal consistency (Cronbach's $\alpha = 0.913$) and temporal stability (ICC $= 0.93$; $p < 0.001$; [31]). Internal consistency in the current sample was good ($\alpha = 0.86$).

Negative affect

We used the 17-items of the fear, guilt and sadness subscales of the Positive and Negative Affect Scale-revised (PANAS-X; [33]) to measure negative affect over the past 3 weeks; higher scores indicate greater negative affect. This subscale has demonstrated good internal consistency in past research (current sample $\alpha = 0.95$).

Table 1 Participant demographics and descriptive statistics for all three samples

| | Study 1 (N = 185) | Study 2 (N = 64) | Study 3 (N = 100) |
	% or M (SD)	%	% or M (SD)
Age	65.91 (5.09)	84.4% (Age 66–75) 15.6% (Age 76+)	60.57 (5.05)
Race/Ethnicity			
Black	9.2%	15.9%	16.8%
White	86.4%	14.3%	72.0%
Hispanic/Latinx	2.2%	65.1%	2.0%
Other/mixed	4.3%	4.8%	9.0%
Level of education			
Grade school or less	–	32.9%	0.0%
Some high school	–	15.6%	0.0%
High school diploma/GED	–	26.6%	5.0%
Some college/technical school	–	23.4%	16.8%
Bachelor's degree	–	1.6%	18.8%
Some graduate school	–	0.0%	9.9%
Master's degree	–	0.0%	34.7%
Doctoral degree	–	0.0%	14.9%
Annual household income			
Under $10,000	–	46.9%	–
$10,000-$40,000	–	37.5%	–
$40,000-$65,000	–	3.1%	–
BMI	28.29 (7.71)	–	26.62 (6.04)
Binge eating	26.5%	20.4%	19.0%
Compensatory behaviors			
Driven exercising	8.7%[a]	12.6%[b]	13.9%[b]
Self-induced vomiting	2.7%[a]	7.9%[b]	1.0%[b]
Laxatives or diuretics	2.7%[a]	11.0%[b]	3.0%[b]

Study 1 = General online sample; Study 2 = Women living with food insecurity; Study 3 = Women with high education levels; BMI = Body mass index; Binge Eating = binge eating at a frequency of weekly or more; Compensatory behaviors = behaviors endorsed for the purpose of weight/shape control

[a] = Endorsed this behavior in the past week

[b] = Endorsed this behavior in the past month

Consumption of nutritious foods

The two-item Eating Behaviors Questionnaire (EBQ; [34]) measured self-reported consumption of nutritious foods. Items inquire how often participants consciously tried to increase micronutrient density in meals and frequency of consuming fresh fruits and vegetables over the past week. The EBQ uses a 5-point Likert scale (1 = *consume at every meal*, 5 = *never*); items are summed, and higher scores indicate less consumption of nutritious foods. Internal consistency in this sample was adequate ($\alpha = 0.63$).

Results

We used descriptive statistics to evaluate BE prevalence and frequency in this sample. Due to the ordinal nature of BE frequency measure, we used Spearman's rho to investigate correlations of BE frequency with BMI, ED symptoms, negative affect, and consumption of nutritious foods. Finally, we used a binomial logistic regression model to investigate the degree to which BE frequency contributed to risk for obesity status while controlling for age, race, and ethnicity. Regarding BE frequency and prevalence (Table 1), 48% of the sample reported never BE. Using the clinical frequency criterion of BE once per week or more, 26.5% of the sample reported BE at least weekly. As a secondary measure of BE frequency in this sample, we examined rates of BE using the BE item on the EDE-Q Short. One participant's answer did not align with their response on the VA-BES, resulting in 25.5% of the sample endorsing at least one BE episode in the past week. BE frequency was correlated with higher BMI ($\rho = 0.40$, $p < 0.01$), more ED symptoms ($\rho = 0.65$, $p < 0.001$), greater negative affect ($\rho = 0.43$, $p < 0.01$), and less frequent consumption of nutritious foods ($\rho = 0.16$, $p < 0.05$). Finally, BE frequency contributed significant risk for obese status based on self-reported BMI ($OR = 2.08$; 95% CI [1.52; 2.82], $p < 0.001$). Age, race, and ethnicity categories were non-significant in the model.

Study 2 (replication): sample living with food insecurity
Participants
This sample consisted of 64 older women (ages 66+) who were clients at food pantries of the local food bank who participated in a larger study of individuals living with food insecurity [35]. Age was only captured in clusters; thus, only women who selected the "age 66 or over" option were included in this study. Younger participants and men were not included. The majority of participants identified as Hispanic (65.1%; Table 1). Over a third (39.1%) reported disabled status, and 48.4% had less than a high school education or equivalent (GED). Almost half (46.9%) reported a household annual income of less than $10,000/year. Access to current health data is often low among individuals living with extreme poverty; scales are considered luxury items and often are not in the home [35]. Thus, requesting current height and weight in this sample was likely to elicit inaccurate data. Therefore, we do not have BMI data in this sample.

Procedure
This study received IRB approval and was run in collaboration with the local food bank. See Becker et al. [35] for details regarding the full study and community partnership. All questionnaires were available in either English or Spanish. Following informed consent, participants completed questionnaires in person; undergraduate research assistants facilitated reading as needed (i.e., read questions aloud in language of choice) and answered questions. Participants received a $5 gift card to a local grocery store as compensation.

Measures
Consistent with working with a marginalized, low-education population and incorporating a socially conscious lens [36, 37], we evaluated survey complexity. Guided by a colleague with extensive experience working with marginalized populations, we employed best practices delineated by Stonewall and colleagues [38] to evaluate and modify questionnaire language. We modified or removed items based on reading level or that may impact comprehension (for detailed rationale and procedure for measures modification, see Becker et al. [35]). This process ensured that our survey used appropriate language in order to be inclusive and culturally sensitive [36].

Food insecurity
To assess severity of food insecurity, we used the Radimer Cornell Food Insecurity Measure (RCFIM; [39, 40]).

This measure uses a Likert scale, and global scores indicate level of food insecurity: (1) not food insecure (i.e., did not meet criteria for food. insecurity); (2) household food insecurity (i.e., anxiety about food, eating the same thing repeatedly due to lack of resources, and food running out but no one going hungry in the home); (3) individual food insecurity (i.e., adult reports being hungry at times because they lack food); and (4) child hunger food insecurity (i.e., adult reports inability to adequately feed their children secondary to lack of resources). For this study, we only included participants in the two highest levels of food insecurity (individual and child hunger), as these are the most severe. Internal consistency was good in our sample (Cronbach's $\alpha = 0.92$).

Binge eating
We used the BE item from the Eating Disorder Diagnostic Scale for DSM 5 (EDDS-5) to assess frequency of BE over the past month [41]. The EDDS is a brief self-report measure designed to assess the spectrum of EDs. The BE item asks, "How many times in the past month (30–31 days) on average have you eaten an unusually large amount of food and experienced a loss of control?" A report of ≥ 4 times in the past month equated to weekly binge eating.

Internalized weight stigma
We used the Weight Self-Stigma Questionnaire (WSSQ) to assess internalization of weight bias [42]. Items are rated on a 7- point Likert scale ($1 = strongly\ disagree$ to $7 = strongly\ agree$), and participants rate their level of agreement with explicit weight bias statements (e.g., "I became fat because I'm a weak person" and "People think that I am to blame for being fat."). Scores are summed for a total score and higher scores indicate greater self-stigma; internal consistency was excellent ($\alpha = 0.97$).

Anxiety
We used eight items from the Penn State Worry Questionnaire (PSWQ; [43]) to assess anxiety/worry. Items are rated on a 5-point Likert scale ($1 = not\ at\ all\ typical\ of\ me$ to $5 = very\ typical\ of\ me$); higher scores indicate more anxiety/worry. Internal consistency for this version of the PSWQ in the current sample was excellent ($\alpha = 0.95$).

Results
Similar to the index study, we used descriptive statistics to evaluate BE prevalence and frequency in this replication sample. We used bivariate correlations of BE frequency with anxiety and internalized weight stigma. Finally, we examined rates of unhealthy weight control behaviors (e.g., self-induced vomiting, use of laxatives/diuretics for weight control) in this sample. Regarding

BE prevalence, 20.4% of this sample reported BE on a weekly or more basis in the past month. Frequency of BE was positively correlated with higher anxiety ($r=0.37$, $p=0.008$) and internalized weight stigma ($r=0.42$, $p=0.002$). Within this sample of older women living with significant food insecurity, 7.9% of women reported self-induced vomiting, and 11% reported use of laxative or diuretics for weight control in the past month.

Study 3 (replication): sample with high education levels
Participants
Participants were 100 women recruited online for a larger study of body image in a diverse sample of adult women. Participant ages ranged from 55–79 years ($M=60.57$, $SD=5.05$) and reported a mean body mass index of 26.62 ($SD=6.04$). The majority (72.0%) self-identified as White; 2.0% identified as Hispanic/Latina, and 72% were currently married (Table 1). Notably, 50% of women in this sample had a Masters or Doctoral degree.

Procedure
IRB approval was granted for this study and participants were recruited via email, social media, personal and professional networks, and by word of mouth. Recruitment emails described the study as exploring body image and wellness in a diverse population of adult women. All emails and posts requested that women forward the study invitation to their own social and professional networks (i.e., snowball sampling). After providing informed consent, participants completed self-report questionnaires online and had the option to provide their email address to enter a raffle for a $200 Amazon gift card.

Measures
Binge eating
We assessed BE with the diagnostic items of the EDE-Q [32], which is a self-report measure of eating behaviors and attitudes over the past 28 days. The BE items inquire about frequency of BE episodes over the past 28 days. A report of ≥ 4 times in the past four weeks (28 days) equated to weekly BE.

BMI
Participants self-reported their height and weight in order to calculate BMI.

Depressive symptoms
We used the Beck Depression Inventory- II (BDI-II; [44]) to measure depressive symptoms. Due to liability in assessing suicidality anonymously and via online survey, we removed the suicidality item from the BDI-II. Thus,

our final measure included 20 items and had good internal validity in the current sample ($\alpha=0.85$).

Body shame
We administered the Shame subscale of the Objectified Body Consciousness Scale (OBCS; [45]). This subscale includes eight items rated from 1 (*strongly disagree*) to 7 (*strongly agree*), with a "not applicable" option for items that do not apply. Higher scores indicate greater shame, and 25% or more of items NA or missing qualifies as missing overall score. In the present sample, internal consistency was good ($\alpha=0.85$).

Results
Similar to the previous studies, we used descriptive statistics to evaluate BE prevalence and frequency in this second replication sample. We used bivariate correlations of BE frequency with BMI, depressive symptoms, and body shame. Finally, we used a binomial logistic regression model to investigate the degree to which BE frequency contributed to risk for obesity status while controlling for age, race, and ethnicity. In this sample of women with high education levels, 19% reported BE weekly or more in the past month. BE frequency was positively correlated with greater depressive symptoms ($r=0.36$, $p<0.001$) and higher body shame ($r=0.44$, $p<0.001$), but was not correlated with BMI ($r=0.20$, $p=0.075$). Finally, BE frequency contributed a small, but statistically significant risk for obesity status ($OR=1.12$; 95% CI [1.00, 1.24], $p=0.04$). Neither age nor race/ethnicity were significant in the model.

Discussion
The index study in this series of studies was designed to examine the frequency, prevalence, and health correlates of binge eating (BE) in a single sample of older women aged 60 and over. Findings from this index study indicated that roughly 26% of older women in our sample reported experiencing BE at a frequency of weekly or more in the past month. Notably, the clinical frequency criterion for a diagnosis of binge eating disorder or bulimia nervosa is BE weekly or more for at least 3 months [4]. Prior research, however, identified lower prevalence rates of weekly BE among midlife and older adult women. For instance, 11% of women in midlife reported regular BE as assessed by self-report with the Bulimia Test-Revised (BULIT-R; [12]). Using a non-validated self-report measure inquiring about frequency of BE episodes, 3.5% of women aged 50+ reported weekly BE [46]. Using a similar assessment measure, a sample of women aged 60–70 years, 3.8% met criteria for an ED,

while another 4.4% endorsed at least one core symptom of an ED [2].

Notably, the vast majority of research examining prevalence rates and types of eating disordered behaviors among older adults used self-report measures, rather than gold standard clinical interviews (e.g., the Eating Disorders Examination; [47]). In one study that utilized a structured clinical interview, 5.6% of women aged 65–94 reported BE episodes in the past month, with mean frequency of 8 episodes/month [1]. Thus, prevalence rates of disordered eating documented in the literature ranged from roughly 4–11% and are smaller than our findings.

Of note, 59.6% of participants in the index study met BMI classification criteria for overweight (i.e., $25 < BMI < 30$) or obese status (i.e., $BMI > 30$). To put this in context, past research investigating BE prevalence in obese patients presenting for weight loss treatment has documented clinically relevant BE at approximately 30% [48–50]. Thus, our observed prevalence rate for weekly BE in the index study was slightly lower than data from general adult patients (i.e., not older adults) presenting for weight loss programs. Our sample was neither a treatment-seeking sample, nor did we conduct targeted recruitment for clinical populations. Thus, the higher prevalence of overweight/obesity may have played a role in the elevated rates of BE in this first sample, as compared to past research and to the other two studies.

Because the prevalence rate of weekly or more BE from this index study was surprisingly high (i.e., a "surprising finding" per Lindsay; [28]), we were concerned about a spurious finding. Specifically, our findings fell into one construct of the "troubling trio" [28] in the replication crisis in psychological science, which raised concerns regarding replicability. Per recommendations from Lindsay [28], such results warrant efforts for replication. Therefore, we sought to replicate our index study results using existing data from two other samples of older adult women that included self-reported BE frequency. Results from both replications using data from two additional independent studies—with notably different demographics—were largely consistent with the index study.

We propose that the combined results suggest that BE rates in older women may be higher than previously thought and are deserving of further research. While these data do not examine the full diagnostic criteria for binge eating disorder, findings across the three studies provide preliminary data supporting the need for more research regarding eating disorders among older adults. The primary strength of the three studies, when viewed collectively, is the ability to refute the argument that the primary findings of the index study (i.e., BE prevalence and frequency) were artificially inflated due to one or more of the following three factors: (1) sampling biases

secondary to recruitment strategy; (2) measurement error (i.e., risk of inherent response biases within one measure); and (3) participant demographics (i.e., limited generalizability). Regarding the first concern of sampling bias, two of the three studies used different types of internet sampling (i.e., snowball sampling, social media, and MTurk), whereas one used in-person recruitment and data collection. Despite the different sampling methods (internet versus in-person/community), prevalence rates of BE were similar across all three studies, suggesting the rates were not unique to one sampling method.

The second potential concern pertains to the way in which BE was assessed. For instance, it could be argued that the primary measurement strategy of the index study (i.e., the VA-BES) was flawed and resulted in inflated estimates of BE in the index sample. However, we used a total of four validated measures of BE across the three studies and findings remained remarkably consistent. Therefore, our findings regarding prevalence rates of BE were not simply due to measurement error. Of note, prior research utilized both validated and non-validated self-report instruments to assess rates of current binge eating among midlife and older women; only one study used a clinical interview.

Finally, one could argue, based on the index study alone, that the representativeness of the index sample in terms of sample characteristics (i.e., participant demographics) led to elevated assessment of BE. This supposition, however, does not appear to hold water when the nature of the three samples are compared. For instance, the community sample collected at local food pantries was predominantly Hispanic (65%), predominantly very low SES (47% reported an annual household income $< \$10,000/$ year) and living with significant food insecurity. Moreover, nearly 50% reported less than a high school degree or equivalent, and nearly 40% reported disabled status. In contrast, both of the internet samples were majority Non-Hispanic White, and one internet sample comprised women with high levels of education (50% Masters or Doctoral Degree). In summary, we found fairly consistent rates of self-reported BE at least weekly (19–26%) across three independent and very different samples in terms of race/ethnicity, education, food security status, measurements used, and data collection methods.

In addition to a high prevalence rate of weekly BE across the three samples, correlational analyses indicated that BE frequency was related to poorer psychological and physical health indices. Specifically, higher BE frequency was positively correlated with greater depression and negative affect, body shame, worry, and internalized weight stigma. Additionally, BE frequency was negatively correlated with frequency of consuming nutrient-dense foods. Lastly, results regarding BMI were mixed across two samples. In our index study, BE frequency was positively correlated with BMI, while this relation was non-significant in the highly educated sample. However, in both samples BE frequency increased risk for obesity status in our binomial logistic regression models. Thus, further investigation into obesity risk as a factor BE among diverse samples of older women is warranted.

Correlational findings from these three studies align with previous research on correlates of BE in younger samples. For instance, BE is consistently linked with depressive symptoms [12] and elevated BMI [51, 52] in prior research. Our correlational findings in this sample of older women are consistent with BE correlates observed in previous BE research conducted with more well-investigated samples (i.e., younger adults). In other words, expected BE and health correlates previously established hold true in this newer population of older adult women, which provides confidence in our interpretation of these data. Finally, these data extend prior research by documenting additional negative health correlates (e.g., internalized weight stigma, worry, and consumption of nutritious foods) of BE in older adult women.

It is important to note that we did not assess the full criteria for a diagnosis of binge eating disorder, per the DSM-5 [4]. Although women across these three separate studies reported BE weekly, this was only assessed in the past month. Additionally, we did not collect information on the emotional/cognitive criteria for binge eating disorder; rather, we only assessed the frequency of the behavior in the past month. Therefore, these findings may reflect a lower level of BE pathology severity in comparison to clinical-level binge eating disorder. Alternatively, our data support the contention that regular BE, regardless of full diagnostic status, is associated with poorer health constructs (e.g., depression/negative affect, less frequent consumption of micronutrients, body shame, worry, internalized weight stigma). Future research is needed to disentangle the potential health impacts of BE behaviors versus clinical threshold binge eating disorder among older adult populations.

There are numerous limitations to the current studies. First, all studies used self-report measures exclusively. Thus, it is entirely possible that results from self-report measures showed a greater frequency of BE as compared to those assessed by structured clinical interview. Further, we did not have objective measures of BMI nor clinical interviews to further explore clinical constructs. Second, although the three studies used different sampling methods, two of the three studies comprised minimal racial/ethnic diversity of participants and were online samples. Future research should use purposeful sampling methodology in order to evaluate more diverse samples of older

adult women and therefore enhance generalizability of findings. Additionally, analyses were cross-sectional and correlative in nature, therefore we are unable to evaluate causality among variables within each study. Future research should include larger sample sizes, incorporate clinical interviews, and utilize longitudinal methodology designed to investigate causality and chronological outcomes. Lastly, future studies should assess the full diagnostic criteria for binge eating disorder, in order to better estimate the prevalence of this pathology among older adult women.

Conclusions

In sum, findings indicated relatively stable rates of weekly or more BE (19–26%) among three independent and very different samples of older adult women. The rates observed across these three samples are higher than those documented in prior research and in younger samples, suggesting that older adult women may be at elevated risk for BE, yet further research is needed to examine the full diagnostic criteria for binge eating disorder. Correlations indicated that BE frequency is linked with negative health constructs, including depression and negative affect, body shame, worry, and internalized weight stigma. Longitudinal research is needed to better investigate the chronological effects of BE among older adult samples, as well as objective or interview methods of data collection.

Abbreviations

BE: Binge eating; BMI: Body mass index; ED: Eating disorder; DSM-5: Diagnostic and Statistical Manual for Mental Disorders, 5th edition; IBR: Institutional Review Board; VA-BES: Veterans Affairs-Binge Eating Screener; EDE-Q: Eating Disorders Examination-Questionnaire; PANAS-X: Positive and Negative Affect Schedule; EBQ: Eating Behaviors Questionnaire; RCFIM: Radimer Cornell Food Insecurity Measure; EDDS-5: Eating Disorders Diagnostic Scale for DSM-5; WSSQ: Weight Self Stigma Questionnaire; PSWQ: Penn State Worry Questionnaire; BDI-II: Beck Depression Inventory-II; OBCS: Objectified Body Consciousness Scale; SES: Socioeconomic status.

Acknowledgements

The authors thank the San Antonio Food Bank and affiliated food pantries, as well as Dr. Keesha Middlemass and Ms. Christina Verzijl, for their contributions to this research.

Authors' contributions

SAW was involved in development, data collection, and data cleaning of Study 3. SAW also was instrumental in writing this manuscript. CBB was PI for Studies 2 and 3 (i.e., study conceptualization, data collection, data analyses), and she was instrumental in writing this manuscript. KEK helped with conceptualization and execution of Study 1 and editing of this manuscript. NM and SEE were both involved with conceptualization, measures selection, and data interpretation for Study 1. They also edited the manuscript. LSK was PI for Study 1 (i.e., conceptualization, data collection, data analyses), conceptualized the current manuscript, conducted data analyses for all three studies, and was instrumental in writing. All authors read and approved the final manuscript.

Competing interests

The authors declare that they have no competing interests.

Author details

[1]Department of Psychology, University of Missouri-Kansas City, Kansas City, MO, USA. [2]Department of Psychology, Trinity University, San Antonio, TX, USA. [3]ReACH Center, UT Health San Antonio, San Antonio, TX, USA. [4]Barshop Institute, UT Health San Antonio, San Antonio, TX, USA. [5]South Texas VA Health System, Audie Murphy Veterans Hospital, San Antonio, TX, USA.

References

1. Conceicao EM, Gomes F, Vaz AR, Pinto-Bastos A, Machado PP. Prevalence of eating disorders and picking/nibbling in elderly women. Int J Eat Disord. 2017;50(7):793–800.
2. Mangweth-Matzek B, Rupp CI, Hausmann A, Assmayr K, Mariacher E, Kemmler G, Whitworth AB, Biebl W. Never too old for eating disorders or body dissatisfaction: a community study of elderly women. Int J Eat Disord. 2006;39(7):583–6.
3. Mangweth-Matzek B, Hoek HW, Pope HG Jr. Pathological eating and body dissatisfaction in middle-aged and older women. Curr Opin Psychiatry. 2014;27(6):431–5.
4. American Psychiatric Association. Diagnostic and statistical manual of mental disorders (DSM-5®). American Psychiatric Pub; 2013.
5. Johnson JG, Spitzer RL, Williams JB. Health problems, impairment and illnesses associated with bulimia nervosa and binge eating disorder among primary care and obstetric gynaecology patients. Psychol Med. 2001;31(8):1455–66.
6. Olguin P, Fuentes M, Gabler G, Guerdjikova AI, Keck PE, McElroy SL. Medical comorbidity of binge eating disorder. Eat Weight Disord. 2017;22(1):13–26.
7. Avena NM, Rada P, Hoebel BG. Sugar and fat bingeing have notable differences in addictive-like behavior. J Nutr. 2009;139(3):623–8.
8. Masheb RM, Dorflinger LM, Rolls BJ, Mitchell DC, Grilo CM. Binge abstinence is associated with reduced energy intake after treatment in patients with binge eating disorder and obesity. Obesity. 2016;24(12):2491–6.
9. Mitchell JE, King WC, Pories W, Wolfe B, Flum DR, Spaniolas K, Bessler M, Devlin M, Marcus MD, Kalarchian M, Engel S. Binge eating disorder and medical comorbidities in bariatric surgery candidates. Int J Eat Disord. 2015;48(5):471–6.
10. Mitchell JE. Medical comorbidity and medical complications associated with binge-eating disorder. Int J Eat Disord. 2016;49(3):319–23.
11. Thornton LM, Watson HJ, Jangmo A, Welch E, Wiklund C, von Hausswolff-Juhlin Y, Norring C, Herman BK, Larsson H, Bulik CM. Binge-eating disorder in the Swedish national registers: somatic comorbidity. Int J Eat Disord. 2017;50(1):58–65.
12. Marcus MD, Bromberger JT, Wei HL, Brown C, Kravitz HM. Prevalence and selected correlates of eating disorder symptoms among a multiethnic community sample of midlife women. Ann Behav Med. 2007;33(3):269–77.
13. Chapman IM. Nutritional disorders in the elderly. Med Clin. 2006;90(5):887–907.
14. Baker JH, Eisenlohr-Moul T, Wu YK, Schiller CE, Bulik CM, Girdler SS. Ovarian hormones influence eating disorder symptom variability during the menopause transition: a pilot study. Eat Behav. 2019;35:101337.
15. Bromberger JT, Matthews KA, Schott LL, Brockwell S, Avis NE, Kravitz HM, Everson-Rose SA, Gold EB, Sowers M, Randolph JF Jr. Depressive symptoms during the menopausal transition: the Study of Women's Health Across the Nation (SWAN). J Affect Disord. 2007;103(1–3):267–72.
16. Dingemans A, Danner U, Parks M. Emotion regulation in binge eating disorder: a review. Nutrients. 2017;9(11):1274.
17. Cerolini S, Ballesio A, Ferlazzo F, Lucidi F, Lombardo C. Decreased inhibitory control after partial sleep deprivation in individuals reporting binge eating: preliminary findings. PeerJ. 2020;8:e9252.
18. Koumoutzis A, Cichy KE. What's eating you? Risk factors for poor health behaviors among family caregivers. Aging Ment Health. 2020. https://doi.org/10.1080/13607863.2020.1805722.
19. Kally Z, Cumella EJ. 100 midlife women with eating disorders: a phenomenological analysis of etiology. J Gen Psychol. 2008;135(4):359–78.
20. Evans WJ, Lexell J. Human aging, muscle mass, and fiber type composition. J Gerontol A Biol Sci Med Sci. 1995;50(Special_Issue):11–6.
21. Šitum M, Buljan M, Čavka V, Bulat V, Krolo I, Lugović ML. Skin changes in the elderly people–how strong is the influence of the UV radiation on skin aging? Coll Antropol. 2010;34(2):9–13.
22. Tchkonia T, Morbeck DE, Von Zglinicki T, Van Deursen J, Lustgarten J, Scrable H, Khosla S, Jensen MD, Kirkland JL. Fat tissue, aging, and cellular senescence. Aging Cell. 2010;9(5):667–84.
23. Gupta MA. Concerns about aging skin and eating disorders. In: Strumia R, editor. Eating disorders and the skin. Berlin: Springer; 2013. p. 97–102.
24. Peat CM, Peyerl NL, Muehlenkamp JJ. Body image and eating disorders in older adults: a review. J Gen Psychol. 2008;135(4):343–58.
25. Stice E. Risk and maintenance factors for eating pathology: a meta-analytic review. Psychol Bull. 2002;128(5):825–48.
26. Kilpela LS, Verzijl CL, Becker CB. Body image in older women: a mediator of BMI and wellness behaviors. J Women Aging. 2021;33(3):298–311.
27. Anderson JE, Aarts AA, Anderson CJ, Attridge PR, Attwood A, Axt J, Babel M, Bahník Š, Baranski E, Barnett-Cowan M, Bartmess E. Estimating the reproducibility of psychological science. Science. 2015;349(6251):1–8. https://doi.org/10.1126/science.aac4716.
28. Lindsay DS. Replication in psychological science. Psychol Sci. 2015;26(12):1827–32.
29. Stunkard AJ, Albaum JM. The accuracy of self-reported weights. Am J Clin Nutr. 1981;34(8):1593–9.
30. Dorflinger LM, Ruser CB, Masheb RM. A brief screening measure for binge eating in primary care. Eat Behav. 2017;26:163–6.
31. Gideon N, Hawkes N, Mond J, Saunders R, Tchanturia K, Serpell L. Development and psychometric validation of the EDE-QS, a 12 item short form of the Eating Disorder Examination Questionnaire (EDE-Q). PLoS ONE. 2016;11(5):e0152744.
32. Fairburn CG, Beglin SJ. Eating disorder examination questionnaire. In: Cognitive behavior therapy and eating disorders. 2008. p. 309–13.
33. Crawford JR, Henry JD. The Positive and Negative Affect Schedule (PANAS): Construct validity, measurement properties and normative data in a large non-clinical sample. Br J Clin Psychol. 2004;43(3):245–65.
34. Becker CB, Verzijl CL, Kilpela LS, Wilfred SA, Stewart T. Body image in adult women: associations with health behaviors, quality of life, and functional impairment. J Health Psychol. 2019;24(11):1536–47.
35. Becker CB, Middlemass K, Taylor B, Johnson C, Gomez F. Food insecurity and eating disorder pathology. Int J Eat Disord. 2017;50(9):1031–40.
36. Belone L, Lucero JE, Duran B, Tafoya G, Baker EA, Chan D, Chang C, Greene-Moton E, Kelley MA, Wallerstein N. Community-based participatory research conceptual model: community partner consultation and face validity. Qual Health Res. 2016;26(1):117–35.
37. Snow ME, Tweedie K, Pederson A. Heard and valued: the development of a model to meaningfully engage marginalized populations in health services planning. BMC Health Serv Res. 2018;18(1):1–3.
38. Roscoe RD, Chiou EK, Wooldridge AR, editors. Advancing diversity, inclusion, and social justice through human systems engineering. Boca Raton: CRC Press; 2019.
39. Kendall A, Olson CM, Frongillo EA Jr. Validation of the Radimer/Cornell measures of hunger and food insecurity. J Nutr. 1995;125(11):2793–801.
40. Radimer KL, Olson CM, Greene JC, Campbell CC, Habicht JP. Understanding hunger and developing indicators to assess it in women and children. J Nutr Educ. 1992;24(1):36S-44S.
41. Stice E, Fisher M, Martinez E. Eating disorder diagnostic scale: additional evidence of reliability and validity. Psychol Assess. 2004;16(1):60.
42. Lillis J, Luoma JB, Levin ME, Hayes SC. Measuring weight self-stigma: the weight self-stigma questionnaire. Obesity. 2010;18(5):971–6.
43. Meyer TJ, Miller ML, Metzger RL, Borkovec TD. Development and validation of the penn state worry questionnaire. Behav Res Ther. 1990;28(6):487–95.
44. Beck AT, Steer RA, Brown GK. Manual for the beck depression inventory-II.
45. McKinley NM, Hyde JS. The objectified body consciousness scale: development and validation. Psychol Women Q. 1996;20(2):181–215.

46. Gagne DA, Von Holle A, Brownley KA, Runfola CD, Hofmeier S, Branch KE, Bulik CM. Eating disorder symptoms and weight and shape concerns in a large web-based convenience sample of women ages 50 and above: results of the gender and body image (GABI) study. Int J Eat Disord. 2012;45(7):832–44.

47. Cooper Z, Fairburn C. The eating disorder examination: a semi-structured interview for the assessment of the specific psychopathology of eating disorders. Int J Eat Disord. 1987;6(1):1–8.

48. Dymek MP, le Grange D, Neven K, Alverdy J. Quality of life and psychosocial adjustment in patients after Roux-en-Y gastric report bypass: a brief report. Obes Surg. 2001;11(1):32–9.

49. Pagoto S, Bodenlos JS, Kantor L, Gitkind M, Curtin C, Ma Y. Association of major depression and binge eating disorder with weight loss in a clinical setting. Obesity. 2007;15(11):2557–9.

50. Conti C, Di Francesco G, Lanzara R, Severo M, Fumagalli L, Guagnano MT, Porcelli P. Alexithymia and binge eating in obese outpatients who are starting a weight-loss program: a structural equation analysis. Eur Eat Dis Rev. 2019;27(6):628–40.

51. Hudson JI, Hiripi E, Pope HG Jr, Kessler RC. The prevalence and correlates of eating disorders in the National Comorbidity Survey Replication. Biol Psychiatry. 2007;61(3):348–58.

52. Udo T, Grilo CM. Prevalence and correlates of DSM-5—defined eating disorders in a nationally representative sample of US adults. Biol Psychiatry. 2018;84(5):345–54.

7

Real-time predictors and consequences of binge eating among adults with type 1 diabetes

Ashley A. Moskovich[1], Natalia O. Dmitrieva[2], Michael A. Babyak[1], Patrick J. Smith[1], Lisa K. Honeycutt[1], Jan Mooney[1] and Rhonda M. Merwin[1*] (iD)

Abstract

Background: Objective binge eating (OBE) is common among individuals with type 1 diabetes (T1D) and may have negative consequences for glycemic control. Recent studies have suggested that diabetes distress (i.e., emotional distress specific to diabetes and living with the burden of management) is a distinct emotional experience among individuals with diabetes. Preliminary studies have found diabetes distress is associated with eating disorder symptoms and poor glycemic control. The aim of the current study was to examine real-time emotional precursors and consequences of OBE in adults with T1D (i.e., general negative affect, specific emotional states and diabetes distress) using ecological momentary assessment methods. We also explore the impact of OBE on 2-h postprandial glycemic control relative to non-OBE eating episodes.

Methods: Adults with T1D ($N = 83$) completed 3-days of ecological momentary assessment assessing mood and eating behavior using a telephone-based survey system. Participants were prompted to rate momentary affect, including level diabetes distress, at random intervals and reported on eating episodes. Participants also wore continuous glucose monitors allowing for ongoing assessment of glycemic control. Multi-level modeling was used to examine between- and within-person effects of momentary increases in emotions prior to eating on the likelihood of OBE and the impact of OBE on postprandial blood glucose. Generalized linear mixed models examined whether change in post-meal affect differed between OBE and non-OBE episodes.

Results: Participants were predominately middle-aged (Mean = 42; SD = 12.43) Caucasian (87%) females (88%) reporting clinically significant eating disorder symptoms (76%). Nearly half of the sample (43%) reported OBE during the 3-day study period. The between-person effect for negative affect was significant (OR = 1.93, $p < .05$), indicating a 93% increased risk of OBE among individuals with higher negative affect compared to individuals with average negative affect. Between-person effects were also significant for guilt, frustration and diabetes distress (OR = 1.48–1. 77, $ps < .05$). Analyses indicated that mean change in post-meal negative affect was significantly greater for OBE relative to non-OBE episodes ($B = 0.44$, $p < .001$). Blood glucose at 120 min postprandial was also higher for OBE than for non-OBE episodes ($p = .03$).

Conclusions: Findings indicate that individuals who tend to experience negative affect and diabetes distress before eating are at increased risk of OBE at the upcoming meal. Results also suggest that engaging in binge eating may result in greater subsequent negative affect, including diabetes distress, and lead to elevated postprandial blood glucose levels. These findings add to a growing literature suggesting diabetes distress is related to eating disordered behaviors among individuals with T1D.

Keywords: Type 1 diabetes, Eating disorders, Binge eating, Ecological momentary assessment, EMA

* Correspondence: rhonda.merwin@duke.edu
[1]Duke University Medical Center, DUMC Box 3842, Durham, NC 27712, USA
Full list of author information is available at the end of the article

Plain english summary

Binge eating is common among individuals with type 1 diabetes (T1D) and may negatively impact glycemic control. Existing eating disorder treatments are less effective for individuals with T1D, suggesting the need to better understand factors that may contribute to binge eating in this population. Previous research indicates that people are more likely to binge eat when they are feeling negative emotions. However, whether there are different emotional antecedents or consequences for T1D patients is not known. The current study tested whether increases in negative affect, including diabetes distress (i.e., emotional distress specific to living with diabetes), increased the likelihood of binge eating among adults with T1D. Eighty-three adults with T1D provided information about their emotions and eating behavior throughout the day for 3 days using a telephone-based survey system. Findings indicated individuals who reported higher levels of guilt, frustration and diabetes distress before eating episodes were more likely to binge eat than individuals who reported average levels of these emotions. Results also indicated that people felt worse (generally and about diabetes) and had higher blood glucose levels after binge eating. Findings suggest that interventions focused on helping individuals cope with negative emotions and diabetes distress may be helpful to incorporate into treatments for binge eating.

Background

Eating problems are common among individuals with type 1 diabetes [1–3]. This includes binge eating, dietary restriction and compensatory behaviors observed in the general population (e.g., self-induced vomiting) along with the unique capacity to restrict insulin for weight control. Studies show that disordered behaviors are associated with poor metabolic control and diabetes complications even when full diagnostic criteria for an eating disorder is not met (e.g., binge eating disorder, bulimia nervosa) [1, 3–5].

Up to 45–80% of young women with type 1 diabetes report binge eating behavior [6, 7], and many engage in this behavior frequently [3]. For example, a recent study found that 56% of adolescents completing a national survey reported binge eating at least once during the past 14 days [3]. Objective binge eating (OBE), defined as a loss of control over eating while consuming an objectively large amount of food [8], makes it challenging to manage diabetes. Most notably, individuals may struggle to accurately count carbohydrate and estimate bolus insulin needs when eating is uncontrolled. Binge eating may also motivate the use of dangerous behaviors to compensate for excessive calories consumed, further disrupting glycemic control (e.g., intentionally restricting insulin to induce glycosuria; the excretion of glucose

into the urine) [9]. Poor glycemic control is associated with an array of diabetes-related medical complications (e.g., neuropathy, retinopathy) [9, 10], highlighting the importance of addressing OBE in this patient population.

Despite the high prevalence and clinical significance of OBE in type 1 diabetes, it remains an understudied problem and effective treatments are lacking. Data suggests that conventional outpatient eating disorder treatments (developed for nondiabetic individuals) are less effective for individuals with type 1 diabetes [11–14]. One treatment study found that individuals continued to binge eat and restrict insulin, even when there were improvements in weight and shape concerns [14]. This indicates the need to better understand the factors associated with OBE in this unique patient population in order to develop more effective interventions.

A large body of empirical work in the general population suggests that negative affect is associated with OBE among individuals without diabetes [15, 16]. Previous studies have demonstrated that individuals who engage in OBE tend to report higher levels of depression and anxiety in general [16–18], and experience momentary increases in negative affect prior to binge eating episodes. When examining specific emotional states, guilt, sadness, and anger tend to be the strongest predictors of binge eating [19–22]. Studies examining affect post binge eating have mixed results. While some studies report that negative affect increases after binge eating [15, 21], others suggest that binge eating may actually temporarily decrease negative affect thereby functioning as a maladaptive emotion regulation strategy [19, 20, 22, 23].

At least one study has found individuals with type 1 diabetes with OBE report greater anxiety and depression than type 1 diabetes patients who do not engage in OBE [24]. However, there are no studies that have tested momentary changes in affect that may precede or follow an episode of binge eating in this high-risk patient population. Thus, whether emotional precursors or consequences of OBE are the same for individuals with type 1 diabetes as in the general population is unknown. This may include differences in general emotional states or more uniquely, diabetes distress (i.e., emotional distress specific to diabetes and living with the burden of management), which has been identified as a distinct emotional state experienced by individuals with diabetes [25–27].

For individuals with diabetes, maintaining control over eating is not only about controlling weight but also about preventing immediately life-threatening circumstances (e.g., diabetic ketoacidosis) and staving off future long-term diabetes-related complications. Thus, mealtimes may be particularly emotionally evocative, evoking negative affect generally, and specifically feelings of fear, anger and guilt associated with diabetes and living with the burden of diabetes management. Diabetes distress is increasingly recognized as a factor associated with poor management in type 1 diabetes [27, 28]. A few studies suggest diabetes distress is associated with eating disorder symptoms and taking less insulin than is needed [26, 29–31]. However, whether diabetes distress is functionally-related to OBE, increasing risk for this behavior in real-time, a consequence of OBE, or neither, has not been determined.

The current study examined real-time precursors and consequences of OBE in adults with type 1 diabetes using ecological momentary assessment methods. We examined general negative affect as a predictor of OBE, as well as specific emotional states and diabetes distress. We also established both the between- and within-person effects in each predictor (i.e., distinguished between individual differences in negative affect from potential additional impact of a momentary increase in negative affect) on OBE episode likelihood. Finally, we examined the impact of binge eating on glycemic control by examining blood glucose 2 h postprandial for OBE episodes versus non-OBE episodes. These findings may shed light on behavior patterns and treatment targets for this high-risk patient population.

Methods
Participants
Participants were recruited from two medical centers in the Southeast United States and the surrounding area as part of a larger study investigating eating disorder symptomatology among individuals with type 1 diabetes (see [31, 32]). Participants were adults between the ages of 18 and 65 years diagnosed with type 1 diabetes without hypoglycemic unawareness (as assessed via the Gold method [33]) or cognitive disabilities that interfered with their capacity to manage diabetes independently. Individuals with clinically significant eating disorder symptomatology (as indicated by a score of ≥20 on the Diabetes Eating Problems Survey-Revised (DEPS-R) [34] described in more detail below) were recruited first to answer primary research questions of the larger investigation (see Merwin et al., 2018 [32]). After the initial recruitment target was surpassed, enrollment was opened to individuals with DEPS-R scores below 20 to capture the full range of eating disorder symptomatology (see Merwin et al., 2015 [31]). The final sample consisted of 83 individuals, including 63 with DEPS-R ≥ 20.

Procedure
As described in previous papers (see [31, 32]), participants completed 3 days of ecological momentary assessment of mood and eating behavior using a telephone-based survey system. Interstitial glucose levels were monitored throughout the assessment period using blinded continuous glucose monitoring (CGM).

Eligible participants presented to the laboratory on two separate days. On Day 1, participants completed self-report measures of their illness history and had a blood draw to determine hemoglobin A_{1c} (HbA_{1c}). They had a glucose sensor placed and were then trained on the momentary assessment procedures which included completing surveys at random intervals throughout the day and initiating survey entries for meals/snacks (described in detail below). Participants returned to the laboratory 3 days later to have their glucose sensor removed and data downloaded using specialized software. They also completed additional self-report measures not relevant to the current study. Procedures were approved by the Duke University Health System Institutional Review Board (IRB) and all participants documented informed consent before participation in the study protocol.

Assessments
Diabetes eating problems survey-revised (DEPS-R; [34])
The DEPS-R is a 16-item self-report assessment of problematic eating attitudes and behaviors specifically tailored to individuals with diabetes. Items measure how often the individual has experienced each attitude and behavior over the past 4 weeks using a 6-point scale ranging from "Never" to "Always". Sample items include "I feel that my eating is out of control", "I would rather be thin than have good control of my diabetes" and "After I overeat, I skip my next insulin dose." DEPS-R scores range between 0 and 80 and scores ≥20 have been associated with higher HbA_{1c} [34]. The DEPS-R has demonstrated excellent internal consistency (Chronbach's α = 0.86–0.89), good construct validity as evidenced by associations with diabetes distress and eating disorder symptoms, and external validity [34, 35].

Ecological momentary assessment (3 days)
Participants received randomly generated phone calls from IfByPhone®, an automated telephone system, at the rate of 1–2 times an hour between the hours of 8 am and 10 pm. Participants also placed calls to the survey system to report meals/snacks and were asked to do so immediately after eating. At each call, participants completed brief surveys (taking less than 1–2 min to complete) on their current emotion or mood and eating and type 1 diabetes management behavior.

At each call, participants were asked to provide momentary ratings of their affective state (*happy, sad, frustrated, angry, anxious or nervous, guilty or disgusted with yourself*) using a scale from 1 to 6 (e.g., "On a scale from 1-6, how *sad* do you feel?"). Current level of diabetes distress was also assessed by the following question: "How upset do you feel about your diabetes or diabetes management?" (1 = Not at All, 6 = Very Much).

For calls reporting eating, participants were also asked to indicate the time they started eating and answer questions about their eating behavior. Relevant to the current study were questions assessing whether or not OBE was present including: "Did you eat a *large amount of food*, more than would be typical of others in a similar situation?" and "Did you experience a *loss of control* over your eating?" . For the first item (Large amount of food), participants responded with key presses indicating 1 = Yes, I ate a large amount of food or 2 = No). For the second item (Loss of control), participants responded using a 6-point Likert scale (1 = Not at all, indicating no loss of control; 6 = Very much). Later, this item was changed to dichotomous for ease of administration and analysis (1 = Yes, loss of control present, 2 = No loss of control). OBE was determined to be present when participants indicated that "Yes" they had eaten a large amount of food for the situation *and* "Yes" they had experienced a loss of control over eating (i.e., reporting anything other than 1 = No loss of control for the scaled item; or "Yes" to the dichotomous item).

Participants received specific training on the study definitions of a "large amount of food" (i.e., an amount of food that is definitely larger than what most individuals would eat in a similar situation) and "loss of control over eating" (i.e., a feeling that one cannot stop or control eating) as defined by the Diagnostic and Statistical Manual of Mental Disorders – 5 [8]. The study coordinator reviewed the definitions with all individuals and provided examples. Participants received a training handbook that included the definitions and examples to refer to as needed throughout the 3-day assessment period.

Continuous glucose monitoring (CGM)

The Medtronic CGMS® iPro™ or iPro2™ was used for CGM. Trained study staff inserted Medtronic glucose sensors under participants' abdominal skin and then connected the sensor to small, lightweight monitors. Monitors lay flat on the skin of abdomen, attached by a small adhesive patch. Participants were able to engage in all normal activities after sensor placement, including swimming and bathing. Sensors sampled interstitial glucose levels continuously and transferred 5-min averages to the monitors for storage. Participants were blinded to their glucose values, but did continue to check their blood glucose with finger sticks a minimum of 3 times a day (as needed for CGM calibration and ongoing management of their diabetes) using a One Touch meter and strips that we provided. The mean absolute difference percentage of 9.9 indicated that CGM calibration accuracy was good. CGM data was downloaded by specialized software after completion of the 3-day assessment period.

Data analytic strategy

Eating reports, random prompts and CGM data were time synced for analyses.

Level of participation

Level of participation during the 3-day assessment period was determined by calculating the percentage of random calls completed and total number of eating episodes reported.

Emotional predictors of binge eating

We used multi-level modeling to examine the effects of momentary increases in emotions prior to eating on the likelihood of OBE episode. This allowed us to examine both within and between-person effects while also accounting for the nesting of observations [36–38]. Analyses were restricted to eating episodes with random prompt affect ratings within 60 min prior to eating. We controlled for the time between the affect report and start of eating. We created a composite negative affect variable by taking the mean responses of *sad, frustrated, angry, anxious or nervous, and guilty or disgusted with self* to first examine the overall effect of negative affect on OBE. All individual emotional states, including happiness and diabetes distress were then examined as independent predictors of OBE.

We used a two-level generalized linear mixed modeling (SAS GLIMMIX) strategy with random intercepts to predict the likelihood of the dichotomous OBE variable. Models were estimated with Maximum Likelihood adaptive Gauss-Hermite quadrature, the logit link function, binary distribution, between-within denominator degrees of freedom.

Change in post-meal affect

Generalized linear mixed models were used to examine whether change in post-meal negative affect differed significantly between OBE and non-OBE episodes. Analyses were constrained to eating episodes with random prompt affect ratings within 60 min before and after eating. We controlled for pre-meal levels of affect. We first compared OBE to non-OBE eating episodes on post-meal negative affect using the composite negative affect variable. Follow-up analyses for individual affect states, including diabetes distress, were then conducted.

OBE and glycemic control

We estimated a two-level linear mixed-model to examine the effect of OBE on 120-min postprandial blood glucose. Predictor variables included OBE (coded as present or absent) and pre-meal blood glucose, with the participant serving as the clustering variable. Thus, our analysis compared the impact of OBE to the impact of all other eating episodes, including normal eating, overeating, and subjective binge eating (i.e., eating events during which an individual experiences a loss of control over eating, but does not consume an objectively large amount of food [39]).

Results

Sample characteristics

Eighty-three adults with type 1 diabetes participated in the current study. The sample was predominately female (88%) and Caucasian (87%) with a mean age of 41.9 (SD = 12.43; Range 18–68). See Table 1 for additional demographic information. Data analyses excluded nine individuals who either did not complete the 3-day assessment (n = 5) or had unusable data due to technical problems (n = 4).

Level of participation

Level of participation was high. Participants on average responded to 96% of the random prompts and reported 4 eating episodes per day. Participants reported eating 1002 eating episodes during the 3-day period, 80 (8%) of which were characterized as OBE episodes. Nearly half of the sample (44%) reported at least one episode of OBE during the 3 days.

Table 1 *Participant Demographics (N = 83)*

Characteristic	Mean (SD) or %
Age (yrs.)	41.89 (12.43)
Sex (% female)	88.00
Race/Ethnicity (%)	
Caucasian/White	86.7
African-American/Black	10.8
Asian/Pacific-Islander	1.2
Hispanic	1.2
Marital Status (%)	
Never Married	22.9
Married	63.9
Separated/Divorced	12.0
Widowed	1.2
Highest Level of Education (%)	
High school graduate or GED	6.0
Some college/technical school	19.3
Bachelor's Degree	54.2
Graduate degree	20.5
Age at Type 1 Diabetes Diagnosis (Yrs.)	18.5 (10.7)
Duration of Type 1 Diabetes (Yrs.)	23.4 (13.4)
Treatment Regimen (%)	
Insulin Pump Therapy	62.7
Multiple Daily Injections	37.3
HbA$_{1c}$ (mean (SD))	8.8 (2.3)

Emotional predictors of binge eating

The current analyses examined the reported eating episodes with random prompt affect ratings within 60 min of eating (n = 659). This included 55 OBE episodes reported by participants. As demonstrated in Table 2,

Table 2 Fixed Effect Estimates for Affect Predicting Subsequent Binge Eating Episode

Parameter	B	SE	Odds Ratio	95% CI
Intercept	− 3.63***	0.5		
Lag Time	1.02	0.7	2.8	0.7–11.2
Negative Affect (BP)	0.66*	0.3	1.9	1.1–3.4
Negative Affect (WP)	−0.43	0.3	0.7	0.4–1.1
Intercept	−3.60***	0.5		
Lag Time	1.01	0.7	2.7	0.7–10.9
Happy (BP)	−0.13	0.2	0.9	0.6–1.4
Happy (WP)	0.06	0.2	1.1	0.8–1.5
Intercept	−3.65***	0.5		
Lag Time	1.03	0.7	2.8	0.7–11.3
Sad (BP)	0.21	0.4	1.2	0.6–2.6
Sad (WP)	−0.42†	0.2	0.7	0.4–1.0
Intercept	−3.58***	0.5		
Lag Time	0.92	0.7	2.5	0.6–10.1
Angry (BP)	0.46	0.2	1.6	0.9–2.9
Angry (WP)	−0.38†	0.3	0.7	0.5–1.0
Intercept	−3.62***	0.5		
Lag Time	1.00	0.7	2.7	0.7–10.9
Frustrated (BP)	1.35*	0.4	1.7	1.1–2.6
Frustrated (WP)	−0.23	0.2	0.8	0.6–1.1
Intercept	−3.65***	0.5		
Lag Time	1.07	0.7	2.9	0.7–11.9
Anxious/Nervous (BP)	0.46†	0.2	1.6	1.0–2.5
Anxious/Nervous (WP)	−0.20	0.2	0.8	0.6–1.2
Intercept	−3.62***	0.5		
Lag Time	1.02	0.7	2.8	0.7–10.9
Guilty/Disgusted With Yourself (BP)	0.57*	0.2	1.8	1.1–2.8
Guilty/Disgusted With Yourself (WP)	0.07	0.2	1.1	0.8–1.4
Intercept	−3.65***	0.5		
Lag Time	1.05	0.7	2.9	0.7–11.4
Upset about Diabetes (BP)	0.40*	0.2	1.5	1.1–2.1
Upset about Diabetes (WP)	0.15	0.2	1.2	0.8–1.7

BP between persons effects, *WP* within-persons effects
$^{\dagger}p$ < .10. *p < .05. **p < .01. ***p < .001

there was a between-person effect for negative affect 60 min prior to a meal predicting OBE ($OR = 1.93$, $p = .02$, 95% CI = 1.09, 3.41), indicating a 93% increased risk of OBE among individuals with higher negative affect compared to individuals with average negative affect. The odds ratio indicates that for every 1-point increase in the negative affect score, the odds of OBE nearly doubled.

Analyses testing specific affect states as predictors of OBE indicated significant between-person effects for *guilty or disgusted with yourself* ($OR = 1.77$, $p = .01$, 95% CI = 1.13, 2.77), *frustrated* ($OR = 1.71$ $p = .01$, 95% CI = 1.13, 2.59), and *diabetes distress* ($OR = 1.48$, $p = .02$, 95% CI = 1.07, 2.07).

There was not a significant within-person effect of negative affect on OBE ($OR = 0.65$, $p = .11$, 95% CI = 0.39, 1.10), indicating that a momentary increase does not confer additional risk over and above the effect of individual differences in negative affect. In exploratory analyses, there were non-significant within-person trends for *sad* ($OR = 0.66$, $p = .07$, 95% CI = 0.42, 1.04) and *angry* ($OR = 0.69$, $p = .08$, 95% CI = 0.45, 1.04). See Table 2.

Change in post-meal affect
Analyses were conducted with the 520 eating episodes that had affect reports within 60 min before and after eating. As shown in Table 3, results indicated that, after controlling for pre-meal negative affect, the increase in negative affect was greater when binge eating occurred than when it did not, $B = 0.44$, $SE = 0.08$ $p < .001$.

Analyses examining specific post-meal affective states indicated that changes in affect were significantly greater for OBE episodes relative to non-OBE episodes for all emotions except *happiness*. After controlling for pre-meal level of affect, individuals reported increased levels of *sadness, anger, frustration, anxiety or nervousness, guilt or disgust with yourself*, and *diabetes distress* following OBE compared to non-OBE episodes (Bs: 0.27–0.60, all ps < .05). The strongest effects were for *frustrated* ($B = 0.60$, $SE = 0.16$, $p < .001$) and *guilty or disgusted with yourself* ($B = 0.59$, $SE = 0.12$, $p < .001$). See Table 3.

OBE and glycemic control
Blood glucose at 120 min postprandial was higher for OBE ($M = 213$ mg/dL, 95% CI = 191, 234), than for non-OBE episodes ($M = 188$ mg/dL, 95% CI = 179, 198), $p = .03$.

Discussion
The current study examined real-time emotional predictors and consequences of binge eating during 3-days of ecological momentary assessment in adults with type 1 diabetes reporting a range of eating disorder symptomatology. Of the 1002 eating episodes reported by participants, 80 were classified as OBE episodes and 43% of participants engaged in binge eating at least once during

Table 3 Fixed Effect Estimates of OBE Episodes Predicting Mean Change in Affect Relative to Non-OBE Episodes

Parameter	B	SE	DF	t
Intercept	1.21***	0.1	75	10.1
Pre Negative Affect	−0.50***	0.1	442	−9.4
Post OBE Δ Negative Affect	0.44***	0.1	442	−5.4
Intercept	1.63***	0.2	74	7.1
Pre Happy	−0.57***	0.1	443	−10.7
Post OBE Δ Happy	−0.13	0.2	443	0.8
Intercept	1.21***	0.1	75	9.4
Pre Sad	−0.59***	0.1	443	−12.9
Post OBE Δ Sad	0.39***	0.1	443	−3.6
Intercept	1.28***	0.1	75	9.4
Pre Angry	−0.71***	0.1	443	−15.3
Post OBE Δ Angry	0.27*	0.1	443	−2.5
Intercept	1.66***	0.2	75	9.2
Pre Frustrated	−0.59***	0.1	442	−11.9
Post OBE Δ Frustrated	0.60***	0.2	442	−3.9
Intercept	1.06***	0.1	75	7.3
Pre Nervous/Anxious	−0.52***	0.1	442	−10.7
Post OBE Δ Nervous/Anxious	0.27*	0.1	442	−2.2
Intercept	1.42***	0.2	75	9.0
Pre Guilty/Disgusted With Yourself	−0.47***	0.1	442	−10.1
Post OBE Δ Guilty/Disgusted With Yourself	0.59***	0.1	442	−4.8
Intercept	1.57***	0.2	75	7.4
Pre Upset About Diabetes	−0.49***	0.1	442	−8.1
Post OBE Δ Upset About Diabetes	0.30*	0.1	442	−2.4

All models control for pre-meal levels of affect. *OBE* objective binge eating
*$p < .05$. **$p < .01$. ***$p < .001$

the 3-day assessment period. Results indicated increased odds of OBE among individuals with higher levels of pre-meal negative affect and increased emotional distress and 2-h postprandial blood glucose following OBE relative to non–OBE episodes.

Elevated blood glucose levels may be the result of difficulty determining amounts of carbohydrate consumed and approximating insulin response to the carbohydrate load or intentional insulin restriction to compensate for calories consumed. Overall, results highlight the importance of helping individuals with type 1 diabetes develop skills to cope with emotional distress in order to manage diabetes and achieve optimal glycemic control.

In the current study, individuals with type 1 diabetes who reported higher average levels of frustration, guilt and diabetes distress within 60 min of eating were more likely to engage in OBE than their peers who scored lower on negative affect. Individuals with elevated levels of negative affect before eating may be struggling to cope with managing a chronic illness that impacts every meal. For example, individuals may feel frustrated about their pre-meal blood glucose and their ability to control their blood glucose and eating well enough to achieve optimal glycemic targets. They may also feel as though they have to impose strict dietary rules to control blood glucose and may feel frustrated that diabetes prevents them from eating what they would like or feel guilt and distress about what they are planning to eat. These individuals may turn toward binge eating as a way to cope with these difficult feelings, or alternatively, give up and abandon efforts at managing diabetes altogether by eating unrestricted amounts of food. Evidence suggests that this leads to more, not less distress (including specifically about diabetes), which may in part be due to the negative impact losing control over eating and consuming large amounts of food (and/or engaging in compensatory weight control behaviors) has on glycemic control and/or one's perceived ability to effectively manage their eating/diabetes.

Past studies have found that diabetes distress is associated with eating disorder symptoms among individuals with diabetes [26, 29–31]. The current study adds to this preliminary data, and expands what is known by suggesting that diabetes distress may not only be a factor that increases risk, but is also a consequence that may maintain these behavior patterns. This may mean that explicitly targeting diabetes distress in eating disorder treatment, rather than narrowly focusing on body weight and shape concerns, could have benefits for this unique patient population.

Diabetes distress was a between-person factor significantly associated with OBE, but momentary elevations in diabetes distress did not explain additional variance in OBE episode risk. In our previous study, we found that diabetes distress tends to have less variability than other negative emotional states with participants' diabetes distress levels remaining relatively constant when assessed multiple times a day [31]. This may indicate that individuals are less sensitive to subtle changes in diabetes distress and may benefit from treatments that increase capacity to observe fluctuations influencing momentary behavior. Diabetes distress may also be conflated with or influence other negative emotional states (or other negative emotional states may influence perceptions of diabetes distress). For example, participants may have been reporting anger when, perhaps with less awareness, underlying distress about diabetes was generating such

anger (e.g., feeling angry that pre-meal blood sugar was out of range).

The results of the current study should be considered in light of its limitations. First, the 3-day assessment period may not have been a sufficient amount of time to capture patterns of emotional antecedents and consequences of binge eating. It may be that with additional time and more episodes of binge eating to analyze (either due to decreases in participant reactivity or simply more opportunities for binge eating to occur), different patterns may emerge. Second, we characterized OBE episodes based on participant report of whether or not an objectively large amount of food was consumed. While participants were trained on parameters defining an objectively large amount of food, patient perception may still have biased results by inaccurately classifying eating episodes. For example, participants who feel a lot of shame for eating may describe an episode as an objectively large amount of food despite it not meeting the provided definition. Third, the impact of OBE on postprandial blood glucose may have been underestimated in this study. We examined the effect of OBE on postprandial blood glucose irrespective of whether or not insulin restriction also occurred. Elevations in postprandial blood glucose may be even higher when insulin restriction follows OBE, which might commonly occur among some individuals. We also compared the effect of OBE episodes on postprandial blood glucose relative to all non-OBE eating episodes combined (i.e., non-OBE episodes included normal eating, overeating and subjective binge eating episodes). This may have further mitigated the relative effects of OBE on postprandial blood glucose by elevating postprandial blood glucose of non-OBE episodes. While an objectively large amount of food is by definition not consumed during subjective binge eating episodes, the experience of losing control over eating may still increase the risk of using insulin restriction for weight control resulting in subsequent postprandial blood glucose elevations [40]. In our previous study, feeling of loss of control over eating (regardless of whether an objectively large amount of food was consumed) was associated with insulin restriction (see Merwin et al., 2015 [31]). Lastly, the sample consisted mostly of White women with type 1 diabetes who reported elevated DEPS-R scores and is not a representative sample. Thus, we cannot say anything about frequency of OBE in the general population of type 1 diabetes patients or whether these patterns would generalize to other type 1 diabetes patients with OBE. This may limit the generalizability of the findings.

Conclusions

Overall, findings indicate that individuals who tend to experience negative affect and diabetes distress before eating are at increased risk of binge eating at the upcoming meal. Engaging in binge eating may result in greater subsequent negative affect, including diabetes distress, and lead to elevated postprandial blood glucose levels. Although the current study cannot speak to causation, it is possible that the negative consequences of OBE may actually be a factor maintaining binge eating behavior. That is, individuals may engage in subsequent binge eating to cope with the emotional distress they experience following previous binge eating episodes (e.g., feeling distressed about elevations in blood glucose and/or their ability to effectively manage their eating/diabetes). These findings add to a growing literature suggesting diabetes distress is related to eating disordered behaviors among individuals with type 1 diabetes and further suggest that it may have a role in maintaining the problem [21, 24–26]. Interventions that focus on helping individuals cope with negative affect and specifically diabetes distress may be helpful to incorporate into treatments for type 1 diabetes patients.

Abbreviations
CGM: continuous glucose monitoring; DEPS-R: Diabetes Eating Problems Survey-Revised; OBE: objective binge eating; T1D: type 1 diabetes

Authors' contributions
AM assisted in data collection and drafted the manuscript. ND, MB and PS conducted the analyses and reviewed/edited the manuscript. LH assisted in the development and execution of study protocols and assisted in manuscript preparation. JM assisted in manuscript preparation. RM developed the research idea, directed all research activities and drafted the manuscript. All authors read and approved the final manuscript.

Competing interests
The authors declare that they have no competing interests.

Author details
[1]Duke University Medical Center, DUMC Box 3842, Durham, NC 27712, USA.
[2]Northern Arizona University, Flagstaff, AZ, USA.

References
1. Toni G, Berioli M, Cerquiglini L, Ceccarini G, Grohmann U, Principi N, et al. Eating disorders and disordered eating symptoms in adolescents with type 1 diabetes. Nutrients. 2017;9(8):906–15.
2. Young V, Eiser C, Johnson B, Brierley S, Elliott J, Heller S. Eating problems in adolescents with type 1 diabetes: a systematic review with meta-analysis. Diabet Med. 2013;30:189–98.
3. Araia E, Hendrieckx C, Skinner T, Pouwer F, Speight J, King RM. Gender differences in disordered eating behaviors and body dissatisfaction among adolescents with type 1 diabetes: results from diabetes MILES youth—Australia. Int J Eat Disord. 2017;50(10):1183–93.
4. Reinehr T, Dieris B, Galler A, Teufel M, Berger G, Stachow R, et al. Worse metabolic control and dynamics of weight status in adolescent girls point to eating disorders in the first years after manifestation of type 1 diabetes mellitus: Findings from the Diabetes Patienten Verlaufsdokumentation registry. J Pediatr. Available online 20 December 2018. DOI: https://doi.org/10.1016/j.jpeds.2018.11.037.
5. Wisting L, Reas DL, Bang L, Skrivarhaug T, Dahl-Jørgensen K, Rø Ø. Eating patterns in adolescents with type 1 diabetes: associations with
6. metabolic control, insulin omission, and eating disorder pathology. Appetite. 2017;114:226–31.
6. Colton PA, Rydall AC, Olmstead MP, Rodin GM, Daneman D. Disturbed eating behavior and eating disorders in preteen and early teenage girls with type 1 diabetes: a case-controled study. Diabetes Care. 2004;27(7):1654–9.
7. Bryden KS, Neil A, Mayou RA, Peveler RC, Fairburn CG, Dunger DB. Eating habits, body weight, and insulin misuse. A longitudinal study of teenagers and young adults with type 1 diabetes. Diabetes Care. 1999;22(12):1956–60.
8. American Psychiatric Association. Diagnostic and statistical manual of mental disorders. 5th ed. (DSM-5®). Am Psychiatric Pub. 2013. p. 350.
9. Crow S, Keel P, Kendall D. Eating disorders and insulin-dependent diabetes mellitus. Psychosomatics. 1998;39:233–43.
10. Nathan DM, DCCT/Edic Research Group. The diabetes control and complications trial/epidemiology of diabetes interventions and complications study at 30 years: overview. Diabetes Care. 2014;37(1):9–16.
11. Rodin G, Olmsted MP, Rydall AC, Maharaj SI, Colton PA, Jones JM, et al. Eating disorders in young women with type 1 diabetes mellitus. J Psychosom Res. 2002;53(4):943–9.
12. Custal N, Arcelus J, Agüera Z, Bove FI, Wales J, Granero R, et al. Treatment outcome of patients with comorbid type 1 diabetes and eating disorders. BMC Psychiatry. 2014;14(1):140–4.
13. Peveler RC, Fairburn CG. The treatment of bulimia nervosa in patients with diabetes mellitus. Int J Eat Disord. 1992;11(1):45–53.
14. Olmsted MP, Daneman D, Rydall AC, Lawson ML, Rodin G. The effects of psychoeducation on disturbed eating attitudes and behavior in young women with type 1 diabetes mellitus. Int J Eat Disord. 2002;32(2):230–9.
15. Haedt-Matt AA, Keel PK. Revisiting the affect regulation model of binge eating: a meta-analysis of studies using ecological momentary assessment. Psychol Bull. 2011;137(4):660–81.
16. Heatherton TF, Baumeister RF. Binge eating as escape from self-awareness. Psychol Bull. 1991;110(1):86–108.
17. Bulik CM, Sullivan PF, Kendler KS. Medical and psychiatric morbidity in obese women with and without binge eating. Int J Eat Disord. 2002;32(1):72–8.
18. Antony MM, Johnson WG, Carr-Nangle RE, Abel JL. Psychopathology correlates of binge eating and binge eating disorder. Compr Psychiatry. 1994;35(5):386–92.
19. Berg KC, Crosby RD, Cao L, Crow SJ, Engel SG, Wonderlich SA, et al. Negative affect prior to and following overeating-only, loss of control eating-only, and binge eating episodes in obese adults. Int J Eat Disord. 2015;48(6):641–53.
20. Smyth JM, Wonderlich SA, Heron KE, Sliwinski MJ, Crosby RD, Mitchell JE, et al. Daily and momentary mood and stress are associated with binge eating and vomiting in bulimia nervosa patients in the natural environment. J Consult Clin Psychol. 2007;75(4):629–38.
21. Wegner KE, Smyth JM, Crosby RD, Wittrock D, Wonderlich SA, Mitchell JE. An evaluation of the relationship between mood and binge eating in the natural environment using ecological momentary assessment. Int J Eat Disord. 2002;32(3):352–61.
22. Berg KC, Crosby RD, Cao L, Peterson CB, Engel SG, Mitchell JE, et al. Facets of negative affect prior to and following binge-only, purge-only, and binge/purge events in women with bulimia nervosa. J Abnorm Psychol. 2013;122(1):111–8.
23. Munsch S, Meyer AH, Quartier V, Wilhelm FH. Binge eating in binge eating disorder: a breakdown of emotion regulatory process? Psychiatry Res. 2012;195(3):118–24.
24. Takii M, Komaki G, Uchigata Y, Maeda M, Omori Y, Kubo C. Differences between bulimia nervosa and binge-eating disorder in females with type 1 diabetes: the important role of insulin omission. J Psychosom Res. 1999;47(3):221–31.
25. Fisher L, Mullan JT, Arean P, Glasgow RE, Hessler D, Masharani U. Diabetes distress and not clinical depression or depressive symptoms is associated with glycemic control in both cross-sectional and longitudinal analyses. Diabetes Care. 2009;33(1):23–8.
26. Polonsky WH, Anderson BJ, Lohrer PA, Welch G, Jacobson AM, Aponte JE, et al. Assessment of diabetes-related distress. Diabetes Care. 1995;18(6):754–60.
27. Fisher L, Polonsky WH, Hessler DM, Masharani U, Blumer I, Peters AL, et al. Understanding the sources of diabetes distress in adults with type 1 diabetes. J Diabetes Complicat. 2015;29(4):572–7.
28. Pallayova M, Taheri S. Targeting diabetes distress: the missing piece of the successful type 1 diabetes management puzzle. Diabetes Spectr. 2014;27(2):143–9.

29. Martyn-Nemeth P, Quinn L, Hacker E, Park H, Kujath AS. Diabetes distress may adversely affect the eating styles of women with type 1 diabetes. Acta Diabetol. 2014;51(4):683–6.

30. Goebel-Fabbri AE, Fikkan J, Franko DL, Pearson K, Anderson BJ, Weinger K. Insulin restriction and associated morbidity and mortality in women with type 1 diabetes. Diabetes Care. 2008;31(3):415–9.

31. Merwin RM, Dmitrieva NO, Honeycutt LK, Moskovich AA, Lane JD, Zucker NL, et al. Momentary predictors of insulin restriction among adults with type 1 diabetes and eating disorder symptomatology. Diabetes Care. 2015; 38(11):2025–32.

32. Merwin RM, Moskovich AA, Honeycutt LK, Lane JD, Feinglos M, Surwit RS, et al. Time of day when type 1 diabetes patients with eating disorder symptoms Most commonly restrict insulin. Psychosom Med. 2018;80(2):222–9.

33. Gold AE, Macleod KM, Frier BM. Frequency of severe hypoglycemia in patients with type I diabetes with impaired awareness of hypoglycemia. Diabetes Care. 1994;17(7):697–703.

34. Markowitz J, Butler D, Volkening L, Antisdel J, Anderson B, Laffel L. Brief screening tool for disordered eating in diabetes. Internal consistency and external validity in a contemporary sample of pediatric patients with type 1 diabetes. Diabetes Care. 2010;33:495–500.

35. Wisting L, Frøisland DH, Skrivarhaug T, Dahl-Jørgensen K, Rø Ø. Psychometric properties, norms, and factor structure of the diabetes eating problem survey–revised in a large sample of children and adolescents with type 1 diabetes. Diabetes Care. 2013;36(8):2198–202.

36. Snijders T, Bosker R. Multilevel Analysis: An introduction to basic and advanced Multilevel modeling. Thousand Oaks, Sage Publications; 2011. p. 200–206.

37. Hoffman L, Stawski RS. Persons as contexts: evaluating between-person and within-person effects in longitudinal analysis. Res Hum Dev. 2009; 6(2–3):97–120.

38. Curran PJ, Bauer DJ. The disaggregation of within-person and between-person effects in longitudinal models of change. Annu Rev Psycho. 2011;62:583–619.

39. Fairburn CG, Cooper Z. The Eating Disorder Examination (12th edition). In: Fairburn CG, Wilson GT, editors. Binge eating: Nature, assessment, and treatment. New York: Guilford Press; 1993. p. 317–60.

40. Mond J, Hay P, Rodgers B, Owen C, Crosby R, Mitchell J. Use of extreme weight control behaviors with and without binge eating in a community sample: implications for the classification of bulimic-type eating disorders. Int J Eat Disord. 2006;39(4):294–302.

Processes and pathways to binge eating: development of an integrated cognitive and behavioural model of binge eating

Amy L. Burton and Maree J. Abbott[*] (iD)

Abstract

Background: There are a number of factors commonly believed to be important to the development and maintenance of binge eating that have been identified across multiple models and theories in the psychological literature. In the present study, we sought to develop and test a psychological model for binge eating that incorporated the main variables identified in the literature to drive binge eating behaviour; specifically, core low self-esteem, negative affect, difficulty with emotional regulation, restricted eating and beliefs about eating.

Methods: Questionnaire data was collected from 760 unselected participants. The proposed model of binge eating was developed, bivariate relationships between the included variables were assessed, and the goodness-of-fit of this new model was evaluated using structural equations modelling.

Result: The results identified significant bivariate relationships between all the included variables. While the originally proposed model did not provide a good fit to the data, the revised version of the model provided a good fit to the data.

Conclusions: Supporting, integrating and building upon the current existing psychological models of binge eating, this study presents a new integrated cognitive and behavioural model of binge eating. The dual-pathway to binge eating identified in the new model provides a different way to understand transdiagnostic binge eating.

Keywords: Binge eating, Model, Cognitive Behavioural, Metacogntive, Eating disorder, Structural equations modelling

Plain English summary

This paper describes the development and assessment of a new way to understand the behaviour of binge eating. Previous research has identified a number of factors that appear to lead to the development of binge eating and have been found to contribute to maintaining binge eating in those with eating disorders. The model presented in this paper considers the role of core low self-esteem, negative emotion (e.g. depression, anxiety and stress), difficulty with emotional regulation, restricted eating (e.g. dieting) and particular unhelpful beliefs about eating. The results of this study provide support for the relationship between binge eating and the included factors (core low self-esteem, negative emotion etc.). In particular, the importance of core low self-esteem for the

development and maintenance of binge eating is highlighted by the results of the paper.

Background

Binge eating involves the sense of 'losing control' over one's eating and consuming a large amount of food within a short duration of time, typically accompanied by feelings of guilt, shame, disgust and depression. Binge eating is a feature of bulimia nervosa (BN), binge eating disorder (BED) and the binge-purge type of anorexia nervosa (AN-BP) [1]. Lifetime and point prevalence data has demonstrated that between 1.5 and 2.9% of people have experienced BN, as many as 2.9 to 5.6% of people have met criteria for BED, and 0.4 to 0.9% of people have experienced anorexia nervosa (AN) [2–6]. Among the general community, studies have found that up to 7.2 to 13% of the population currently engage in regular binge eating episodes and the prevalence of binge eating in

* Correspondence: maree.abbott@sydney.edu.au
School of Psychology, The University of Sydney, Camperdown, NSW, Australia

the community is increasing over time [3, 7]. Binge eating is associated with obesity, a number of chronic physical and mental health conditions, poorer quality of life, and impaired social functioning [4, 5, 8–10]. Given the high prevalence and seriousness of associated comorbid conditions, a sound understanding of the causes and maintenance of binge eating is required so that effective and affordable treatments can be developed.

A number of cognitive and behavioural models of binge eating have been proposed (see Williamson, White, York-Crowe and Stewart, 2004 [11] and Burton & Abbott, 2017 [12] for a comprehensive summary of the existing models). Many of these models overlap in hypothesised constructs; reviews of existing models have identified a number of features common among the leading psychological models of binge eating [11, 12]. A number of theories and models have hypothesised that the factors of dietary restraint, negative affect, poor emotional regulation skills, low self-esteem and the presence of thoughts/beliefs about food and eating play an important role in the development and maintenance of binge eating [12].

Dietary restraint

One of the earliest models to account for binge eating was that of the 'dietary restraint theory' [13, 14]. This theory was based on both clinical observation and animal studies and proposed that a combination of dieting and restrictive eating is a precipitating factor that causes people to engage in binge eating [14]. Since it was first proposed, a growing body of evidence has supported the causal link between dietary restraint and binge eating [15], and dietary restraint has been included as a precipitating factor in many of the theories and models of binge eating that have since been developed [12]. Of note, the importance of dietary restraint is emphasised in the influential cognitive-behavioural model of BN by Fairburn, Cooper, and Cooper [16], the transdiagnostic model of eating disorders [17], the dual-pathway model [18], and the functional analysis of binge eating [19]. However, the presence of dietary restraint on its own does not account for the development of all binge eating; because of this, the dietary restraint model has received criticism for being oversimplified and for not providing an explanation for the maintenance of binge eating that occurs in those who do not engage in restrained eating [19, 20].

Negative affect and emotional regulation

Many psychological models have proposed that binge eating is preceded by the experience of negative affect in the form of distress or depression and that binge eating is used as a way to cope with or to avoid these negative emotions [12]. This idea is explored in the escape theory proposed by Heatherton and Baumeister [21], which predicts that binge eating occurs as a way for the individual to 'escape' from aversive emotional states. In this way, binge eating can be seen as a coping mechanism and/or a way to avoid unpleasant emotions that can be used by individuals who experience difficulty with regulating their emotional state. In addition to the escape theory, poor emotional regulation skills in combination with the experience of negative affect are hypothesised to lead to binge eating across a number of current binge eating models, including McManus and Waller's functional analysis of binge eating [19], Fairburn and colleagues' cognitive behavioural model [22] and the transdiagnostic model of eating disorders [17], and the cognitive model of BN [23]. Evidence from clinical observation, naturalistic and observational studies, and experimental laboratory studies has supported the link between negative affect, difficulty with emotional regulation and binge eating [24–28].

Low self-esteem

Another reliable predictor of binge eating is the presence of low self-esteem, also described as negative self-schemas in the schema framework, and negative self-beliefs or negative core beliefs about the self in the cognitive-behavioural framework [12]. Low self-esteem is hypothesised to be related to binge eating across a number of leading binge eating models, including the cognitive-behavioural model of BN [16], the transdiagnostic model of eating disorders [17], the cognitive model of BN [23], the functional analysis of binge eating [19], the escape theory [21], and the schema model of binge eating [29]. Research investigating the relationship between the presence and strength of negative self-schemas and eating disordered behaviours have consistently found that individuals with BED or BN have a higher level of negative self-schemas compared to community controls [29–31].

Thoughts and beliefs about Food & Eating

In addition to negative self-beliefs, poor emotional regulation and negative affect, the cognitive model of BN developed by Cooper et al. [23] emphasises the role of specific beliefs about eating in the maintenance of binge eating. These specific eating beliefs have been categorised into three sets of beliefs:

(1) Positive beliefs about eating; beliefs related to the role of eating in self-soothing, e.g., "eating makes me feel better"
(2) Negative beliefs about eating; beliefs related to the negative consequences of eating, e.g., "I'll get fat if I eat"
(3) Permissive thoughts; thoughts that allow the person to engage in the binge episode, e.g., "it's okay to eat when I feel stressed", or thoughts related to the loss of control, e.g., "I can't control my eating" ('no control' beliefs)

Cooper et al. [23] hypothesised that these eating beliefs are triggered by the experience of negative affect and that the positive, negative, and permissive beliefs interact and ultimately lead to a binge eating episode. Bergin and Wade [32] used multiple regression analyses and structural equation modelling (SEM) to test the predictions of the cognitive model of BN. Results of these analyses identified an association between negative self-beliefs and negative affect, an association between negative affect and eating beliefs, and an association between both positive and permissive beliefs and binge eating. There was no association between the negative beliefs and binge eating, although an association between negative beliefs and compensatory behaviours was identified.

The most influential psychological models of binge eating differ from each other in a number of significant ways, yet they share a number of predictive variables that have demonstrated associations with binge eating. In this paper, we draw upon the evidence-based literature to formulate a new model of the maintaining factors of binge eating based on the key overlapping constructs from existing conceptualisations of binge eating.

Hypothesised model
The authors developed a model of binge eating that focused on five variables of interest which were believed to maintain binge eating [12]. These variables were based on a review of the relevant literature which found that these following five main variables were commonly agreed to be important predisposing, precipitating and perpetuating/maintaining factors of binge eating psychopathology:

(1) core low self-esteem/negative beliefs about the self.
(2) the presence of negative affect/distress.
(3) poor emotional regulation.
(4) dietary restraint/restriction.
(5) beliefs about eating, or 'eating beliefs'.

In the hypothesised model, individuals who have negative core beliefs about the self, or *core low self-esteem*, are predisposed to engage in binge eating (vulnerability factor). When the core beliefs are triggered, *negative affect* (low mood, anxiety, and/or stress) is experienced. Individuals who experience *difficulty with emotional regulation* feel intolerant of such negative affect and wish to find a way to neutralise the emotion. This discomfort with the negative affect is addressed by engaging in *dietary restraint* (which serves to distract from or control the emotion) and/or experiencing thoughts about food and eating (*eating beliefs*), such as positive beliefs about eating ("eating helps to control my emotions"), negative beliefs about eating ("I can't control my eating because am weak"), and permissive beliefs about eating ("I deserve to have a pleasure like binge eating"). It is hypothesised that when these eating beliefs are triggered,

binge eating occurs. The hypothesised model is presented in Fig. 1.

Aims and hypotheses
The aim of this study was to develop and test a psychological model for binge eating that incorporated the main common variables identified across a number of existing cognitive and behavioural theories of binge eating. Based on the literature, we predicted that the variables of core low self-esteem, negative affect, difficulty with emotional regulation, dietary restraint, and beliefs about eating would be positively correlated with the behavioural symptom of binge eating. Additionally, we hypothesised that a model based on these five variables would provide an acceptable fit to the data.

Methods
Participants
Participants were recruited from a sample of first year psychology students at the University of Sydney. A total of 767 students participated in the study (71.2% female, mean age = 19.37 years, SD = 3.46 years, mean BMI = 21.99, SD = 3.52). For analyses performed in this study, a data set with no missing data was required. Consequently, the data from 7 participants who had missing data was removed from further analysis. Therefore, the complete data for 760 participants was used for the analyses reported (n = 760, 71.1% female, mean age = 19.37, SD = 3.47, mean BMI = 21.99, SD = 3.53). Of these 760 participants, 62% self-reported that they had never suffered from or been treated for a psychological condition such as depression, anxiety, psychosis, or an eating

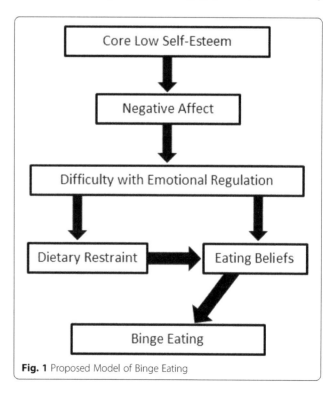

Fig. 1 Proposed Model of Binge Eating

disorder. Lifetime prevalence rates of eating disorders amongst the participant sample closely resembled previously reported Australian prevalence rates (Wade et al., 2006); 2.8% of participants reported that they had suffered from or been treated for anorexia nervosa, 2.9% for bulimia nervosa, 3% for binge eating disorder, and 2.1% for an atypical eating disorder (e.g., EDNOS or OSFED). Of the 760 participants, 22.1% ($n = 168$) self-reported that they had experienced at least four binge eating episodes that were paired with a sense of loss of control over the previous 28 days, with the total sample reporting an average of 2.43 (SD = 5.09) binge eating episodes with loss of control over the previous 28 days (Range = 0 to 50). Informed consent was obtained from all individual participants included in the study.

Procedure

Participants were asked to provide demographic information (age, gender, height, weight, previous or current mental health diagnoses) and to complete a series of questionnaires online that focused on eating behaviours and their beliefs about eating using the Qualtrics online questionnaire program.

Measures

Eating disorder symptoms: dietary restraint and binge eating

The Eating Disorder Examination Questionnaire (EDE-Q) [33] version 6.0 was used to collect information on possible eating disorder symptoms and behaviours such as binge eating and restrictive eating practices. The EDE-Q is a self-report questionnaire that asks respondents to record information regarding the frequency and severity of eating and body image-related concerns and behaviours experienced over the past 28 days. The EDE-Q is a valid and reliable measure with demonstrated psychometric properties [34]. A composite of two items was used in this study as the measure of 'binge eating': item 14, which assesses the number of occasions over the past 28 days that the respondent has eaten "what other people would regard as an unusually large amount of food (given the circumstances)" and experienced "a sense of having lost control over your eating (at the time)"; and item 15, which assesses the number of days over the past 28 days that "such episodes of over eating occurred (i.e., you have eaten an unusually large amount of food and had a sense of loss of control at the time)". This composite score gives an overall assessment of the severity of binge eating, with higher scores indicating increased severity of binge eating. A composite score was chosen to measure the construct of binge eating rather than a single item as the use of multiple items to measure a constructs reduces the effect of item-specific measurement error and therefore leads to more accurate research findings [35]. The restraint subscale was used as the measure of 'dietary restraint' in this study. The restraint subscale contains 5 items that assess the presence of fasting, dieting, calorie restriction and strict rules about food and eating. In the present study, the EDE-Q global score had a Cronbach's alpha (α) of .94, and α = .80 for the restraint subscale.

Negative affect

The Depression Anxiety Stress Scales Short Form (DASS-21) [36] was included to measure the negative affect currently experienced by respondents. The DASS-21 is a self-report questionnaire used to assess depression, anxiety, and stress symptoms that have been experienced over the past week. The DASS-21 is a valid and reliable self-report instrument [37]. A total score based on all 21 items was used as the measure of 'negative affect' in this study. In the present study, the DASS-21 total score had a Cronbach's alpha of .93.

Core low self-esteem

The Eating Disorders Core Beliefs Questionnaire (ED-CBQ) [38] was used to assess the presence of core beliefs about the self relevant to eating disorders. In the development paper, the ED-CBQ demonstrated contruct validity and internal consistency [38]. Items on the self-loathing subscale, such as "I am repulsive", were used to assess core low self-esteem. In the present study, the Cronbach's alpha of the ED-CBQ total was α = .92, and α = .93 for the self-loathing subscale.

Poor emotional regulation

The Difficulty in Emotion Regulation Scale (DERS) [39] is a 36-item self-report questionnaire used to assess difficulties with emotion regulation. The DERS assesses different aspects of emotional regulation including non-acceptance of emotional responses, difficulty engaging in goal-directed behaviour, impulse control difficulties, lack of emotional awareness, limited access to emotional regulation strategies, and lack of emotional clarity; higher scores reflect poorer emotion regulation. The DERS has demonstrated good internal consistency, construct and predictive validity and test-retest reliability [39]. The total score of the DERS was used as a measure of difficulty with emotional regulation in this study. The DERS total score demonstrated Cronbach's alpha of .89 in the present study.

Eating beliefs

The Eating Beliefs Questionnaire (EBQ-18) [40] is an 18-item self-report measure that assesses three types of beliefs about food and non-hungry eating: positive beliefs such as "eating helps me cope with negative feelings", 'no control' beliefs such as "once I start eating, I can't stop", and permissive beliefs such as "I deserve to have a pleasure like binge eating". The EBQ-18 is a valid and reliable measure with demonstrated psychometric properties [40, 41]. The total score of the EBQ-18 was used as the measure of eating beliefs in this study. The EBQ-18 total score demonstrated a Cronbach's alpha of .92 in the present study.

Statistical analyses

The SPSS v22 program was used to generate descriptive statistics such as means, standard deviations and Cronbach's alphas. Structural equations modelling was conducted using the AMOS version 22 program [42]. The overall fit of the models was assessed using a number of known indicators of goodness-of-fit; the goodness-of-fit index (GFI), the comparative fit index (CFI), the Tucker-Lewis index (TLI), the incremental fit index (IFI), the root mean square error of approximation (RMSEA), and the p of close fit statistic (PCLOSE). According to Hu and Bentler [43], values over .95 on the CFI, TLI, and IFI are indicative of an acceptable model fit, and RMSEA values of less than 0.06 indicate an acceptable fit. A non-significant PCLOSE statistic (>.05) indicates a 'close' fit of the model to the data [44].

Results

The means and standard deviations for the included variables, and the bivariate relationships among the included variables, are presented in Table 1, with all correlations significant at $p < .05$.

Structural equations modelling

The hypothesised model (Model 1; see Fig. 1) was fitted to the data using the AMOS program. The regression weights for the hypothesised model are shown in Table 2; the pathway between 'Dietary Restraint' and 'Eating Beliefs' was not significant ($p = .60$). However, all other pathways described in Table 2 were significant. This model did not demonstrate acceptable fit across a number of the goodness-of-fit indices (see Table 3).

Inspection of the regression weights, covariances, and correlations, as well as a discussion of the theoretical meaning of the pathways in the model between the authors, led to a series of changes to the model for the purpose of improving the fit. The authors removed the non-significant pathway from 'Dietary Restraint' to 'Eating Beliefs' and a pathway from 'Dietary Restraint' to 'Binge Eating' was added (Model 2); this revised model demonstrated improved fit across the indices (see Table 3).

Again, upon close inspection of the fit statistics, covariances, correlations, and discussion of the theoretical value of each pathway, three more changes were made, and each revision resulted in an improvement of fit: first, a path from 'Core Low Self-Esteem' to 'Difficulty with Emotional Regulation' was added (Model 3); then a path from 'Core Low Self-Esteem' to 'Eating Beliefs' was also included (Model 4). Model 4 demonstrated acceptable fit across most of the goodness-of-fit indices, however, the χ^2/df value and the RMSEA value were higher than optimal. Finally, a path from 'Core Low Self-Esteem' to 'Dietary Restraint' was added (Model 5). The final model (Model 5) demonstrated good fit to the data across all the goodness-of-fit indicators (see Table 3). The regression weights for the final model are presented in Table 4 (all significant) and the pathways of the final model as shown in Fig. 2.

Discussion

The aim of the present study was to develop and test a new psychological model of binge eating which included variables hypothesised by the leading existing cognitive and behavioural theoretical models on the maintenance of binge eating. In particular, our model bears a number of shared variables with the models of functional analysis of binge eating [19], the transdiagnostic model of eating disorders [17], and the cognitive model of BN [23].

The included variables of Core Low Self-Esteem, Negative Affect, Difficulty with Emotional Regulation, Dietary Restraint, and Eating Beliefs were all found to be positively correlated with Binge Eating. In addition, significant bivariate relationships were found amongst all the included variables. The originally hypothesised model did not demonstrate acceptable fit to the data, and the pathway between dietary restraint and eating beliefs was not found to be significant. Once this non-significant pathway was removed and a number of additional pathways between variables that had strong covariances were added, a modified model demonstrated good fit to the data. Therefore, the results indicated that the final revised model (Model 5; refer to Fig. 2) provided the best fit to the data. We present this final model as a new way to conceptualise the maintaining factors for binge eating; that is, the integrated cognitive and behavioural model of binge eating.

Table 1 Descriptive Statistics and Bivariate Relationships for all Included Variables

	Mean	SD	1	2	3	4	5
1. Core Low Self-Esteem	18.47	10.84					
2. Negative Affect	36.90	11.02	.55*				
3. Difficulty with Emotional Regulation	88.38	23.43	.55*	.71*			
4. Dietary Restraint	2.23	1.29	.23*	.30*	.30*		
5. Eating Beliefs	38.72	12.55	.41*	.39*	.49*	.16*	
6. Binge Eating	5.09	9.23	.30*	.29*	.30*	.27*	.46*

*= $p < .05$

Table 2 Unstandardised and Standardised Regression Weights for Hypothesised Model (Model 1) (Standard Errors in Brackets)

Pathway	Unstandardised Estimate	Standardised Estimate	p
Core Low Self-Esteem → Negative Affect	.55 (.03)	.55	<.001
Negative Affect → Difficulty with Emotional Regulation	1.51 (.05)	.71	<.001
Difficulty with Emotional Regulation → Dietary Restraint	.02 (.002)	.30	<.001
Difficulty with Emotional Regulation → Eating Beliefs	.262 (.02)	.49	<.001
Dietary Restraint → Eating Beliefs	.168 (.32)	.017	.60
Eating Beliefs → Binge Eating	.34 (.02)	.46	<.001

The results of this study provide further support for the relationship between the predicted variables (Core Low Self-Esteem, Negative Affect, Difficulty with Emotional Regulation, Dietary Restraint, and Eating Beliefs) and the outcome of binge eating. In particular, the role of Core Low Self-Esteem has been highlighted as particularly important, with the significant pathways from Core Low Self-Esteem to Binge Eating being mediated through a number of direct (via Dietary Restraint or Eating Beliefs) and indirect (via negative affect or Difficulty with Emotional Regulation) pathways. Also of interest is the strength of the bivariate relationship between Eating Beliefs and Binge Eating, as well as the strength of the relationship between Eating Beliefs and the two predicted preceding variables: Core Low Self-Esteem and Difficulty with Emotional Regulation. Of the included variables, Eating Beliefs showed the least amount of existing evidence supporting its role in the maintenance of binge eating in the literature due to its relative novelty in the field, being first proposed in 2004 whilst the other variables first appeared in the literature in between 1975 and 1991. These findings regarding Eating Beliefs (comprised of positive beliefs, permissive beliefs, and 'no control' beliefs) are in line with those reported in Bergin and Wade [32] who found that positive and permissive/no control thoughts predicted binge eating.

Furthermore, the results of this study provide support for the role of dietary restraint as an important predictive factor for binge eating. Of particular interest is the non-significant pathway between Dietary Restraint and Eating Beliefs indicating that these two variables act independently from one another. As a result, the final model includes a 'dual pathway' to binge eating; either via Dietary Restraint or via the activation of Eating Beliefs. In fact, it is possible that this 'dual pathway' may indicate two separate types of binge eating. The first, mediated by Dietary Restraint, more closely resembles the pathways to binge eating hypothesised in the transdiagnostic

model [17]. This first pathway could represent the type of binge eating that is more strongly maintained by a sense of loss of control and may be more commonly observed in people with restrictive eating disorders such as AN-BP and certain cases of BN. The second, mediated by Eating Beliefs, more closely resembles the pathway to binge eating proposed in the cognitive model of BN [23]. This second type of binge eating could represent the type of binge eating that is more strongly maintained by its function to comfort and self-soothe, and may be more commonly observed in people who do not restrict their eating such as BED, certain cases of BN, and sub-clinical binge eating.

Similarities to other models
The new model presented in this paper posits that core low self-esteem is a major underlying predisposing factor for binge eating. This is in line with the functional analysis of binge eating [19], the transdiagnostic model [17], the cognitive model of BN [23], and a number of other binge eating models [12] that also identify low self-esteem as an important predisposing factor for the development of binge eating. The new model proposes that when core low self-esteem is triggered (experienced as a range of feelings and beliefs, measured by negative statements about the self), negative affect is experienced (in line with the cognitive model of BN [23]). The new model then suggests that a difficulty with regulating the negative affect is experienced, and as such, the individual responds in one of two ways:

(1) They engage in, or attempt to engage in, restrictive eating practices as a way to cope with the negative affect attempting to gain 'affective' control, and this restrained eating then triggers binge eating (as in the dietary restraint theory, functional analysis of binge eating, transdiagnostic model of eating disorders, and many others [12]).

Or

(2) Beliefs about eating are activated and themselves trigger binge eating as a means of functionally coping with negative affect (as in the cognitive model of BN [23]).

Table 3 Goodness-of-Fit Indices for Models

Model	χ²/df	GFI	CFI	TLI	IFI	RMSEA (90% CI)	PCLOSE
1	17.363	0.94	0.895	0.826	0.896	.147 (.127 to .167)	.000
2	13.08	0.956	0.923	0.871	0.923	.126 (.106 to .147)	.000
3	7.612	0.975	0.962	0.93	0.963	.093 (.072 to .116)	.001
4	4.716	0.986	0.982	0.96	0.982	.070 (.047 to .095)	.074
5	2.781	0.993	0.992	0.981	0.992	.048 (.022 to .077)	.487

Table 4 Unstandardised and Standardised Regression Weights for Final Model (Model 5) (Standard Errors in Brackets)

Pathway	Unstandardised Estimate	Standardised Estimate	p
Core Low Self-Esteem → Negative Affect	.55 (.03)	.54	<.001
Core Low Self-Esteem → Difficulty with Emotional Regulation	.49 (.06)	.23	<.001
Core Low Self-Esteem → Dietary Restraint	.02 (.01)	.17	<.001
Core Low Self-Esteem → Eating Beliefs	.23 (.04)	.20	<.001
Negative Affect → Difficulty with Emotional Regulation	1.25(.06)	.59	<.001
Difficulty with Emotional Regulation → Dietary Restraint	.01 (.002)	.20	<.001
Difficulty with Emotional Regulation → Eating Beliefs	.207 (.02)	.39	<.001
Dietary Restraint → Binge Eating	1.435 (.23)	.20	<.001
Eating Beliefs → Binge Eating	.315 (.02)	.43	<.001

Unique contributions

In addition to synthesising the main evidence-based variables hypothesised to lead to and maintain binge eating, the new model presented in this paper also offers some unique insights into the way in which these variables relate to one another to lead to binge eating, above and beyond what has already been demonstrated in previous studies. Most important is the dual pathway to binge eating identified in this model, indicating the possibility of two different 'types' of binge eating which are maintained by different processes. The relevance and necessity of dietary restraint in the development and maintenance of binge eating has been contested in the literature and amongst clinicians [19, 45]; the dual pathway presented in this new model provides an alternative in that binge eating can be triggered either by restrained eating or by the activation of particular beliefs about eating. Furthermore, the new model presented in this paper provides an integrated cognitive-behavioural model of binge eating

which is transdiagnostic, and focused on behavioural symptoms rather than simply the presence or absence of a diagnosis.

Limitations

It is important to note that the results of this study need to be interpreted in the context of a number of limitations. Firstly, the results are limited by the instruments used to measure the variables and associated constructs. For example, both binge eating and dietary restraint were measured by the same instrument, the EDE-Q, and therefore it is possible that the relationship between these two variables might have been artificially enhanced due to the fact that they were measured together. Also, the instruments used assess different time periods, for example, while the EDE-Q assesses symptoms experienced over the previous 28-days, the items in the DASS-21 refer to the past week. Therefore, in order to be able to more accurately assess if binge eating behaviours are occurring at the

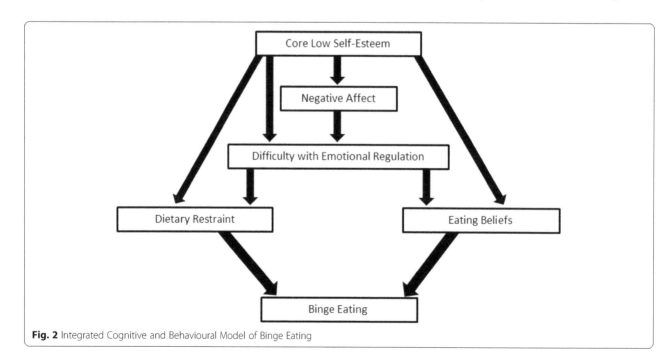

Fig. 2 Integrated Cognitive and Behavioural Model of Binge Eating

same time as negative affect it is recommended that future studies utilise measures referring to the same period of time and to test the model with a range of different measures for each factor. Future research should also assess the stability of the model fit if alternative questionnaires are used to measure the proposed predictive variables. This is especially important with regard to the measurement of binge eating, as the EDE-Q has received some criticism with regard to the accuracy of the measurement of binge eating [33, 34, 46]. Secondly, the participants included in this study were non-clinical, and the eating disorder symptoms (including binge eating) were based on a self-report measure. Future studies investigating the new model should test the fit of the model to a clinical sample whose binge eating status and/or eating disorder diagnosis has been assessed by a trained clinician using semi-structured interviews such as the Eating Disorders Examination [22]. Furthermore, it is important to emphasise that this paper represents a preliminary investigation of this new model, and further research is required to assess the utility and validity of this new model in longitudinal research and in intervention-based research.

Conclusion

Based on the existing literature, a cognitive and behavioural model of transdiagnostic binge eating was developed and tested. The resultant model provides a good fit to the data and offers a novel way to conceptualise binge eating that supports, integrates, and builds upon the current existing psychological models of binge eating. The model can provide a framework for understanding the causal and maintenance factors of binge eating and provides several areas for intervention. Based on the model, treatments that target the core low self-esteem and improve emotional regulation skills are likely to lead to reductions in binge eating. Depending on whether the individual's binge eating is usually triggered by dietary restraint or usually triggered by the activation of eating beliefs, or if their binge eating can be triggered by either of these factors, then treatment approaches can be personalised to focus more on addressing the dietary restraint, addressing unhelpful beliefs about eating, or on addressing both. Results presented here are preliminary, and further investigation is required to assess the accuracy and the clinical utility of the model for individuals seeking treatment for binge eating.

Abbreviations
AN: Anorexia Nervosa; AN-BP: Anorexia Nervosa (binge/purge subtype); BED: Binge Eating Disorder; BMI: Body Mass Index; BN: Bulimia Nervosa; CFI: Comparative Fit Index; CI: Confidence Intervals; DASS-21: Depression Anxiety Stress Scales; DERS: Difficulty in Emotion Regulation Scale; df: degrees of freedom; EBQ-18: Eating Beliefs Questionnaire (18 items); ED-CBQ: Eating Disorders Core Beliefs Questionnaire; EDE-Q: Eating Disorders Examination Questionnaire; EDNOS: Eating Disorder Not Otherwise Specified; GFI: Goodness of Fit Index; IFI: Incremental Fit Index; OSFED: Other Specified Feeding or Eating Disorder; RMSEA: Root Mean Square Error of Approximation; SD: Standard Deviation; SEM: Structural Equations Modelling; SPSS: Statistical Package for Social Sciences; TLI: Tucker-Lewis Index

Acknowledgements
We thank Matthew Modini for his support and advice.

Authors' contributions
AB prepared the manuscript. MA and AB were involved in the conception and design of the study, the analysis and interpretation of the data. MA contributed to the revision of the manuscript. All authors read and approved the final manuscript.

Competing interests
The authors declare that they have no competing interests.

References
1. American Psychiatric Association. Diagnostic and statistical manual of mental disorders (DSM-5). Washington, DC: American Psychiatric Publishing; 2013.
2. Hay P, Girosi F, Mond J. Prevalence and sociodemographic correlates of DSM-5 eating disorders in the Australian population. J Eat Disord. 2015;3(1):19.
3. Hay P, Mond J, Buttner P, Darby A. Eating disorder behaviors are increasing: findings from two sequential community surveys in South Australia. PLoS One. 2008;3(2):e1541.
4. Hudson JI, Hiripi E, Pope HG, Kessler RC. The prevalence and correlates of eating disorders in the National Comorbidity Survey Replication. Biol Psychiatry. 2007;61(3):348–58.
5. Kessler RC, Berglund PA, Chiu WT, Deitz AC, Hudson JI, Shahly V, Aguilar-Gaxiola S, Alonso J, Angermeyer MC, Benjet C. The prevalence and correlates of binge eating disorder in the World Health Organization world mental health surveys. Biol Psychiatry. 2013;73(9):904–14.
6. Wade TD, Bergin JL, Tiggemann M, Bulik CM, Fairburn CG. Prevalence and long-term course of lifetime eating disorders in an adult Australian twin cohort. Aust N Z J Psychiatry. 2006;40(2):121–8.
7. Mitchison D, Touyz S, González-Chica D, Stocks N, Hay P. How abnormal is binge eating? 18-year time trends in population prevalence and burden. Acta Psychiatr Scand. 2017.
8. Mustelin L, Bulik CM, Kaprio J, Keski-Rahkonen A. Prevalence and correlates of binge eating disorder related features in the community. Appetite. 2017;109:165–71.
9. Wilfley DE, Friedman MA, Dounchis JZ, Stein RI, Welch RR, Ball SA. Comorbid psychopathology in binge eating disorder: relation to eating disorder severity at baseline and following treatment. J Consult Clin Psychol. 2000;68(4):641.
10. Wilfley DE, Wilson GT, Agras WS. The clinical significance of binge eating disorder. Int J Eat Disord. 2003;34(S1):S96–S106.
11. Williamson DA, White MA, York-Crowe E, Stewart TM. Cognitive-behavioral theories of eating disorders. Behav Modif. 2004;28(6):711–38.
12. Burton AL, Abbott MJ. Conceptualising binge eating: a review of the theoretical and empirical literature. Behav Chang. 2017;34(3):168–98.
13. Herman CP, Mack D. Restrained and unrestrained eating. J Pers. 1975; 43(4):647–60.
14. Polivy J, Herman CP. Dieting and binging: A causal analysis. Am Psychol. 1985;40(2):193.
15. Stice E, Burger K. Dieting as a risk factor for eating disorders. *The Wiley handbook of eating disorders*. 2015:312–323.
16. Fairburn CG, Cooper Z, Cooper PJ. The clinical features and maintenance of bulimia nervosa. In: *Handbook of Eating Disorders: Physiology, Psychology and Treatment of Obesity, Anorexia and Bulimia*. Edn. Edited by Brownell KD, Foreyt JT. New York, NY: Basic Books; 1986: 389–404.
17. Fairburn CG, Cooper Z, Shafran R. Cognitive behaviour therapy for eating disorders: a "transdiagnostic" theory and treatment. Behav Res Ther. 2003;41(5):509–28.
18. Stice E, Shaw H, Nemeroff C. Dual pathway model of bulimia nervosa: longitudinal support for dietary restraint and affect-regulation mechanisms. J Soc Clin Psychol. 1998;17(2):129–49.
19. McManus F, Waller G. A functional analysis of binge-eating. Clin Psychol Rev. 1995;15(8):845–63.
20. Waller G, Dickson C, Ohanian V. Cognitive content in bulimic disorders: Core beliefs and eating attitudes. Eat Behav. 2002;3(2):171–8.

21. Heatherton TF, Baumeister RF. Binge eating as escape from self-awareness. Psychol Bull. 1991;110(1):86.

22. Fairburn CG, Wilson GT, Schleimer K. Binge eating: nature, assessment, and treatment. New York, NY: Guilford Press; 1993.

23. Cooper MJ, Wells A, Todd G. A cognitive model of bulimia nervosa. Br J Clin Psychol. 2004;43(1):1–16.

24. Danner UN, Sternheim L, Evers C. The importance of distinguishing between the different eating disorders (sub) types when assessing emotion regulation strategies. Psychiatry Res. 2014;215(3):727–32.

25. Engelberg MJ, Steiger H, Gauvin L, Wonderlich SA. Binge antecedents in bulimic syndromes: an examination of dissociation and negative affect. Int J Eat Disord. 2007;40(6):531–6.

26. Lavender JM, Wonderlich SA, Engel SG, Gordon KH, Kaye WH, Mitchell JE. Dimensions of emotion dysregulation in anorexia nervosa and bulimia nervosa: a conceptual review of the empirical literature. Clin Psychol Rev. 2015;40:111–22.

27. Leehr EJ, Krohmer K, Schag K, Dresler T, Zipfel S, Giel KE. Emotion regulation model in binge eating disorder and obesity-a systematic review. Neurosci Biobehav Rev. 2015;49:125–34.

28. Munsch S, Meyer AH, Quartier V, Wilhelm FH. Binge eating in binge eating disorder: a breakdown of emotion regulatory process? Psychiatry Res. 2012;195(3):118–24.

29. Waller G, Ohanian V, Meyer C, Osman S. Cognitive content among bulimic women: the role of core beliefs. Int J Eat Disord. 2000;28(2):235–41.

30. Talbot D, Smith E, Tomkins A, Brockman R, Simpson S. Schema modes in eating disorders compared to a community sample. J Eat Disord. 2015;3(1):41.

31. Waller G. Schema-level cognitions in patients with binge eating disorder: a case control study. Int J Eat Disord. 2003;33(4):458–64.

32. Bergin JL, Wade TD. A cross-sectional analysis of the cognitive model of bulimia nervosa. Int J Eat Disord. 2012;45(6):776–86.

33. Fairburn CG, Beglin SJ. Assessment of eating disorders: interview or self-report questionnaire? Int J Eat Disord. 1994;16(4):363–70.

34. Burton AL, Abbott MJ, Modini M, Touyz S. Psychometric evaluation of self-report measures of binge eating symptoms and related psychopathology: a systematic review of the literature. Int J Eat Disord. 2016;49:123–40.

35. Boateng GO, Neilands TB, Frongillo EA, Melgar-Quiñonez HR, Young SL. Best practices for developing and validating scales for health, social, and behavioral research: a primer. Front Public Health. 2018;6.

36. Lovibond PF, Lovibond SH. The structure of negative emotional states: comparison of the depression anxiety stress scales (DASS) with the Beck depression and anxiety inventories. Behav Res Ther. 1995;33(3):335–43.

37. Antony MM, Bieling PJ, Cox BJ, Enns MW, Swinson RP. Psychometric properties of the 42-item and 21-item versions of the depression anxiety stress scales in clinical groups and a community sample. Psychol Assess. 1998;10(2):176.

38. Fairchild H, Cooper M. A multidimensional measure of core beliefs relevant to eating disorders: preliminary development and validation. Eat Behav. 2010;11(4):239–46.

39. Gratz KL, Roemer L. Multidimensional assessment of emotion regulation and dysregulation: development, factor structure, and initial validation of the difficulties in emotion regulation scale. J Psychopathol Behav Assess. 2004;26(1):41–54.

40. Burton AL, Abbott MJ. The revised short-form of the eating beliefs questionnaire: measuring positive, negative, and permissive beliefs about binge eating. J Eat Disord. 2018;6(1):37.

41. Burton AL, Mitchison D, Hay P, Donnelly B, Thornton C, Russell J, Swinbourne J, Basten C, Goldstein M, Touyz S, Abbott MJ. Beliefs about binge eating: psychometric properties of the eating beliefs questionnaire (EBQ-18) in eating disorder, obese, and community samples. Nutrients. 2018;10(9):1306.

42. Arbuckle J. AMOS 22. Chicago, IL: SmallWaters Corporation; 2013.

43. Hu Lt BPM. Cutoff criteria for fit indexes in covariance structure analysis: conventional criteria versus new alternatives. Struct Equ Model Multidiscip J. 1999;6(1):1–55.

44. Kenny DA. Measuring model fit. In.; 2015.

45. Waller G. The psychology of binge-eating. In: *Eating Disorders and Obesity: A Comprehensive Handbook (2nded)*. Edn. Edited by Fairburn CG, Brownell KD. New York, NY: Guildford Press; 2002: 98–102.

46. Luce KH, Crowther JH, Pole M. Eating disorder examination questionnaire (EDE-Q): norms for undergraduate women. Int J Eat Disord. 2008;41(3):273–6.

9

Does binge-eating matter for glycemic control in type 2 diabetes patients?

Marcelo Papelbaum[1,2]*, Rodrigo de Oliveira Moreira[1], Walmir Ferreira Coutinho[1], Rosane Kupfer[1], Silvia Freitas[1], Ronir Raggio Luz[3] and José Carlos Appolinario[1,2]

Abstract

Background: Eating behavior is an important aspect related to type 2 diabetes mellitus (T2DM) treatment and may have an impact on glycemic control. Previous reports showed elevated prevalence of eating disordered behaviors, especially binge eating disorder in clinical samples of type 2 diabetes patients. However, results regarding the impact of an eating disorder on the glycemic and clinical control of T2DM is inconsistent. The purpose of this study was to assess the impact of a comorbid eating disorder on glycemic control (GC) in a group of patients with T2DM.

Methods: Eating behaviors of 70 consecutive patients with T2DM were assessed using a Structured Clinical Interview for DSM-IV and the Binge Eating Scale. The GC was examined with fasting blood glucose (FBG) and glycated hemoglobin (A1c) levels. In addition, secondary clinical variables were assessed, including body mass index (BMI) and lipids. Chi-square and Student's T tests were used to compare clinical and psychopathological characteristics of patients with and without an ED. In order to evaluate the relationship between GC and eating disorder (ED) a linear regression analysis was performed, controlling for BMI. A significance level of 5% was adopted.

Results: Seventy-seven percent of the sample (n = 54) were female and 50% were obese. Fourteen patients exhibited an ED, mostly binge eating disorder (BED). In a regression analysis, both FBG (beta coefficient = 47.4 (22.3); p = 0.037) and A1c (beta coefficient = 1.12 (0.57); p = 0.05) were predicted by the presence of an ED. However, the presence of an ED lost its impact on glycemic control outcomes after the addition of the BMI in the models.

Conclusions: Eating psychopathology is frequently observed in patients with T2DM. Among individuals with T2DM, co-morbid ED is associated with a poorer glycemic control in the presence of a higher BMI. The presence of an eating disordered behavior in patients with T2DM seems to have clinical relevance in the usual care of patients with diabetes. Therefore, we recommend eating psychopathology should be routinely assessed in T2DM patients.

Keywords: Binge eating disorder, Diabetes mellitus, Glycemic control

Plain English summary

Eating behavior is an important aspect related to diabetes treatment. Indeed, previous studies had already observed higher rates of eating disordered behaviors, specifically binge eating disorder, in type 2 diabetes mellitus (T2DM) patients. Whether the presence of eating psychopathology has a negative impact on glycemic control of T2DM patients is a subject of controversy. Our study evaluated the relationship between eating disorder (ED) and glycemic control (and other metabolic outcomes) in patients with type 2 diabetes. We found that patients who exhibited binge eating-related eating psychopathology had worse glycemic levels than those without an ED in the presence of a higher BMI. In the usual care of people with type 2 diabetes we therefore recommend routine screening for eating disorder symptoms.

Background

Binge-eating related psychopathology has been associated with increased risk for a variety of clinical comorbidities, not necessarily associated with overweight and obesity [1]. For instance, some reports showed binge-eating behaviors, especially binge eating disorder (BED),

* Correspondence: marcelo.papelbaum@gmail.com
[1]State Institute Diabetes and Endocrinology, Rio de Janeiro, Brazil
[2]Group of Obesity and Eating Disorders, Institute of Psychiatry of the Federal University of Rio de Janeiro and State Institute Diabetes and Endocrinology, Avenida Ataulfo de Paiva 204, 707, Leblon, Rio de Janeiro 22440-033, Brazil
Full list of author information is available at the end of the article

to be associated with increased risk of hypertension, gastrointestinal disorders and fibromyalgia [2]. In this respect, the comorbidity between type 2 diabetes mellitus (T2DM) and BED has been consistently found in prevalence studies [2, 3].

Eating behavior in T2DM might be influenced by several factors. Firstly, both eating psychopathology and type 2 diabetes could be associated with weight [4]. In addition, a restricted diet, with limited consumption of carbohydrates, is commonly prescribed as nutritional strategy for glycemic control in diabetes [5]. Lastly, binge-eating behavior might be a consequence of hypoglycemia, although it is less frequently seen in type 2 when compared to type 1 diabetes mellitus [6]. Because of the importance of eating behavior in the metabolic control of diabetes, several studies have investigated the epidemiology of the association between T2DM and eating psychopathology [7].

Herpertz et al. [8] conducted the first large multicenter study to investigate the prevalence of ED in a sample of type 1 (n = 341) and type 2 (n = 322) diabetes patients. Although the authors found similar ranges of ED prevalence between both samples, the distribution of the ED categories differed between them. In the T2DM group there was 12.6% lifetime prevalence in females (2.4% BN; 7.1% BED; 3% EDNOS) and 7.1% in males (1.3% BN; 4.5% BED; 1.3% EDNOS). In the type 1 diabetes mellitus (T1DM) group there was, for instance, 16.5% lifetime prevalence of ED, with predominance of anorexia nervosa and bulimia nervosa (BN). The most observed ED associated with type 2 diabetes was BED, with a lifetime prevalence of 5.9%. Subsequently, Kenardy et al. [9] investigated the prevalence of BED in 50 newly diagnosed T2DM patients compared to case-matched control without diabetes. A greater number of patients with type 2 diabetes (14%) reported episodes of binge eating compared to control subjects (4%). However, the diagnostic of BED did not differ between the two samples. In this way, another study also observed higher levels of regular binge eating (greater or equal twice per week over the past six months) in female (11%) and male (18%) T2DM patients [10]. Indeed, although other studies confirmed this clinical comorbidity, differences in the prevalence of ED in T2DM has varied according to the population studied, type of measurement of ED and presence of other confounding factors, especially overweight and obesity. Mannucci et al. [11], using a structured interview (Eating Disorder Examination [EDE]), found lower levels of BED in T2DM. In addition, the authors concluded that obesity, rather T2DM per se, might be a more important risk factor for eating psychopathology in T2DM. Nicolau et al. [12] also observed a positive correlation between eating psychopathology and body mass index in a sample of T2DM patients.

Although the comorbidity of an ED and T2DM has been observed across studies, the impact of this association on the clinical control of diabetes has been less consistent. Most studies investigating the clinical control of T2DM in patients with eating psychopathology focused exclusively on glycemic control, frequently using glycated hemoglobin (A1c) as the primary outcome [9, 11, 13, 14]. Two studies did not show difference on A1c between type 2 diabetes patients with and without regular binge (at least twice a week over the last 6 months) or BED, respectively [9, 14]. However, as the studies were designed specifically to investigate the prevalence of abnormal eating behavior in a diabetic population as the primary outcome, it might have lacked the power to detect a difference in the glycemic control. On the other hand, positive correlation was found between Binge Eating Scale (BES) and EDE scores and glycemic control [11, 13]. Also, only one study evaluated this impact using a longitudinal design, not showing differences on glycemic control associated with disordered eating behavior with a follow-up of 2.2 years [15].

Considering the lack of consensus regarding the impact of an eating disordered behavior on the clinical control of T2DM, the main purpose to the article was to investigate metabolic control in a clinical sample of type 2 diabetes patients with and without an ED.

Research design

Seventy outpatients with T2DM, aged 18 to 65 years, were assessed consecutively at the Diabetes and Endocrinology State Institute of Rio de Janeiro. Diabetes was diagnosed according to the American Diabetes Association criteria [16]. Patients with T1DM, gestational diabetes, secondary diabetes due to another disease or using medication likely to affect food intake (antidepressants, anti-obesity agents) were excluded from the analysis. Patients who met the inclusion criteria were consecutively evaluated after informed consent was obtained.

Methodology
Clinical examination

Screened patients were asked to come to a scheduled visit. Anthropometric examinations and laboratory tests were obtained in the same day, early in the morning, to assess the metabolic control of diabetes. Weight was measured in light street clothes, without shoes, on a calibrated balance-beam scale and, subjects' heights were measured using a stadiometer. Body mass indices (BMI) were calculated by dividing weight (kg) by height squared (m2). Glycemic control of diabetes was assessed measuring the levels of fasting blood glucose (FBG) and A1c. FBG was measured using a colorimetric enzymatic method, and A1c levels were determined using high-performance liquid chromatography (HPLC; Variant turbo,

Bio-Rad, National Glycohemoglobin Standardization Program). Clinical characteristics of diabetes were collected from the medical records, including duration of diabetes, insulin and oral anti-diabetics use and the presence of microvascular complications related to diabetes (retinopathy, nephropathy and neuropathy).

Psychiatric instruments

All subjects were interviewed by a psychiatrist (MP) trained in the use of the Structured Clinical Interview for DSM-IV, patient edition (SCID-P) [17]. This instrument was used for the diagnosis of ED. The BES was also applied to provide a measure of severity of eating psychopathology [18]. This instrument has been translated into Portuguese, presenting good reliability [19, 20].

Data analysis

Continuous variables were expressed as means and standard deviations, and categorical data were described as absolute and relative frequencies. Patients with ED were compared to those with no eating psychopathology in terms of clinical and psychopathological characteristics using non-paired t tests to compare means of continuous variables and the Chi-square test to analyze categorical variables. In order to analyze the relationship between diabetes glycemic control and eating psychopathology, a linear regression was performed. Two different models were considered, using A1c and FBG as the main outcome (dependent variables) and eating disorder diagnosis status as an independent variable. Also, the BMI was later added in both models as an independent variable to evaluate possible confounding factor. A significance level of 5% was adopted. The statistical analysis was conducted using SPSS software.

Results

A total of 113 diabetes outpatients were consecutively screened. After the observance of exclusion criteria, our final sample consisted of 70 T2DM individuals. All individuals who met the inclusion criteria agreed to participate in the evaluation. Our study sample consisted mostly of females (77%), married individuals (70%) and individuals who had less than nine years of schooling (71%) with a mean age was 52.9 ± 6.8 years. Mean BMI was $30.6 \pm 5.2 \, \text{kg/m}^2$. Half of the individuals were obese (mean BMI = $34.8 \pm 3.5 \, \text{kg/m}^2$), 22 were overweight (mean BMI = $27.9 \pm 1.1 \, \text{kg/m}^2$) and 13 exhibited normal weight (mean BMI = $23.6 \pm 1.2 \, \text{kg/m}^2$). The sample consisted of patients with a long illness duration (13.33 ± 7.55 years), with high rates of neuropathy (22%), retinopathy (42%) and nephropathy (52%). In addition, 51% of the patients were using insulin regularly.

The prevalence of ED was 20%. The most frequently observed condition was BED, observed in 7 of the 14 the participants with an ED. In addition, BN was diagnosed in 3 patients, and 4 individuals exhibited an eating disorder not otherwise specified (EDNOS), with subclinical BED. Because of the low number of bulimic and subclinical BED individuals, it was decided to analyze the group as a whole, with a binge eating-related ED. The rate of an ED varied according to BMI status. Specifically, normal-BMI individuals exhibited a rate of ED of 8%, contrasted with a 26% prevalence of ED in obese patients. In addition, there was a positive correlation between eating psychopathology severity (using BES scores) and BMI (r = 0.24; p = 0.04) However, patients with ED did not differ from those without an ED diagnosis regarding to the presence of insulin use (50% vs 52%; p = 0.9). In addition, the presence of a binge-eating related disorder did not have an impact on metformin mean dosage use (2007.1 ± 514.3 mg vs. 2030.3 ± 628.9 mg; $p > 0.05$).

Table 1 shows the comparison of clinical and psychopathological features between patients with and without a ED. None of those characteristics was associated with the presence of an ED. In addition, the subjects with T2DM and a co-existing ED exhibited higher levels of eating psychopathology severity, measured by BES scores, compared to those without an ED.

In a regression analysis (Table 2), ED status predicted both FBG and A1c levels. However, the addition of the BMI in the two models had an impact on the results

Table 1 Clinical and psychopathological comparison between type 2 diabetes patients with and without eating disorders

	T2DM	T2DM	T2DM	p value
	Total sample	Without eating disorder	With eating disorder	
	n = 70	n = 56	n = 14	
Age (years)	52.9 ± 6.8	53.2 ± 6.9	51.8 ± 6.8	0.50
Diabetes duration (years)	13.4 ± 7.5	13.6 ± 7.5	12.2 ± 8.0	0.52
Body mass index (kg/m2)	30.6 ± 5.2	30.0 ± 5.2	32.6 ± 4.8	0.09
Total cholesterol (mg/dl)	199.8 ± 44.2	199.1 ± 44.5	202.3 ± 44.5	0.81
Triglycerides (mg/dl)	131.9 ± 55.5	128.4 ± 50.3	145.0 ± 72.8	0.34
Binge eating scale	12.8 ± 10.3	9.5 ± 8.1	25.6 ± 8.1	< 0.001

Data are presented as mean (SD). *T2DM* Type 2 diabetes mellitus

Table 2 Regression analysis of glycated hemoglobin ang fasting blood glucose according to the presence of an eating disorder before and after controlling for body mass index

Model	R	Unstandardized Beta Coefficients (Std. error)	p value
1- Dependent Variable: A1c			
ED	0.25	1.12 (0.57)	0.05
ED	0.28	0.99 (0.58)	0.09
BMI		0.05 (0.05)	0.32
2- Dependent Variable: FBG			
ED	0.26	47.4 (22.3)	0.037
ED	0.29	42.3 (22.7)	0.067
BMI		1.9 (1.8)	0.274

A1c Glycated hemoglobin, *BMI* Body mass index, *ED* Eating disorder, *FBG* Fast blood glucose

and, therefore, the presence of an ED lost its influence on glycemic control outcomes.

Discussion

In our study, 20% of patients with T2DM had an ED, predominantly BED. Also, those with an ED had higher levels of obesity. In addition, patients with comorbid ED had a poorer glycemic control compared to those with normal eating behaviors, not related specifically to age or duration of diabetes. However, when including BMI in the regression model, the impact of eating psychopathology on A1c and FBG disappeared, showing that body weight may play a major role modulating the relationship between ED disturbances and glycemic control.

Elevated rates of eating psychopathology in type 2 diabetes individuals has been found in several studies. However, heterogeneity of results could be influenced by the clinical characteristics of the sample and the instruments used for ED diagnosis. Evaluating those who displayed regular binge eating episodes or presented with one or more positive response as per Questionnaire of Eating and Weight Pattern scoring criteria, rates of eating psychopathology found in type 2 diabetes patients were 14 and 40%, respectively [9, 13]. On the other hand, the use of a more restrictive diagnostic instrument may have led to lower estimates of ED numbers. For instance, using the EDE, Mannucci et al. [11] found low rates of BED (2.5%) in T2DM female patients with obesity. In the Look AHEAD trial [21] 14% of the 845 T2DM patients were screened positive for BED (using Eating Disorder Examination Questionnaire) or night eating syndrome (NES), using NES questionnaire. When using the EDE interview or the Night Eating Syndrome History and Inventory (NESHI) to confirm the diagnosis, only 5.2% of those were diagnosed an ED. The results of our study corroborate the high rate of eating psychopathology seen across studies. Although we also used a semi-

structured interview for ED diagnosis, the longer duration of diabetes and the high mean age of the patients could have influenced the prevalence of ED found in our study, as it was higher from those studies that used more structured interviews. Indeed, Gagnon et al. [10] showed that ED-T2DM patients had a younger onset of diabetes than the type 2 diabetes subjects without ED.

Previous studies that investigated metabolic control in the comorbidity between T2DM and ED were heterogeneous and showed different results. A poorer glycemic control in T2DM exhibiting an ED was also observed in other studies. However, different from our investigation, they did not use a semi-structured interview for the diagnosis of ED. Mannucci et al. [11], evaluating eating psychopathology in 156 T2DM patients, observed a positive correlation between A1c levels and EDE scores. More recently, Meneghini et al. [13], evaluating a multi-ethnic sample of T2DM patients, found statistically higher levels of A1c in patients who exhibited binge-eating episodes compared to those who did not ($p = 0.027$). On the other hand, other investigations did not observe this association. Nicolau et al. [12] found similar levels of A1c and FBG in T2DM patients despite the presence of a comorbid ED. Crow et al. [22] evaluated eating psychopathology in 43 consecutive T2DM patients. Patients with type 2 diabetes who exhibited binge eating showed no differences in A1c levels compared to their non-binge eating counterparts ($p = 0.553$). Similarly, Kenardy et al. [9] investigated the binge-eating diagnosis in 215 females with T2DM. No difference was observed in mean A1c levels in T2DM patients who binged regularly compared to those who displayed no eating psychopathology. Herpertz et al. [23] also found no difference in A1c levels in TD2M patients with an ED compared to those who exhibited no eating psychopathology ($p = 0.26$). Finally, Ryan et al. [10] found similar A1c levels in type 2 diabetes patients who exhibited abnormal eating behaviors compared to those who had normal eating behaviors. These conflicting results could reflect differences in regard to sample size, duration of diabetes and assessment of an ED and its severity.

In our study, the levels of A1c and FBG were predicted according to ED occurrence. However, after controlling for BMI these associations lost statistical significance. In fact, our results are in line with previous notion that weight is a major contributor to metabolic and glycemic control in individuals with type 2 diabetes [24]. Indeed, some authors struggled to demonstrate an independent impact of eating psychopathology on glycemic control, when controlling for weight status [11]. As a matter of fact, the relationship between eating behavior and weight is so intrinsic that both variables should be accounted together when evaluating glycemic control. Nevertheless, it is not possible to rule out that diabetes-specific treatment features and the intermittent natural course of binge-eating psychopathology could also have influenced some of the results.

Generally, levels of A1c and FBG should share a similar trend when evaluating glycemic control. However, is important to note that they measure different aspects of glycemic control. The American College of Endocrinology guidelines for glycemic control states that periodic measurements of A1c levels (which represent a 2- to 3-month average blood glucose concentrations) should be made. In addition, regular measurements of FBG (which indicates acute glycemic control) should also be included [22]. However, it is not uncommon for clinicians who treat people with diabetes to find individuals in whom A1c and FBG do not match [25]. Different from previous studies, we decided to evaluate the relationship between binge-eating related psychopathology with both A1c and FBG in order to assess specific aspects of glycemic evaluation. Although it is not possible to address any interpretation with the data presented, it seems interesting to discuss that, regarding to BED patients, the presence of late evening binge eating (raising FBG) coupled with daytime food restriction (lowering A1c) could result in some discrepancy between FBG and A1c levels. Nevertheless, in order to address this hypothesis specific methodological procedures would be necessary, for instance, the use of 24-h food diaries. In addition, evaluation of glycemic variability, with continuous glucose monitoring, could help understand differences between FBG and A1c and investigate a possible role of binge eating on dysglycemia (peaks and nadirs) [26].

Although glycemic control has been the gold-standard when investigating the impact of eating psychopathology on T2DM, other diabetes-related variables could be secondarily analyzed. For instance, although Crow et al. [14] did not find worse clinical control of T2DM in patients with ED compared to those without ED, the authors observed that patients who exhibited regular binge eating episodes used a greater number of medications for diabetes management than did those who did not binge frequently. The same situation occurred in the study by Kenardy et al. [9], who observed that the percentage of T2DM patients who used insulin or more than one hypoglycemic drug was higher in those patients who binged regularly than in those who did not. In addition, those patients who binged had a lower adherence to diabetes diet and exercise recommendations. Finally, Nicolau et al. [12] observed higher triglycerides levels in T2DM patients with an ED compared to those without an eating abnormality. Differently from Kenardy et al., our study did not find an association between insulin use and ED diagnosis. Overall, our findings are consistent with the majority of previous research that did not find an association between eating psychopathology and general diabetes clinical or treatment features.

Some limitations of this study must be discussed. As this was an exploratory study, sample size calculation was not made and might have limited the power to detect some of the associations. Also, control for multiple variables was avoided due to sample size. The term ED was used to refer to binge eating-related diagnosis and, as only 3 patients were diagnosed with bulimia, analysis by ED category was not possible. In addition, it could be argued that the inclusion of 4 patients with EDNOS with subclinical BED (which would be characterized in DSM-5 as either BED or other specified feeding or eating disorder [BED type]) could have limited the severity of eating psychopathology and, subsequently, the power to detect associations. However, the sample of ED individuals seemed to reflect well the presence of eating psychopathology as BES scores were markedly high and differed between those with and without ED. Nevertheless, it is not possible to rule out that subjects with more severe ED could have been selected out, as those taking psychotropics were excluded. The use of a broader multidimensional evaluation, including food diary, general psychopathology and diabetes-specific quality of life measures could have added information regarding other aspects of the clinical control of diabetes. On the other hand, the use of a semi-structured interview for ED diagnosis, associated with a self-report instrument to assess severity of eating psychopathology should be considered one strength in methodology, especially compared to most of the studies in this field.

Conclusions

The pool of evidence regarding the association between ED and T2DM seems to justify screening diabetic patients for abnormal eating behaviors. In addition, when obesity is present, eating psychopathology investigation is even more recommended, since it may disrupt obesity treatment and indirectly affect diabetes control.

Although the objective negative clinical impact of an ED on type 2 diabetes control is yet to be confirmed, is possible to speculate that the remission of binge episodes could play a major role in diabetes treatment. The clinical control of eating psychopathology could enhance nutritional recommendations adherence and may diminished post-prandial glycemic peaks. Nevertheless, although the spectrum of the clinical significance of the comorbidity of ED and T2DM has not been extensively studies, treatment of binge-eating related disorders could improve perception of self-efficacy of patients toward the diabetes dietary carbohydrate goals and, ultimately improved diabetes-related quality of life.

Abbreviations
A1c: Glycated hemoglobin; ADA: American Diabetes Association; BDI: Beck depression inventory; BES: Binge Eating Scale; BMI: Body mass index; ED: Eating disorder; EDE: Eating Disorder Examination; FBG: Fasting blood glucose; GC: Glycemic control; NES: Night eating syndrome; SCID-P: Structured Clinical Interview for DSM-IV, patient edition; T2DM: Type 2 diabetes mellitus

Acknowledgements
Not applicable.

Authors' contributions
MP, ROM and JCA participated in the design of the study and ROM, RRL and MP performed the statistical analysis. RK and SF participated in its design and coordination and WC helped to draft the manuscript. All authors read and approved the final manuscript.

Authors' information
State Institute Diabetes and Endocrinology, Rio de Janeiro. Group of Obesity and Eating Disorders, Institute of Psychiatry from the Federal University of Rio de Janeiro and State Institute Diabetes and Endocrinology.

Competing interests
The authors declare that they have no competing interests.

Author details
[1]State Institute Diabetes and Endocrinology, Rio de Janeiro, Brazil. [2]Group of Obesity and Eating Disorders, Institute of Psychiatry of the Federal University of Rio de Janeiro and State Institute Diabetes and Endocrinology, Avenida Ataulfo de Paiva 204, 707, Leblon, Rio de Janeiro 22440-033, Brazil. [3]Institute for Studies in Public Health, Federal University of Rio de Janeiro, Rio de Janeiro, Brazil.

References
1. Thornton LM, Watson HJ, Jangmo A, Welch E, Wiklund C, von Hausswolff-Juhlin Y, et al. Binge-eating disorder in the Swedish national registers: somatic comorbidity. Int J Eat Disord. 2017;50(1):58–65.
2. Javaras KN, Pope HG, Lalonde JK, Roberts JL, Nillni YI, Laird NM, et al. Co-occurrence of binge eating disorder with psychiatric and medical disorders. J Clin Psychiatry. 2008;69(2):266–73.
3. Kessler RC, Berglund PA, Chiu WT, Deitz AC, Hudson JI, Shahly V, et al. The prevalence and correlates of binge eating disorder in the World Health Organization world mental health surveys. Biol Psychiatry. 2013;73(9):904–14.
4. Daousi C, Casson IF, Gill GV, MacFarlane IA, Wilding JPH, Pinkney JH. Prevalence of obesity in type 2 diabetes in secondary care: association with cardiovascular risk factors. Postgrad Med J. 2006;82(966):280–4.
5. Vetter ML, Amaro A, Volger S. Nutritional management of type 2 diabetes mellitus and obesity and pharmacologic therapies to facilitate weight loss. Postgrad Med. 2014;126(1):139–52.
6. Mannucci E, Ricca V, Rotella CM. Clinical features of binge eating disorder in type I diabetes: a case report. Int J Eat Disord. 1997;21(1):99–102.
7. García-Mayor RV, García-Soidán FJ. Eating disoders in type 2 diabetic people: brief review. Diabetes Metab Syndr. 2017;11(3):221–4.
8. Herpertz S, Wagener R, Albus C, Kocnar M, Wagner R, Best F. Diabetes mellitus and eating disorders: a multicenter study on the comorbidity of the two diseases. J Psychosom Res. 1998;44(3/4):503–15.
9. Kenardy J, Mensch M, Bowen K, Pearson S. A comparison of eating behaviors in newly diagnosed NIDDM patients and case-matched control subjects. Diabetes Care. 1994;17(10):1197–9.
10. Ryan M, Gallanagh J, Livingstone MB, Gaillard C, Ritz P. The prevalence of abnormal eating behaviour in a representative sample of the French diabetic population. Diabetes Metab. 2008;34:581–6.
11. Mannucci E, Tesi F, Ricca V, Pierazzuoli E, Barciulli E, Moretti S, et al. Eating behavior in obese patients with and without type 2 diabetes mellitus. Int J Obes Relat Metab Disord. 2002;26:848–53.
12. Nicolau J, Simo R, Sanchís P, Ayala L, Fortuny R, Zubillaga I, et al. Eating disorders are frequent among type 2 diabetic patients and are associated with worse metabolic and psychological outcomes: results from a cross-sectional study in primary and secondary care settings. Acta Diabetol. 2015; 52(6):1037–44.
13. Meneghini LF, Spadola J, Florez H. Prevalence and associations of binge eating disorder in a multiethnic population with type 2 diabetes. Diabetes Care. 2006;29(12):2760.
14. Crow S, Kendall D, Praus B, Thuras P. Binge eating and other psychopathology in patients with type II diabetes mellitus. Int J Eat Disord. 2001;30:222–6.
15. Herpertz S, Albus C, Kielmann R, Hagemann-Patt H, Lichtblau K, et al. Comorbidity of diabetes mellitus and eating disorders: A follow-up study. J Psychosom Res. 2001;51:673–8.
16. American Diabetes Association. Diagnosis and classification of diabetes mellitus. Diabetes Care. 2010;33:S62–9.
17. First MB, Spitzer RL, Gibbon M, Williams JB. Structured clinical interview for DSM-IV-TR Axis I disorders, research version, patient edition (SCID-I/P). New York: Biometrics Research, New York State Psychiatric Institute; 2002.
18. Gormally J, Black S, Daston S, Rardin D. The assessment of binge eating severity among obese persons. Addict Behav. 1982;7(1):47–55.
19. Freitas S, Lopes CS, Coutinho W, Appolinario JC. Translation and adaptation into Portuguese of the binge-eating scale. Rev Bras Psiquiatr. 2001;23(4): 215–20.
20. Freitas SR, Lopes CS, Appolinario JC, Coutinho W. The assessment of binge eating disorder in obese women: a comparison of the binge eating scale with the structured clinical interview for the DSM-IV. Eat Behav. 2006;7(3): 282–9.
21. Allison KC, Crow SJ, Reeves RR, Foreyt JP, DiLillo VG, Wadden TA, et al. Binge eating disorder and night eating syndrome in adults with type 2 diabetes. Obesity. 2007;15:1287–93.
22. American College of Endocrinology Consensus Statement on Guidelines for Glycemic Control*. Endocr Pract. 2002;8(Suppl 1):5–11.
23. Herpertz S, Albus C, Wagener R, Kocnar M, Henning A, Best F. Comorbidity of diabetes and eating disorders: does diabetes control reflect disturbed eating behavior? Diabetes Care. 1998;21(7):1.110–6.
24. Franz MJ, Boucher JL, Rutten-Ramos S, VanWormer JJ. Lifestyle weight-loss intervention outcomes in overweight and obese adults with type 2 diabetes: a systematic review and meta-analysis of randomized clinical trials. J Acad Nutr Diet. 2015;115(9):1447–63.
25. Cohen RM, Lindsell CJ. When the blood glucose and the HbA1c don't match: turning uncertainty into opportunity. Diabetes Care. 2012;35(12): 2421–3.
26. Satya Krishna SV, Kota SK, Modi KD. Glycemic variability: clinical implications. Indian J Endocrinol Metab. 2013;17(4):611–9.

10

Binge eating symptoms prevalence and relationship with psychosocial factors among female undergraduate students at Palestine Polytechnic University

Manal M. Badrasawi*⬤ and Souzan J. Zidan

Abstract

Background: Eating disorders pose a serious challenge to health services due to psychosocial and medical problems. Binge eating disorder (BED) is characterized as a pattern of overeating episodes followed by shame, distress and guilty feelings. Among eating disorders, BED has the highest prevalence, especially among females. The literature reported that BED is associated with nutritional status, socio-demographic factors, and psychological factors in different countries. This study aims to examine the prevalence of binge eating symptoms and its relationship with selected variables (i.e. socio-demographics, nutritional status and dietary habits).

Methods: One hundred fifty-four female undergraduate students, from three different faculties at Palestine Polytechnic University, participated in the study. All the students who consented to join the study were assessed in terms of weight status using body mass index, dietary habits and medical profile. The screening for presence of binge eating symptoms was done using BEDS-7. The psychosocial factors were assessed by validated Arabic version of DASS-21.

Results: Half of the participants (50%) had binge eating symptoms. No association between binge eating symptoms and socio-demographic variables was found. Similarly, binge eating symptoms was not related to body weight status, however, it was associated with eating between meals and number of snacks. A significantly higher score on depression, stress and anxiety was found among binge eaters than non-binge eaters.

Conclusion: It was concluded that binge eating symptoms have considerable prevalence among the study participants, and it was significantly correlated with psychosocial factors. Future studies are needed to examine other risk factors and correlations. Educational programs are also recommended to increase the awareness of eating disorders as well as to promote healthy eating patterns.

Keywords: Binge eating disorder, Prevalence, Risk factors, University students, Depression

* Correspondence: m.badrasawi@najah.edu
Department of Nutrition and Food technology, Faculty of Agriculture and
Veterinary Medicine, An-Najah National University, TulkarmWest Bank, PO Box
7Palestine

Plain English summary

Binge eating is an eating disorder characterized by frequent episodes of out-of-control eating large quantities of food (often very quickly and to the point of discomfort) followed by shame, distress and guilty feelings. The prevalence of binge is the highest as compared to other eating disorders. There is evidence that there is association between binge eating symptoms and nutritional status, social factors, self-esteem, depression, anxiety and stress. The outcomes of the current study showed that half of the female participants have experienced binge eating symptoms. There was also a significant relationship between psychosocial factors and binge eating symptoms.

Introduction

Eating disorders are a group of mental disorders recognized by abnormal eating habits [1]. These disorders most often occur during the late stage of adolescence or early adulthood, and are associated to the social, physical, and psychological maturation of adolescents [2]. These disorders involve anorexia nervosa (AN), bulimia nervosa (BN), and binge eating disorder. AN is characterized by extreme weight loss, irrational fears of weight gain and obesity, and poor body image, whereas BN is known as a repeated bouts of uncontrolled, quick consumption of large amounts of food followed by self-induced vomiting, diuretics or laxative use, fasting, or vigorous exercise in order to avoid weight gain [3]. The focus of this research is on binge eating disorder (BED). The DSM-5 criteria since 2013 defined binge eating episode as a disorder occurs, on average, at least once per week for the past 3 months [4]. An episode of binge eating is recognized by eating abnormally large amounts of food over a limited period of time while experiencing feelings of loss of control [4]. Table 1 summarizes the diagnostic criteria for binge eating disorder.

Binge eating disorder seems to be the most common eating disorder, with estimates of the lifetime prevalence of binge eating disorder ranging from 1.9 to 2.8% [5] and according to some studies, it was found that binge eating disorder is more prevalent among women than males [6], this higher prevalence in males may be explained by males explicate binge eating symptoms in different way as compared to females [7]. Hudson and his colleagues found that there was no gender differences in the prevalence of subthreshold BED and binge eating behavior [8].. It also appears to be more prominent among overweight samples (30%) than among community samples (5% of females and 3% of males). In a college-student sample, the rate of binge eating disorder was 2.6% [3, 9]. This disorder is often linked with obesity even though a considerable rate of individuals (17–30%) have normal body weight [9].

Table 1 Diagnostic criteria for binge eating disorder [a]

A. Recurrent episodes of binge eating, an episode being characterized by:

1) Eating, in a discrete period of time (e.g., in any 2-h period), an amount of food that is definitely larger than most people would eat during a similar period of time

2) A sense of lack of control during the episodes, e.g., a feeling that one can't stop eating or control what or how much one is eating

B. During most binge episodes, at least three of the following behavioural indicators of loss of control:

1) Eating much more rapidly than usual

2) Eating until feeling uncomfortably full

3) Eating large amounts of food when not feeling physically hungry

4) Eating large amounts of food throughout the day with no planned mealtimes

5) Eating alone because of being embarrassed by how much one is eating

6) Feeling disgusted with oneself, depressed, or feeling very guilty after overeating

C. Marked distress regarding binge eating.

D. The binge eating occurs, on average, at least once per week for the past 3 months.

E. The binge eating is not associated with the recurrent use of inappropriate compensatory behavior as in bulimia nervosa and does not occur exclusively during the course of bulimia nervosa or anorexia nervosa

[a] Reprinted with permission from the *Diagnostic and Statistical Manual of Mental Disorders*, Fifth Edition (©2013). American Psychiatric Association [1]

The etiology of binge eating disorder is multifactorial. Cultural and social impacts are defined as one of the risk factors associated with binge eating [10]. Besides it is confirmed that individual's with eating disorders can suffer from mental problems such as alcohol dependence, depression, social stress, daily activity-related stress and other anxiety issues [10]. Former studies have found that most individuals with binge eating experience higher rates of depression than normal individuals [10]. Other research has found that people with binge eating often suffer from several types of anxiety disorders [11].

Binge eating disorder is accompanied by multiple co-morbidities including; psychiatric and medical comorbidities, and a higher mortality rates in comparison to subjects without eating disorders [12]. Moreover, binge-eaters are at a higher risk of developing dyslipidemia, hypertension, type 2 diabetes and metabolic syndrome compared with individuals who are not experiencing eating disorders. They may also have higher rates of sleeping problems when compared to subjects without eating disorders [12]. Psychiatric comorbidities are further related to binge eating disorder. Another study has found, 10 out of 14 studies confirmed a link between depression and binge eating disorder [13]. Former studies have noted that about 30–80% of binge-eaters have lifetime comorbid anxiety or mood disorders. Other personality problems and psychiatric comorbidities might be found in subjects with binge eating disorder including substance abuse, bipolar disorder, and gambling problems, as well as borderline personality disorders, avoidant, and obsessive-compulsive [12].

According to a recent study performed at Palestine, the prevalence of disordered eating attitudes is considerably high among female Palestinian university students [14]. In other research, it was reported that the rate of females at risk of eating disorders in Palestine was estimated to be 38.9% [15]. This could be an indication of the prevalence of binge eating symptoms among female university students in Palestine. However, no reliable research exist about the prevalence of binge eating symptoms among university female students.

To our knowledge, no study has yet assessed the prevalence of binge eating symptoms among female university students. The findings of the present study will add to the literature on binge eating symptoms among Arab female adolescents and young adults, which will help inform the design of educational programs to increase the undergraduate students' awareness on eating disorders to promote healthy eating styles among them and the entire community as well. Furthermore, this study will determine the association between the presence of binge eating symptoms with depression, anxiety and stress among undergraduate students.

Methods
Study design
This study utilized a cross sectional design and aimed to determine the prevalence of binge eating symptoms among female undergraduate students in Palestine Polytechnic university- Hebron – West bank, Palestine, and to determine the relationship between binge eating symptoms and psychosocial factors. The study participants were selected from the three faculties in Palestine polytechnic University (Engineering, Applied Science and human Sciences). Participants were recruited by convenience sampling after personal invitation from the research team. The sample size was determined using Cochran formula for sample size calculation in a survey research [16]. The inclusion criteria included female participants who are doing their undergraduate degree in Palestine Polytechnic University. Participants were excluded if their age is less than 18 years old, have chronic diseases which can affect their dietary intake or nutritional status and participants who were pregnant during the data collection.

Data collection and research tools
The data collection started in March 2018–May 2018. All participants were briefed about the study design and objectives, and they were informed about the type of data that would be collected, with affirmation on the optional participation. Participants who agreed to sign the

consent form were included in the data collection. The local ethics committee of Palestine Polytechnic University approved and supported the current study.

The collected data included socio demographic characteristics; age, area of living, university discipline, academic achievement and self-reported medical history and smoking. Screening for binge eating symptoms was done using Binge Eating Disorder Screener-7 (BEDS-7) for use with adults. The BEDS-7 is a self-report screening tool that is designed to screen for BED symptoms rather than to make a diagnosis. It has been validated against DSM-5 diagnostic criteria [17]. BEDS-7 consists of 7 items asking about episodes of overeating during the last three months and the feelings after these episodes. Depending on the answers, participants are categorized into two categories (presence of binge eating symptoms or normal) following the suggested algorithms. The psychometric properties of BEDS-7; 100% sensitivity and 38.7% specificity [17]. The participants body mass index was assessed using anthropometric measurement (weight and height) following the standard methods reported by Lee and Nieman [18]. The measurements were measured in duplicate then the mean was recorded. The body mass index was calculated from the weight and height then categorized according to WHO cut off points [19]. Dietary intake was assessed using a validated food frequency questionnaire [20]. The Arabic version of the questionnaire consists of a total of ninety-eight food types in thirteen food groups. These foods correspond to items consumed in the Mediterranean region in general and in Palestine in particular. Nutrisuvey software was used to analyze the nutrients content of the selected foods to determine the intake. Participants were asked to answer the frequency of the consumption in addition to describe the portion size of the reported food [20]. The psychological parameters were assessed using the validated Arabic version of Depression Anxiety Stress Scales (DASS). The short form of DASS composed of 21 instrument measuring current ("over the past week") symptoms of depression, anxiety, and stress. Participants were asked to use a 4-point combined severity/frequency scale to rate the extent to which they have experienced each item over the past week. The scale ranges from 0 (did not apply to me at all) to 3 (applied to me very much, or most of the time). Scores for depression, anxiety, and stress were calculated by summing the scores for the relevant items [21].

Statistical analysis
All statistical analysis was carried out using the Statistical Package for Social Sciences (SPSS) software version 22. An alpha level of (0.05) was considered for all the statistical tests used in the study. Two-sided p values of

(0.05) and (80%) power were statistically significant. The data were analyzed according to variable types. The descriptive analysis for the prevalence of presence of binge eating symptoms was done by calculating the frequencies and percentages. The association between the incidences was analyzed using Chi square tests because the variables are of categorical type including area of living, faculty, marital status and body mass index. The mean difference between the groups was done either by independent t-test (depression, anxiety, stress and diet intake).

Results

Subject Charactersitics

Subjects characteristics are presented in Table 2. A total of 154 females were included in the study. The mean age of the sample was (19.64 ± 1.170) and the mean of their academic achievment was (80.07 ± 7.130) out of 100. The procedure of recruiting females is described in Fig. 1.

Subjects' body mass index

The results reveled that majority of the participants (68.1%) are considered normal weight, 9.2% underweight, 19.9% overweight and 2.8% are underweight.

Prevalence of binge eating symptoms and its relationship with socio-demographic variables

Half of the participants (50%) showed positive binge eating symptoms. The relationships between binge and socio-demographic variables; area of living, marital status were not significant, similarly there were no significant

relationship with faculties, years of study or academic achievement ($p > 0.05$).

The relationship between body mass index, dietary habits with presence of binge symptoms

Figure 2 illustrates that there was no association between presence of binge eating symptoms and BMI using Chi square test. Moreover, the results show a higher prevalence of Binge eating symptoms is associated with eating between meals χ^2 (1, $n = 154$, p value = 0.035) and number of snacks χ^2 (1, n = 154, p value = 0.045), while it was not associated with meal skipping, eating fast food, eating alone or with family. Similarly, it was not associated with weight satisfaction.

Relationship between presence of Binge Eating Symptoms & Dietary Intake

Table 3 demonstrates that there was no significant association between presence of binge eating symptoms and dietary intake ($p < 0.05$).

Relationship between presence of binge eating symptoms & psychosocial variables

Table 4 demonstrates that individuals with binge eating symptoms had significantly higher scores on depression, stress and anxiety that those without symptoms ($p < 0.05$).

Discussion

The aim of this study was to determine the prevalence of binge eating symptoms and its relationship with selected variables (i.e. socio-demographics, nutritional status and dietary habits) among undergraduate students at Palestine Polytechnic University, and to investigate the presence of psychological symptoms in subjects with binge eating symptoms.

In the present study, the results reveal that the prevalence of binge eating symptoms among female university students (50%) was relatively higher than the rates obtained in Iceland (0.6%) [22], Netherland (2.3%) [23], Canada (0.7%) [24], USA (3.0%) [25], Italy (0.6%) [26]. This higher rate could be due to different tools used to define the presence of binge eating symptoms. In addition, they could be due to different study aims as this study aimed to examine the presence of binge eating symptoms rather than make a diagnosis of binge eating disorder.

Till this date, cultural theories concerning the influence of Western exposure on the risk of eating disorder have concentrated on factors specific to eating disorders, e.g., media influences, body image ideals, and peer and familial pressures on appearance. Moreover, the exposure to Western countries is correlated with high risk for a broad range of other psychiatric problems such as

Table 2 Subject characteristics presented in numbers and percentages n (%)

Variable		n	%
Faculties	Sciences	71	46.1
	Engineering and technology	39	25.3
	Human Sciences	44	28.6
Years of study	1st year	41	26.6
	2nd year	59	38.3
	3rd year	32	20.7
	(4 + 5) th year	22	14.3
State	Single	138	89.6
	Married + otherwise	16	10.4
Area of living	City	94	61.1
	Village + camp	60	38.9
Monthly Family income	< 3000	41	26.6
	3000–5000	77	50
	> 5000	36	23.4
Type of housing	With family	128	83.2
	University hostels	26	16.8

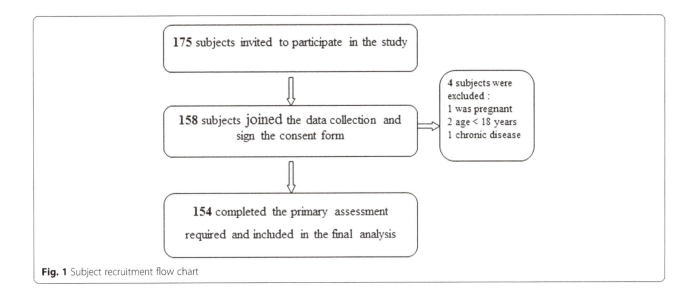

Fig. 1 Subject recruitment flow chart

binge eating disorder [27]. The outcome of higher prevalence in this research could be assigned to media exposure which could be influencing opinions related to body weight and body image. Palestinian females who are not exposed to the Israeli society in a direct way still have the chance to be exposed to Israeli media through social media, television, and other means of communication. Lately, there has also been a growing exposure to Turkish media. Such TV shows and movies may also affect the attitudes and behaviors of Palestinian females, given that Turkish culture is not as conservative as Palestinian culture [14].

Even though obesity is linked with binge eating disorder, it is not included as a diagnostic criteria for binge eating disorder, which is distinguished from obesity [1]. Binge eating disorder is found across the body mass spectrum but is frequently found in individuals with obesity (36.2–42.4%) [28]. A small percentage of people attempting to lose weight were diagnosed with binge eating disorder (13%–27%) [28–30] In the current study,

it was found that there is no association between weight status and binge eating symptoms. Unlike former research where it was noted that overweight/obesity was highly linked to binge eating among adolescents from a high SES population [31]. The difference may be because the current study examined binge eating symptoms rather than examining binge eating disorder diagnosis. This presence is alarming sign for developing the disorder which is associated with obesity and overweight.

The current research indicates that binge eating symptoms is significantly related to stress. This finding is supported by the liturature [32–36]. Since 1959, case reports of Stunkard elucidated that binge-eaters was experiencing marked distress. Elevated levels of distress associated with binge eating are stated in binge-eaters who have either normal weight or obesity, proposing that the distress is not an outcome of comorbid obesity [37]. The current outcomes also confirm that binge-eating is significantly correlated with anxiety, and this

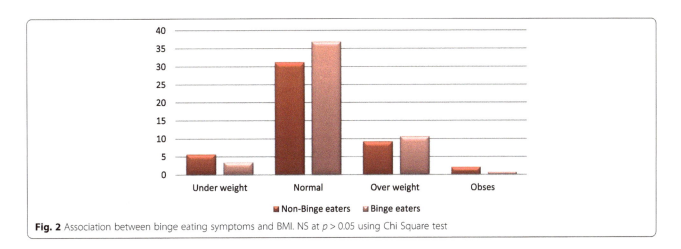

Fig. 2 Association between binge eating symptoms and BMI. NS at $p > 0.05$ using Chi Square test

Table 3 The relationship between presence of binge eating symptoms and Dietary intake

	Unite	Binge eaters	Non-binge eaters	t	CI	P value
Total calories	Kcal /day	2709 ± 800	2410 ± 759	−2.72	− 511.2230.4	0.19
Carbohydrate	gm/day	335 ± 140	310 ± 146	−0.748	−69.5- 28.4	0.23
Protein	gm/day	105 ± 34	100 ± 42	−0.830	−23.3-9.66	0.11
Fat	gm/day	111 ± 46	104 ± 34	−0.817	−16.8- 10.31	0.204
Fiber	gm/day	19.5 ± 8	20 ± 9	−0.476	−2.25- 3.7	0.13
Sugar	gm/day	81 ± 42	78 ± 41	0.487	−11.1-17.08	0.53

N.S using independent t-test

outcome is consistent by previous study performed by Jung and his colleagues [2].

In addition, we have noticed in the current study that there is significant association between binge eating and depression, and this result is consistent with former studies. For instance; Carriere and his colleagues have observed that subjective binge eating was significantly associated with depression [38]. In another study, it was stated that the more severe the depression, the more the severe the binging [39]. French and his colleagues stated that binge-eaters have higher levels of stressful life events and depression in comparison with non-binge eaters [40].

Our study reveals that binge eaters have a slightly distinct eating behavior beyond binge eating. As it was observed that binge-eaters consumed a slightly higher amount of total calories (300 kcal more), which is supported by the literature [41], and a higher amount of calories as a fat when compared to non-binge eaters, however, the differences are insignificant. Overall, little data is available about the eating habits of females who binge eat. Former studies have found few macronutrient variations among binge and non-binge eaters on regular intake at meals. But there is some evidence of elevated fat intake during binge episodes [42, 43]. In a laboratory setting, it was noticed that obese subjects with binge eating disorder consume more calories and a higher amount of calories as a fat than obese subjects without binge eating disorder [42, 43]. Our results also indicate that there are no differences between binge-eaters and non-binge eaters in the consumed

amounts of carbohydrates, protein, sugar, and fiber. This finding is confirmed by former studies as well [42, 43].

There is a complexity in illustrating eating data among females who binge eat, since habitual patterns of eating are typically estimated. Episodes of binge eating may not be reflected by using regular dietary intake questionnaires, especially if the occurrence of binge is low. Furthermore, it is unclear how individuals are stating eating habits that surround their binge eating. For instance, do they integrate these eating episodes into their average habit reports, or are these episodes are excluded from the 'average' habit, because they are seen as uncommon and not representative of their usual patterns? Moreover, embarrassment or shame could result in the elimination of these episodes from self-reports of eating habit. Limited sources are available that resolve these methodological issues [40].

There are a few limitations in the current study. The study only included participants from one university which means that these results are not representative for females' university students in Palestine. Nevertheless, the current study provides for the first-time worthy data on the prevalence of binge eating disorder in Palestine and its association with psychosocial variables.

Conclusion

The present study reveals that the prevalence of binge eating symptoms is relatively high among female Palestinian university students. It was further demonstrated that there is no association between the disorder and body weight status. It also affirms that binge eating symptoms is associated with psychosocial factors such as depression, stress, and anxiety. Future research, that take into consideration a great number of psychological and demographic factors, is needed. According to this study, it is recommended to develop educational programs to increase the level of awareness regarding appropriate nutrition in relation to body weight, and it is possible that a general university optional course would be useful in this regard.

Table 4 The relationship between presence of binge eating symptoms and psychosocial variables presented in mean ± sd

	Binge eaters	Non-binge eaters	T	CI	P value
Depression	7.8 ± 4.6	5.9 ± 3.8	4.21	0.501–3.254	0.007*
Stress	10.1 ± 4.5	8.3 ± 3.9	1.39	0.43–3.100	0.011*
Anxiety	8.6 ± 4.8	6.2 ± 3.9	8.81	0.99–2.88	0.002*

*significant p < 0.05 using independent t-test

Abbreviations
AN: Anorexia nervosa; BN: Bulimia nervosa

Acknowledgments
We are grateful to the participated females for consenting to participate in this study. Correspondence concerning this article should be addressed to Manal M Badrasawi. Department of Nutrition and Food technology, Faculty of Agriculture and Veterinary Medicine, An-Najah National University, Tulkarm, West Bank PO. Box 7, Palestine. E-mail: m.badrasawi@najah.edu

Authors' contributions
MB is the principle investigator proposed the study design, coordinated data collection, and conducted statistical analysis. SZ interpreted the data and drafted the initial manuscript. All authors have read and approved the final version of the manuscript and agree with the order of presentation of the authors.

Competing interests
The authors declare that they have no competing interests.

References
1. American Psychiatric Association. Diagnostic and statistical manual of mental disorders. 5th ed. Washington, DC: American Psychiatric Association; 2013.
2. Jung J-Y, Kim K-H, Woo H-Y, Shin D-W, Shin Y-C, Oh K-S, Shin E-H, Lim S-W. Binge eating is associated with trait anxiety in Korean adolescent girls: a cross sectional study. BMC Womens Health. 2017;17:8.
3. Brown JE, Lechtenberg E. Nutrition through the life cycle. 6th ed. Boston: Cengage Leaning; 2017.
4. Dingemans A, Danner U, Parks M. Emotion regulation in binge eating disorder: a review. Nutrients. 2017;9(11):1274.
5. Kessler RC, Berglund PA, Chiu WT, Deitz AC, Hudson JI, Shahly V, Aguilar-Gaxiola S, Alonso J, Angermeyer MC, Benjet C, Bruffaerts R, de Girolamo G, de Graaf R, Maria Haro J, Kovess-Masfety V, O'Neill S, Posada-Villa J, Sasu C, Scott K, Viana MC, Xavier M. The prevalence and correlates of binge eating disorder in the World Health Organization world mental health surveys. Biol Psychiatry. 2013;73(9):904–14.
6. Hutson PH, Balodis IM, Potenza MN. Binge-eating disorder: clinical and therapeutic advances. Pharmacol Ther. 2018;182:15–27.
7. Lee-Winn AE, Reinblatt SP, Mojtabai R, Mendelson T. Gender and racial/ethnic differences in binge eating symptoms in a nationally representative sample of adolescents in the United States. Eat Behav. 2016;22:27–33.
8. Hudson JI, Hiripi E, Pope HG Jr, Kessler RC. The prevalence and correlates of eating disorders in the National Comorbidity Survey Replication. Biol Psychiatry. 2007;61(3):348–58.
9. Eisenberg D, Nicklett EJ, Roeder K, Kirz NE. Eating disorder symptoms among college students: prevalence, persistence, correlates, and treatment-seeking. J Am Coll Heal. 2011;59(8):700–7.
10. Wiederman MW, Pryor TL. Body dissatisfaction, bulimia, and depression among women: the mediating role of drive for thinness. Int J Eat Disord. 2000;27(1):90–5.
11. Javaras KN, Pope HG, Lalonde JK, Roberts JL, Nillni YI, Laird NM, Bulik CM, Crow SJ, McElroy SL, Walsh BT, Tsuang MT, Rosenthal NR, Hudson JI. Co-occurrence of binge eating disorder with psychiatric and medical disorders. J Clin Psychiatry. 2008;69(2):266–73.
12. Kornstein SG, Kunovac JL, Herman BK, Culpepper L. Recognizing binge-eating disorder in the clinical setting: a review of the literature. Prim Care Companion CNS Disord. 2016;18(3):10.
13. Araujo DM, Santos GF, Nardi AE. Binge eating disorder and depression: a systematic review. World J Biol Psychiatry. 2010;11(2 Pt 2):199–207.
14. Saleh RN, Salameh RA, Yhya HH, Sweileh WM. Disordered eating attitudes in female students of an-Najah National University: a cross-sectional study. J Eat Disord. 2018;6:16.
15. Musaiger AO, Al-Mannai M, Tayyem R, Al-Lalla O, Ali EYA, Kalam F, Benhamed MM, Saghir S, Halahleh I, Djoudi Z, Chirane M. Risk of disordered eating attitudes among adolescents in seven Arab countries by gender and obesity: a cross-cultural study. Appetite. 2013;60(1):162–7.
16. Bartlett JE, Kotrlik JW, Higgins CC. Organizational research: determining appropriate sample size in survey research appropriate sample size in survey research. Inf Technol Learn Perform J. 2001;19(1):43–50.
17. Herman BK, Deal LS, DiBenedetti DB, Nelson L, Fehnel SE, Brown TM. Development of the 7-item binge-eating disorder screener (BEDS-7). Prim Care Companion CNS Disord. 2016;18(2):10.
18. Lee RD, Nieman DC. Nutritional assessment. 6th ed. New York: McGraw Hill; 2013.
19. WHO. Body mass index – report. 2018. http://www.euro.who.int/en/health-topics/disease-prevention/nutrition/a-healthy-lifestyle/body-mass-index-bmi. Assessed 15 May 2019.
20. Hamdan M, Monteagudo C, Lorenzo-Tovar M-L, Tur J-A, Olea-Serrano F, Mariscal-Arcas M. Development and validation of a nutritional questionnaire for the Palestine population. Public Health Nutr. 2014;17(11):2512–8.
21. Moussa MT, Lovibond P, Laube R, Megahead HA. Psychometric properties of an Arabic version of the depression anxiety stress scales (DASS). Res Soc Work Pract. 2017;27(3):375–86.
22. Thorsteinsdottir G, Ulfarsdottir L. Eating disorders in college students in Iceland. Eur J Psychiat. 2008;22(2):107–15.
23. Smink FRE, van Hoeken D, Oldehinkel AJ, Hoek HW. Prevalence and severity of DSM-5 eating disorders in a community cohort of adolescents. Int J Eat Disord. 2014;47(6):610–9.
24. Flament MF, Buchholz A, Henderson K, Obeid N, Maras D, Schubert N, Paterniti S, Goldfield G. Comparative distribution and validity of DSM-IV and DSM-5 diagnoses of eating disorders in adolescents from the community. Eur Eat Disord Rev. 2015;23(2):100–10.
25. Stice E, Marti CN, Rohde P. Prevalence, incidence, impairment, and course of the proposed DSM-5 eating disorder diagnoses in an 8-year prospective community study of young women. J Abnorm Psychol. 2013;122(2):445–57.
26. Favaro A, Ferrara S, Santonastaso P. The Spectrum of eating disorders in young women. Psychosom Med. 2003;65(4):701–8.
27. Swanson SA, Saito N, Borges G, Benjet C, Aguilar-Gaxiola S, Medina-Mora ME, Breslau J. Change in binge eating and binge eating disorder associated with migration from Mexico to the US. J Psychiatr Res. 2012;46(1):31–7.
28. Barnes RD, White MA, Martino S, Grilo CM. A randomized controlled trial comparing scalable weight loss treatments in primary care. Obesity (Silver Spring). 2014;22(12):2508–16.
29. Kolotkin RL, Westman EC, Østbye T, Crosby RD, Eisenson HJ, Binks M. Does binge eating disorder impact weight-related quality of life? Obes Res. 2004;12(6):999–1005.
30. Sandberg RM, Dahl JK, Vedul-Kjelsås E, Engum B, Kulseng B, Mårvik R, Eriksen L. Health-related quality of life in obese Presurgery patients with and without binge eating disorder, and subdiagnostic binge eating disorders. J Obes. 2013;2013:1–7.
31. West CE, Goldschmidt AB, Mason SM, Neumark-Sztainer D. Differences in risk factors for binge eating by socioeconomic status in a community-based sample of adolescents: findings from project EAT. Int J Eat Disord. 2019;52(6):659–68.
32. Bentley C, Gratwick-Sarll K, Harrison C, Mond J. Sex differences in psychosocial impairment associated with eating disorder features in adolescents: a school-based study. Int J Eat Disord. 2015;48(6):633–40.
33. Colles SL, Dixon JB, O'Brien PE. Loss of control is central to psychological disturbance associated with binge eating disorder. Obesity (Silver Spring). 2008;16(3):608–14.
34. Mitchell KS, Neale MC, Bulik CM, Aggen SH, Kendler KS, Mazzeo SE. Binge eating disorder: a symptom-level investigation of genetic and environmental influences on liability. Psychol Med. 2010;40(11):1899–906.
35. Striegel-Moore RH, Dohm FA, Solomon EE, Fairburn CG, Pike KM, Wilfley DE. Subthreshold binge eating disorder. Int J Eat Disord. 2000;27(3):270–8.
36. Stunkard AJ. Eating patterns and obesity. Psychiatr Q. 1959;33:284–95.
37. Goldschmidt AB, Le Grange D, Powers P, Crow SJ, Hill LL, Peterson CB, Crosby RD, Mitchell JE. Eating disorder symptomatology in Normal-weight vs. obese individuals with binge eating disorder. Obesity (Silver Spring). 2011;19(7):1515–8.
38. Carriere C, Michel G, Féart C, Pellay H, Onorato O, Barat P, Thibault H. Relationships between emotional disorders, personality dimensions, and binge eating disorder in French obese adolescents. Arch Pediatr. 2019;26(3):138–44.

39. Berkowitz R, Stunkard AJ, Stallings VA. Binge-eating Disorder in Obese Adolescent Girls. Ann N Y Acad Sci. 1993;699(1 Prevention an):200–6.

40. French S, Jeffery R, Sherwood N, Neumark-Sztainer D. Prevalence and correlates of binge eating in a nonclinical sample of women enrolled in a weight gain prevention program. Int J Obes Relat Metab Disord. 1999;23(6):576–85.

41. Vannucci A, Tanofsky-Kraff M, Crosby RD, Ranzenhofer LM, Shomaker LB, Field SE, Mooreville M, Reina SA, Kozlosky M, Yanovski SZ, Yanovski JA. Latent profile analysis to determine the typology of disinhibited eating behaviors in children and adolescents. J Consult Clin Psychol. 2013;81(3):494–507.

42. Raymond NC, Bartholome LT, Lee SS, Peterson RE, Raatz SK. A comparison of energy intake and food selection during laboratory binge eating episodes in obese women with and without a binge eating disorder diagnosis. Int J Eat Disord. 2007;40(1):67–71.

43. Yanovski SZ, Leet M, Yanovski JA, Flood M, Gold PW, Kissileff HR, Walsh BT. Food selection and intake of obese women with binge-eating disorder. Am J Clin Nutr. 1992;56(6):975–80.

11

Self-directed behaviors differentially explain associations between emotion dysregulation and eating disorder psychopathology in patients with or without objective binge-eating

Elin Monell[1,2]*, David Clinton[1,2,3] and Andreas Birgegård[1,2]

Abstract

Background: Emotion dysregulation and negative self-directed behaviors are key characteristics of eating disorders (EDs), but their interaction in relation to ED psychopathology is insufficiently explored, and empirically robust and clinically relevant models are needed.

Methods: This study examined whether the association between emotion dysregulation and ED psychopathology was mediated by different negative self-directed behaviors in 999 ED patients divided into two sub-samples based on absence or presence of objective binge-eating episodes (OBE). Several simple and extended mediation models were examined using the Difficulties in Emotion Regulation Scale (DERS) as independent variable, the Structural Analysis of Social Behavior (SASB) as mediator, and the Eating Disorder Examination Questionnaire (EDE-Q) as dependent variable.

Results: An associational pathway was found where higher emotion dysregulation was associated with more negative self-directed behaviors, which in turn was associated with higher ED psychopathology. Self-directed behaviors of importance differed between patient groups. In participants without OBE, lower self-love and higher self-attack were influential, whereas in participants with OBE, lower self-affirmation and higher self-blame were influential.

Conclusions: Self-directed behaviors may help to explain the association between emotion dysregulation and ED psychopathology. Our findings have both theoretical and clinical implications that are pathology-specific. Addressing specific self-directed behaviors could be an important way of helping patients deal with their emotions in relation to ED psychopathology.

Keywords: Eating disorders, Emotion dysregulation, Self-directed behaviors, Mediation analysis, Objective binge-eating episodes, DERS

* Correspondence: elin.monell@ki.se
[1]Centre for Psychiatry Research, Department of Clinical Neuroscience, Karolinska Institute, and Stockholm Health Care Services, Stockholm County Council, Norra Stationsgatan 69, SE-11364 Stockholm, Sweden
[2]Department of Medical Epidemiology and Biostatistics, Karolinska Institutet, Stockholm, Sweden
Full list of author information is available at the end of the article

Plain English summary

Eating disorders are complex serious psychiatric conditions but the understanding of how they develop and are maintained is unclear, while treatment outcomes are mixed. This study examined difficulties understanding and managing emotions (emotion dysregulation) and the habitual way an individual internally treats and regulates him–/herself (self-directed behaviors), in relation to eating disorder psychopathology among 999 patients with eating disorders. We found that higher emotion dysregulation, such as difficulties focusing on and understanding emotions, was associated with negatively attuned self-directed behaviors, for instance with harsh self-criticism, which in turn was associated with greater body, shape and weight concerns. We found that in participants who did not have objective binge-eating episodes, higher emotion dysregulation seemed to be associated with less self-love and more self-attack in relation to eating disorder symptoms. In participants who did have objective binge-eating, higher emotion dysregulation was associated with less self-affirmation and more self-blame. Our results suggest that negative types of self-directed behaviors may maintain problematic patterns of emotional difficulties and eating disorder symptoms and that this needs to be addressed in treatment.

Introduction

Eating disorders (EDs) are complex psychiatric conditions associated with high rates of psychiatric and medical comorbidity, life-disruptions, and significant suffering [1], but the etiology of EDs is unclear [2] and treatment outcomes are mixed [3]. In order to improve our understanding and treatment of EDs we need to identify empirically robust and clinically relevant models of etiology and maintenance. Previous research suggests that EDs are characterized by emotion dysregulation and negative self-directed behaviors [4, 5]. Emotion dysregulation refers to difficulties understanding and managing emotions [6], while self-directed behaviors refers to dimensions of self-control vs. spontaneity and self-affiliation vs. self-attack [7]. Independently, these factors impact symptoms, but their interaction in relation to ED psychopathology remains insufficiently explored. Recently, Monell, Högdahl, Forsén Mantilla, and Birgegård [8] suggested that the effect of emotion dysregulation on ED psychopathology in female students was mediated through more negative self-directed behaviors. Increased emotion dysregulation (e.g., losing control over one's behavior when in distress) was associated with negative self-directed behavior (e.g., harsh self-criticism), which in turn was associated with greater ED psychopathology. The present study aims to replicate and extend these findings in a large clinical ED sample, hoping to identify

potential intervention targets that closely reflect patients' experience of emotion dysregulation.

Dimensions of emotion dysregulation and associations with ED pathology

Emotion dysregulation is associated with ED pathology [9, 10] and ED outcome [11]. Further, behavioral ED symptoms may represent dysfunctional emotion regulation strategies in response to negative affect [12]. However, 'emotion dysregulation' as a concept is imprecise as it has been given different meanings and has been measured using a variety of instruments. Converging on a common model, several recent ED studies have employed the multidimensional model of Gratz and Roemer and the Difficulties in Emotion Regulation Scale (DERS) [6]. This model was developed to capture the following four dimensions.

Reduced emotional awareness and clarity describes an inability (or unwillingness) to focus on emotional signals and an insufficient understanding of them, resembling alexithymia (i.e., difficulties identifying and describing emotions) [13]. Alexithymic traits are considered key characteristics of restrictive ED pathology [14]. However, research indicates its relevance across the entire ED diagnostic spectrum [15], and difficulties in emotional awareness and clarity may distinguish ED patients generally from controls [9]. *Non-acceptance of emotional distress* describes tendencies to respond with negative secondary emotions (e.g., self-directed anger, shame) towards one's own distress. It has been argued that non-acceptance and avoidance of emotions is a key maintaining factor in anorexia nervosa (AN) [16]. Non-acceptance is associated with both overall ED psychopathology [9] and restraint [17]. *Difficulties maintaining impulse control and goal-directed behaviors when upset* refers to difficulties controlling, or fear of losing control, over one's reactions and behavior when in distress. This resembles negative urgency (i.e., engaging in rash and impulsive behavior when distressed), particularly relevant for patients with binge-eating [5, 18]. *Perceived lack of emotion regulation strategies when upset* describes a sense of emotional helplessness and a tendency to surrender to negative emotions when upset. It has the strongest unique association with ED psychopathology in both mixed clinical EDs and controls [9, 19]; improvement in this dimension has been associated with better treatment outcome for binge-eating patients [20].

In summary, lower emotional awareness and clarity may differentiate patients from controls, difficulties maintaining impulse control and goal-directed behaviors when upset may characterize binge-eating pathology, and higher levels of perceived emotional helplessness are associated with higher ED psychopathology regardless of diagnostic status.

Self-directed behaviors and associations with ED pathology

Low self-esteem is characteristic of EDs [21], and patients' sense of self-worth is often determined by body weight and shape [22]. However, while the sense of self is a complex phenomenon, most self-related concepts and measures capture unidimensional aspects of self-evaluation and self-directed feelings (i.e., approve-disapprove, like-dislike etc.). In interpersonal theory, the self is conceptualized in terms of the habitual way an individual internally relates to him–/herself [7], and thus it refers to self-directed behaviors. The Structural Analysis of Social Behavior (SASB) model and its accompanying measure [23] organizes self-directed behaviors in a circumplex (see Fig. 1). The horizontal *Affiliation* axis captures affective valence, while the vertical *Autonomy* axis captures self-regulation; combinations of these axes form different types of self-directed behaviors, grouped into the following eight clusters.

Self-emancipation describes spontaneous/free self-regulation as opposed to strict *self-control*. Control and compulsivity are central themes in EDs, particularly AN [24]. ED symptoms have been described as strategies to manage perceived lack of self-control [25], while actual loss of control (over eating) is central in binge-eating

pathology. In AN, self-emancipation and spontaneity seems decreased [26, 27], while self-control is higher relative to other EDs [26]. Higher self-control in AN is associated with worse 3-year outcome [28] and increased 12-month suicidal ideation [29]. *Self-affirmation* describes a friendly, accepting, and curious stance toward the self. Self-affirmation, often strikingly limited in EDs, has received increased attention in novel treatments [30]. *Self-blame* instead describes harsh and hostile self-regulation. Self-blame strongly resembles self-criticism and maladaptive perfectionism, both common ED traits [21]. Low self-affirmation and high self-blame are associated with higher ED psychopathology in clinical, high-risk and normal samples [4]. *Self-love* and *self-attack* are most similar to self-esteem. Lower self-love is associated with higher ED psychopathology [4]. Higher initial self-hate predicts worse outcome in various EDs [28, 31], while higher initial self-love predicts better outcomes in all EDs [31]. *Self-protection* describes active engagement in activities perceived as beneficial for the self and protection of self-interests, while *self-neglect* describes negative autonomy, such as ignoring one's own needs. Although self-protection can be considered a positive behavior, it predicts negative outcome in AN [28], possibly because some patients may perceive their

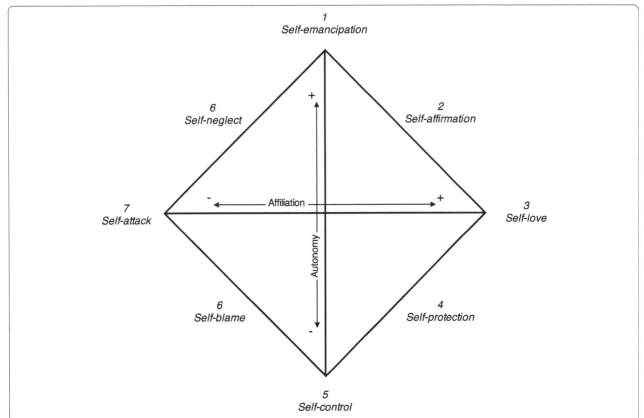

Fig. 1 Structural Analysis of Social Behavior Intrex model Cluster version. From: Benjamin LS. Interpersonal Diagnosis and Treatment of Personality Disorders, 2nd ed. New York: The Guilford Press, 1996

symptoms as the best way of taking care of their needs. More intuitively, higher self-neglect predicts worse outcome in AN [28, 31].

In summary, lower self-affirmation and higher self-blame have strong concurrent associations with higher ED psychopathology in various samples, while lower self-love and higher self-attack predict outcome in several EDs. The associations with self-protection and self-control is distinctive of AN.

Pathways whereby emotion dysregulation and self-directed behaviors may influence ED psychopathology

Several ED etiology and maintenance models include both emotion and self-related aspects [32]. These include for instance the transdiagnostic maintenance model of EDs [21], i.e., 'mood intolerance', 'clinical perfectionism', and 'core low self-esteem'; the cognitive-interpersonal maintenance model of AN [33], i.e., alexithymia, avoidant emotion processing, and compulsivity; and the model underlying integrative cognitive-affective therapy for bulimia nervosa (BN) [34], i.e., emotion dysregulation, self-directed behaviors, and self-discrepancy. An additional model highlights shame, self-criticism, and lack of self-compassion [35].

Evidence for how various emotion dysregulation dimensions and specific self-directed behaviors may influence ED psychopathology is however lacking. Existing models use different terms, study isolated aspects of emotion regulation (e.g., alexithymia) and self-related cognition/behavior (e.g., self-esteem), and few examine a wide range of such constructs simultaneously. Due to different focus on risk versus maintenance factors, they are also difficult to compare and evaluate in terms of potential association chains; one factor being associated with another that in turn might be associated with symptom expression. Mediation models can help delineate such association pathways by which emotion dysregulation and self-directed behaviors could be associated with ED psychopathology. Since the DERS and SASB models encompass important concepts in several theoretical models, their combination may provide an opportunity to integrate existing models, disentangle association pathways, and increase model specificity.

To our knowledge, only our own previous study has concurrently used the DERS and the SASB in relation to ED pathology [8]. Here, we found that higher emotion dysregulation, mediated by negative self-directed behaviors, was associated with greater ED psychopathology in female students [8]. However, this study neither examined ED patients nor specified different emotion dysregulation dimensions or types of self-directed behaviors. Clinically, it may be useful to know if different emotion dysregulation dimensions are associated with ED psychopathology through distinctive types of self-directed

behaviors in ED patients. For instance, perceptions such as "my emotions are shameful and I hate to have them" might be associated with "I'm useless and I need more discipline". This, in turn, may fuel attitudes such as "I have to control my ugly body". Empirically disentangling potential significant association chains between emotion dysregulation, self-directed behaviors, and ED psychopathology could help therapists approach clinical phenomena accurately while remaining close to patients' subjective experiences.

Aims

Given the diagnostic diversity of eating EDs it is important to study mediational pathways in groups of patients with or without particular core symptoms. However, diagnostic migration is common within EDs [36], so specific ED diagnoses may have low clinical and predictive validity [37]. Therefore, diagnosis-specific models may be overly narrow and of limited clincal utility. Even so, there appears to be some differences in emotion and self-related processes between primarily restricting patients and those with loss of control binge-eating, possibly reflecting underlying differences in impulsivity [38]. Such differences may entail differential risk for specific core symptoms; impulse control difficulties and negative urgency seemingly more associated with binge-eating [39–41], whereas over-controlled regulation and compulsivity instead seem more associated with pathological restrictive eating without binge-eating [24, 42]. The current study will therefore group EDs into broader categories depending on presence or absence of loss of control binge-eating (defined as objective binge-eating episodes; OBE) in order to capture a wider and more ecologically valid clinical picture.

We tested whether the association between emotion dysregulation and ED psychopathology is mediated by negative self-directed behaviors in ED patients with or without OBE, expecting to replicate the main finding by Monell et al. [8] in both groups. We also extend our previous work by exploring whether particular emotion dysregulation dimensions are mediated by distinct self-directed behaviors. Here, we had no specific hypotheses regarding which self-directed behaviors would be mediators in which model, or if there would be differences between groups.

Method

Participants

The sample was drawn from a clinical database covering specialized ED units in Sweden (the Stepwise database) [43]. Stepwise inclusion criteria are self- or medical referral to a treatment unit, an ED according to the Diagnostic and Statistical Manual of Mental Disorders 4th version (DSM-IV) [22], and intent to treat from the unit.

Stepwise includes patients with the full range of DSM-IV EDs of all ages entering treatment since 2005. Stepwise initial assessment, performed by trained ED professionals by the patients 3rd visit to the unit, includes semi-structured interviews, clinical ratings and self-ratings (both mandatory and optional, all in Swedish), and takes around 45 min. DSM-IV ED diagnoses are based on the Structured Eating Disorder Interview (SEDI) [44] with good validity. The present sample consisted of 999 female patients aged 16–72 years (M = 24.8, SD = 8.4) with AN restrictive subtype (AN-R; n = 172), AN binge/purge subtype (AN-BP; n = 64), BN (n = 350), binge eating disorder (BED; n = 40), and other specified feeding and EDs (OSFED; n = 373).

Data were extracted on October 30th 2016; extraction procedure, exclusions, and rationale for re-categorization from DSM-IV into DSM 5th version (DSM-5) diagnoses [45] are reported in detail elsewhere [9]. The Eating Disorder Examination Questionnaire (EDE-Q) and the SASB are mandatory in the Stepwise assessment while the DERS was included in Stepwise in 2014 as an optional instrument at the individual patient level (i.e., clinicians decided whether to include DERS or not). DERS was administered to 37% of patients during this study time frame. Patient characteristics (e.g., ED pathology, anxiety, depression, age, ED-duration) did not seem to influence if they were administered the DERS or not; instead, clinician/clinic variables seemed more influential (for more details, see Monell et al.) [9]. Additionally, SASB variables did not differ between patients with or without DERS-ratings (using independent t-tests; ps > .01).

The sample was then split into two groups depending on presence/absence of OBE. Patients with AN-R were categorized into non-OBE EDs; patients with BN and BED into OBE EDs. For patients with AN-BP and OSFED, symptoms can include OBE (in AN-BP, the binge/purge may in some cases refer to purging only), and self-rated presence of OBE in the last month (using self-rated ED-pathology, see measures) decided their group. The study was approved by the Stockholm regional ethics committee (2015/928–31/4).

Measures

The DERS [6] measures self-rated emotion dysregulation in 36 items scored 1–5, providing a Total score and six subscales: Non-Acceptance, Goals, Impulse, Awareness, Strategies, and Clarity. Items are summed to form subscales and the Total score is the sum of all scores; higher scores indicate more emotion dysregulation. The validity and psychometric properties of the subscales are debated [46], and item content might not always match intended theoretical concept [47]. Based on such criticism, rather than using the six subscales and in order to increase

specificity, this study focused on item content in subscales corresponding to the original four dimensions in the extension analyses.

Subscales Awareness and Clarity were summed to form the first dimension (range 11–55). As shown using bifactor modelling, Awareness and Clarity capture high degrees of unique information beyond a general emotion dysregulation factor (48, using largely the same sample as this; 50) and have been combined in previous research [13, 48]. They also correlate strongly, primarily with each other in our sample (see Tables S1 and S2). Non-Acceptance alone formed the second dimension (range 6–30), and Goals and Impulse were summed to form the third (range 11–55). Goals and Impulse capture similar low degrees of unique information [46, 49] and correlate strongly with each other in our sample (Tables S1 and S2). Strategies, that captures the least unique information [46, 49], and thus corresponds to a general emotion dysregulation factor, formed the fourth dimension (range 8–40). The Total score (range 36–180) was used in replication analyses. Apart from the debate on the subscales, the DERS has shown good internal consistency and good test-retest reliability [6]. The Swedish DERS has adequate psychometric properties [46]. In this sample, internal consistency was excellent for Impulse/Goals (α = .927), and good for the other dimensions (αs = .869 to .895).

The SASB intrex version [50] Introject measures self-directed behaviors using 36 items scored 0–100 (10-point increments) providing eight clusters (subscales): 1. Self-emancipation; 2. Self-affirmation; 3. Self-love; 4. Self-protection; 5. Self-control; 6. Self-blame; 7. Self-attack; and 8. Self-neglect (see Fig. 1). Six clusters (2-4 and 6-8) form the Affiliation score ranging from −100 – 100; lower scores indicate more self-attack, -blame and -neglect and higher scores indicate more self-love, -acceptance and -protection. The Affiliation score was used in replication analyses while cluster scores were used in extension analyses. The American version of SASB intrex has shown good psychometric properties [50]. The Swedish SASB intrex has shown good internal consistency (Cronbach's α = .87, Armelius, unpublished manuscript, 2001). In this sample, internal consistency was good for Clusters 3 and 7 (αs = .845 and .830), acceptable for Clusters 2, 4, 6 and 8 (αs = .717–.789), questionable for Cluster 5 (α = .644), and poor for Cluster 1 (α = .594) which was therefore dropped from further analyses.

The EDE-Q [51] version 4.0 measures self-rated ED pathology in the last 28 days, with 36 items scored 0–6 providing four subscales where higher scores indicate more severe pathology, and one mean Global Score, used as outcome in mediation analyses. The EDE-Q also measures ED related behaviors. We used item 18 (frequency of OBE) to categorize AN-BP and OSFED patients (no such episode = non-OBE EDs; one or more = OBE EDs). The original EDE-Q has shown good psychometric properties [52] as has The Swedish EDE-Q [53]. In this sample, internal consistency was excellent for EDE-Q Global Score (α = .927).

Statistical analysis

Prior to analyses (using SPSS version 24 for Mac), Mahalanobis' distance was used to examine potential multivariate outliers in each ED group separately. No outliers were observed for the simple mediation model variables (model description below), whereas for the parallel mediation model variables, some outliers were observed (a maximum of 2, i.e., < 1%) in each group and excluded from the respective analysis. All variables were z-standardized by group, making path coefficients interpretable using effect size conventions for Pearson coefficients (small $\geq$ .1; medium $\geq$ .3; large $\geq$ .5). PROCESS macro version 2.16.3, Model 4 [54] was used for all mediation analyses. Statistical inference for indirect effects (mediation) was conducted by bias-corrected bootstrap confidence intervals (CI) based on 10,000 bootstrap samples. All mediation analyses were adjusted for age and BMI. To avoid Type-I error due to multiple testing, we set alpha for main analyses to $p < .001$ and used 99% bootstrap CI:s for indirect effects.

Simple mediation models

The effect of independent variable X (DERS Total) on dependent variable Y (EDE-Q Global), mediated by mediator M (SASB Affiliation) was examined in both ED groups separately (see Fig. 2 for depiction of mediation

model components). The opposite direction (i.e., X = SASB; M = DERS) was also examined to investigate which model best fit the data, similar to Monell et al. [9]. Simple mediation analysis yields regression coefficients for each model path: first X on M (path a), M on Y adjusted for X (path b), X on Y (total effect; path c), X on Y adjusted for M (direct effect; path c'), and lastly X through M on Y which is the product of path a and b (indirect effect; path ab). The direct and indirect effects are of greatest importance in this type of analysis; the significance of path a and b independently are of minor importance while their signs (positive vs. negative association) tells the direction of the indirect effect.

Extended parallel mediation models

Four parallel mediation models (X = 4 DERS dimensions, Y = EDE-Q Global, mediated by mediators M_{1-7} = SASB Clusters 2–8; Cluster 1 excluded due to poor reliability) were examined in both ED groups separately, regarding the total effect, direct effect (adjusted for all Ms), and seven specific indirect effects (all specific indirect effects adjusted for the others).

Results

After describing sample characteristics, simple mediation results will be presented (one hypothesized and one alternate in each group), followed by the extended mediation models (four in each group); results in participants without OBE are reported prior to results in participants with OBE.

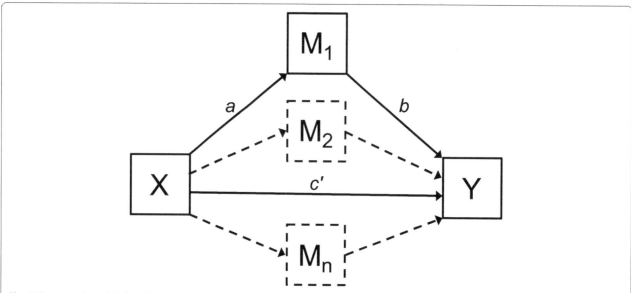

Fig. 2 Conceptual model of mediation analysis; indirect effect of X on Y through mediator M. Components a, b and c' are regression coefficients. Dashed lines indicate an extended parallel mediation model; specific indirect effects through more than one mediator

Sample characteristics

Non-OBE EDs ($n = 439$) consisted of AN-R participants ($n = 172$), and AN-BP and OSFED participants lacking OBE ($n = 35$ and 232, respectively). OBE EDs ($n = 560$) consisted of BN ($n = 350$) and BED participants ($n = 40$), as well as AN-BP and OSFED participants with OBE ($n = 29$ and 141, respectively). Descriptive data on background variables and main measures and group comparisons are presented in Table 1. Since these comparisons were intended to describe and compare the subsamples, differences at $p < .01$ are reported. Participants without OBE were significantly younger, had shorter ED duration (small effects), and lower BMI than those with OBE (large effect). For the main measures, participants without OBE reported lower EDE-Q (medium effect), higher self-affirmation, lower self-neglect, higher overall Affiliation, less difficulties in goal-directed behavior and impulse control when upset, less emotional helplessness when upset, and lower overall emotion dysregulation (small effects) than participants with OBE.

Simple mediation models

DERS Total had an indirect effect on EDE-Q Global through SASB Affiliation in both groups (Table 2), such that higher levels of emotion dysregulation were associated with more negative self-directed behaviors, which in turn was associated with higher ED psychopathology. DERS had no direct effect on EDE-Q when SASB Affiliation was accounted for (sometimes referred to as "full mediation"). Descriptively, associations were slightly stronger in non-OBE than in OBE EDs. There was no evidence of the alternate indirect effect in either ED group; SASB Affiliation had significant strong direct effects on EDE-Q Global in both samples, whereas indirect effects through DERS were negligible and CI:s included zero (see Table 2).

Extended parallel mediation models in EDs without OBE

All models were significant ($ps < .001$; $R^2s = .46$) where DERS dimensions and the majority of SASB clusters were moderately to strongly and significantly associated (a-paths, see all paths for all models in Fig. 3), whereas there were only a few small significant associations between SASB clusters and ED psychopathology when controlling for DERS-dimensions (b-paths). In all models, each emotion dysregulation dimension first had significant moderate associations with ED psychopathology (c-paths; total effects), but when controlling for

Table 1 Descriptives for EDs without OBE ($n = 439$) and EDs with OBE ($n = 560$) on background variables and all main measures, and independent t-test comparisons. Cohen's d (small $\geq .02$, medium $\geq .05$, large $\geq .08$) computed for $p < .01$ differences

Variable	Non-OBE EDs		OBE EDs		t-value	p	Cohen's d
	M (SD)	Min - Max	M (SD)	Min - Max			
Age	23.46 (7.90)	16–66	25.83 (8.61)	16–72	− 4.487	<.001	.287
ED-duration	7.49 (8.12)	0–44	10.04 (8.70)	0–56	−4.739	<.001	.303
BMI	18.78 (3.91)	12.7–43.0	24.29 (6.24)	12.3–53.9	− 16.185	<.001	1.059
EDE-Q Global Score	3.50 (1.35)	0–5.8	4.15 (0.99)	0.2–6	− 8.713	<.001	.545
DERS dimensions:							
1. Awareness/Clarity	32.43 (8.80)	11–55	32.63 (8.68)	11–55	−.355	.723	
2. Non-Acceptance	15.91 (6.16)	6–30	16.61 (6.25)	6–30	−1.747	.081	
3. Goals/Impulse	29.64 (10.47)	11–55	32.28 (10.42)	11–55	− 3.972	<.001	.253
4. Strategies	20.33 (7.81)	8–40	22.15 (7.57)	8–40	−3.715	<.001	.236
DERS Total	98.31 (26.80)	38–176	103.66 (26.07)	38–169	−3.180	.002	.202
SASB clusters:							
1. Self-emancipation	30.36 (17.35)	0–82	32.28 (16.23)	0–90	−1.803	.072	
2. Self-affirmation	32.15 (21.85)	0–100	27.77 (18.17)	0–100	3.454	.001	.218
3. Self-love	32.18 (21.20)	0–100	29.00 (18.23)	0–88	2.542	.011	
4. Self-protection	42.41 (21.04)	0–100	39.71 (19.15)	0–95	2.114	.035	
5. Self-control	59.77 (17.55)	0–100	55.44 (18.06)	0–100	3.814	<.001	.243
6. Self-blame	56.48 (24.64)	0–100	59.20 (22.70)	0–100	−1.808	.071	
7. Self-attack	41.01 (26.02)	0–100	44.71 (23.80)	0–100	−2.342	.019	
8. Self-neglect	36.59 (22.46)	0–100	42.33 (21.57)	0–98	−4.094	<.001	.261
SASB Affiliation	−9.06 (39.37)	−92.5 – 99.2	−16.41 (34.01)	−89.5 – 84.3	3.162	.002	.200

BMI body mass index, *DERS* Difficulties in Emotion Regulation Scale, *ED* eating disorder, *EDE-Q* Eating Disorder Examination Questionnaire, *OBE* objective binge-eating episode, *SASB* Structural Analysis of Social Behavior

Table 2 Simple mediation models examining the hypothesized model and an alternative model in EDs without OBE (*n* = 439) and EDs with OBE (*n* = 560), using standardized variables and 99% CI:s using 10,000 bootstrap samples. All models adjusted for age and BMI

Group	Path *a*	Path *b*	Total effect (*c*)	Indirect effect (*ab*)	99% CI	Direct effect (*c'*)	Model *R²*
Hypothesized direction (DERS Total - > SASB Affiliation - > EDE-Q Global)							
Non-OBE EDs	−.718***	−.631***	.451***	.453	.351–.564	−.002 (n.s.)	.414***
OBE EDs	−.654***	−.479***	.417***	.313	.221–.419	.104*	.304***
Alternative direction (SASB Affiliation - > DERS Total - > EDE-Q Global)							
Non-OBE EDs	−.709***	−.002 (n.s.)	−.630***	.002	−.089–.095	−.631***	.414***
OBE EDs	−.652***	.104*	−.547***	−.068	−.152–.013	−.479***	.304***

BMI body mass index, *DERS* Difficulties in Emotion Regulation Scale, *CI* confidence interval, *ED* eating disorder; *EDE-Q* Eating Disorder Examination Questionnaire, *OBE* objective binge-eating episode, *SASB* Structural Analysis of Social Behavior
*p < .05; ***p < .001

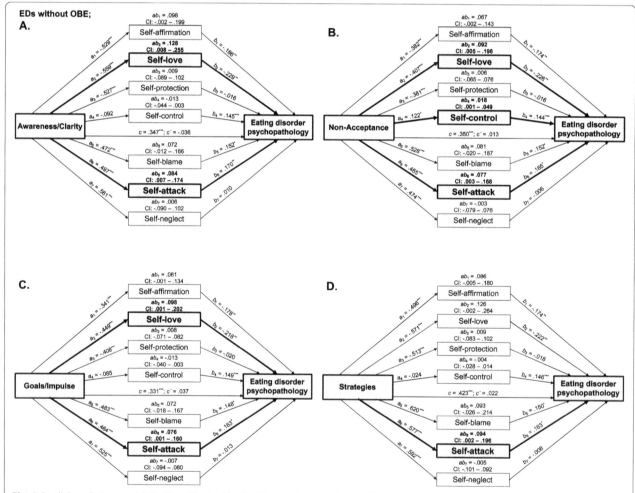

Fig. 3 Parallel mediation models in EDs without objective binge-eating episodes positing emotion dysregulation dimensions as independent variables (**a**. Awareness/Clarity; **b**. Non-Acceptance; **c**. Goals/Impulse; **d**. Strategies), self-directed behaviors as mediators, and ED psychopathology as dependent variable. All effects are adjusted for age and BMI. Bold style and grey boxes indicate indirect effects different from zero. Path coefficients are based on standardized variables; examination of indirect effects is based 99% confidence intervals using 10,000 bootstrap samples. *= p < .05; **= p < .01; ***= p < .001

self-directed behaviors, these associations were non-significant (c´-paths; direct effects); they were instead mediated by different SASB clusters.

Awareness/Clarity had an indirect effect on EDE-Q such that higher difficulties in emotional awareness and clarity through lower levels of self-love and higher self-attack was associated with higher ED psychopathology. No other indirect effects had CI's entirely above zero. *Non-acceptance* had an indirect effect on EDE-Q where higher emotional non-acceptance through lower self-love, higher self-control, and higher self-attack was associated with higher ED psychopathology. No other indirect effects had CI's entirely above zero. *Goals/Impulse* had an indirect effect on EDE-Q where higher difficulties maintaining impulse control and goal-directed behaviors when in distress through lower self-love and higher self-attack was associated with higher ED psychopathology. *Strategies* had an indirect effect on EDE-Q where higher

emotional helplessness through higher self-attack was associated with higher ED psychopathology. No other indirect effects had CI's entirely above zero.

Extended parallel mediation models in EDs with OBE

Again, all models were significant (ps < .001; R^2s = .34) where DERS dimensions and the majority of SASB clusters had significant moderate to strong associations (a-paths, see all paths for all models in Fig. 4), with only a few small significant associations between SASB clusters and ED psychopathology when controlling for DERS-dimensions (b-paths). The DERS-dimensions had small to moderate significant associations with ED psycho-pathology (c-paths), which were reduced when controlling for self-directed behaviors (c´-paths; direct effects), i.e., these effects were mediated by SASB clusters, albeit different ones compared to non-OBE EDs.

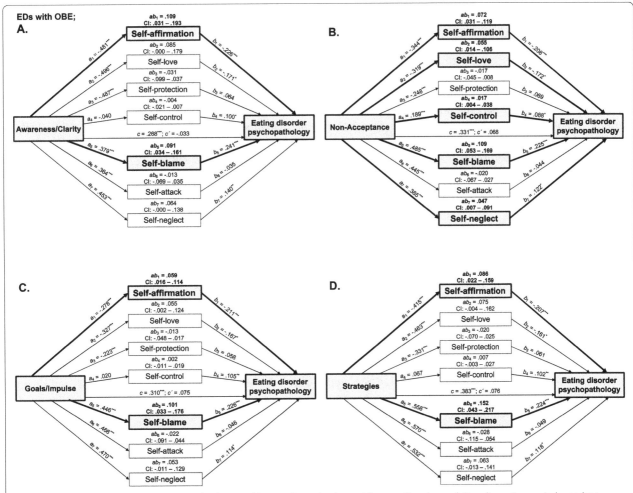

Fig. 4 Pabrallel mediation models in EDs with objective binge-eating episodes positing emotion dysregulation dimensions as independent variables (a: Awareness/Clarity; b. Non-Acceptance; c. Goals/Impulse; d. Strategies), self-directed behaviors as mediators, and ED psychopathology as dependent variable. All effects are adjusted for age and BMI. Bold style and grey boxes indicate indirect effects different from zero. Path coefficients are based on standardized variables, examination of indirect effects is based 99% confidence intervals using 10,000 bootstrap samples. * = p < .05; ** = p < .01; *** = p < .001

Awareness/Clarity had an indirect effect on EDE-Q such that higher difficulties in emotional awareness and clarity through lower self-affirmation and higher self-blame was associated with higher ED psychopathology. No other indirect effects had CI's entirely above zero. *Non-acceptance* had an indirect effect on EDE-Q where higher emotional non-acceptance through lower self-affirmation, lower self-love, higher self-control, higher self-blame, and higher self-neglect was associated with higher ED psychopathology. No other indirect effects had CI's entirely above zero. *Goals/Impulse* had specific indirect effects on EDE-Q where higher difficulties maintaining impulse control and goal-directed behaviors when in distress through lower self-affirmation and higher self-blame was associated with higher ED psychopathology. No other specific indirect effects had CI's entirely above zero. *Strategies* had an indirect effect on EDE-Q where higher emotional helplessness through lower self-affirmation and higher self-blame was associated with higher ED psychopathology. No other indirect effects had CI's entirely above zero.

Discussion

The present study examined associations between trait-level emotion dysregulation, self-directed behaviors, and ED psychopathology in patients who were grouped according to absence or presence of OBE. We found that emotion dysregulation was associated with ED psychopathology through pathology specific self-directed behaviors. The simple mediation results will be summarized and discussed first, followed by the extended mediation results. Thereafter, the theoretical and clinical implications of these results will be discussed.

As hypothesized, our previous mediation finding in a sample of female students [8] was replicated in ED patients. Emotion dysregulation was strongly associated with negative self-directed behavior in both ED groups, and independently, both concepts were moderately (emotion dysregulation) and strongly (self-directed behaviors) associated with ED psychopathology, in line with prior findings [32, 55]. However, emotion dysregulation only had an indirect effect on ED psychopathology through self-directed behaviors, while self-directed behaviors had a strong association with ED psychopathology independent of emotion dysregulation. Associations were generally slightly stronger in the present sample compared to the students [8], and slightly stronger in participants without OBE. Of note, these participants scored somewhat lower ED psychopathology, overall emotion dysregulation, and negative self-directed behaviors although scoring higher self-control, the latter in line with previous findings [26]. Regarding emotion dysregulation, binge-eating participants specifically scored slightly more emotional helplessness, and

difficulties focusing and maintaining control when upset, the latter in line with previous research [18].

Among participants without OBE, the most prominent mediators concerned affiliation (i.e., decreased active self-love and increased self-attack). In participants with OBE, both affiliation and autonomy were involved (i.e., decreased self-affirmation and increased self-blame). Self-blame, -love, and -affirmation have previously shown strong associations with ED psychopathology [4], but their function as potential mechanisms between emotion dysregulation dimensions and ED psychopathology are novel findings.

Although mediators differed between groups based on symptomatology, they diverged surprisingly little between models within each group. Prior work on the DERS suggests that Awareness tends to diverge, for instance by showing weaker relations with other psychopathology and the other subscales except with Clarity [46, 49]. Even so, mediators in this model were similar to the other models within each group; different emotion dysregulation dimensions seem associated with ED psychopathology through similar self-directed behaviors within each ED pathology type. Only the Non-acceptance models included additional mediators: higher self-control among participants without OBE; lower self-love, higher self-control, and higher self-neglect among participants with OBE. However, these indirect effects were smaller than others, and although SASB self-control has showed clinically relevant associations in EDs [28, 29], our self-control results needs to be interpreted with caution due to questionable scale reliability.

Possibly, other ways of grouping patients, for instance by directly assessed impulsivity, compulsivity, or overall psychiatric symptom load; or by narrowing the groups even further (e.g., contrasting highly restrictive patients with multi-impulsive ones), might have generated higher specificity, as well as clarifying the clinical relevance of the differences we saw.

Theoretical and clinical implications

Our overall results suggest that emotion dysregulation only has an indirect effect on ED psychopathology through self-directed behaviors, whereas self-directed behaviors have a substantial direct effect on ED psychopathology. Therefore, self-directed behaviors should likely always be addressed in treatment, both independently and as an important process whereby patients may currently attempt to manage their emotions. Patterns of emotion (dys) regulation and self-directed behaviors develop in childhood within attachment relationships where the child's emerging sense of self as capable or deficient, and worthy of encouragement and care, or of criticism and neglect, is formed in ongoing interactions. These interactions with significant others are *introjected* and become future self-directed behaviors [7], also forming the foundation of emotion regulation abilities [56, 57].

The specific indirect effects indicate differing processes and needs depending on ED presentation. Among participants without loss of control binge-eating, emotion dysregulation was associated with *lower self-love* and *higher self-attack*, which in turn was associated with greater ED psychopathology. Experiencing emotions as unacceptable was additionally associated with somewhat *higher self-control* in relation to pathology. Self-love reflects secure attachment and the experience that someone important provides safety, love, and understanding when needed. Such an experience may be particularly important when emotions are undifferentiated, uncomfortable, or feel out of control. Our results suggest that in such situations, patients who do not lose control over eating may tend to believe that they will not be met with loving care. For these patients, ED psychopathology might serve to cut them off from themselves and others, thereby suppressing the hope for love, but preserving a coherent albeit pathological sense of self. In interpersonal theory, self-hate is understood as introjected interactions characterized by attacking and recoiling, taking the form of aggressive efforts to either master, or gain distance from, perceived threats [7]. Speculatively, in these patients, emotions could represent such threats, evoking aggressive attack towards the body by engagement in ED pathology, thereby concretizing self-attack.

This perspective adds to existing models of primarily restrictive patients, such as the functional emotional avoidance model [16] and the cognitive-interpersonal maintenance model [33], both of which highlight the avoidant/alexithymic emotional processing style in restrictive patients. Our results indicate that therapists who treat restrictive EDs with cognitive-behavioral therapy (CBT) may need to help patients understand how problems regulating emotions could be translated into self-attack and lack of self-love. Interventions based on self-compassion [35] may benefit these patients if delivered with an explicit focus bridging the gap between feelings and symptoms. Psychodynamic and interpersonal therapists who may already be attending to attachment issues, may nevertheless need to place increased focus on patients' sense of security when exploring emotional awareness and instances of self-attack, especially in the context of the therapeutic relationship.

Participants who had loss of control binge-eating displayed a more complex pattern. All emotion dysregulation dimensions were associated with *lower self-affirmation,* which in turn was associated with greater ED psychopathology. Since emotion dysregulation thereby may entail concomitant perceptions of not being met with openness and acceptance, distress tolerance and the possibility of disentangling emotional interpersonal situations may become reduced, thereby increasing the risk for patients to resort to symptoms as a form of distraction. All emotion dysregulation dimensions were also associated with *higher self-blame*; difficulties in emotional acceptance additionally implied *higher self-neglect, higher self-control* and *lower self-love,* in turn associated with greater ED psychopathology. While both self-blame and self-neglect are hostile, self-blame also encompasses aspects of control whereas self-neglect implies relinquishing control. In interpersonal theory, self-blame parallels interpersonal interactions characterized by blaming and appeasing; self-neglect parallels ignoring and walling off. Trying to appease a hostile and controlling other (internally or externally perceived) may necessitate hypervigilance until whatever is perceived as threatening has receded, either by aggressive actions or depressive withdrawal [7]. In the context of threatening emotions, these patients may anxiously oscillate between hostile self-control or by giving up. The former might spur increased efforts of perfectionistic restraint, whereas the latter might spur further loss-of-control symptoms (cf. the "what-the-hell effect" where minor violations of a perfectionistic dietary rule leads to overindulgence) [58]. However, as we only modelled global ED psychopathology, such differentiated outcomes are only speculations.

These findings contribute to dysregulation models of binge-eating pathology [5, 21, 34] by suggesting inclusion of self-blame and spontaneity (in both positive and negative ways) as key processes to highlight in treatment, in that they may represent subjectively valid links between emotions and symptoms. In CBT, learning to tolerate anxiety, disentangling distressing events, and increasing curiosity towards one's mental states, while neither trying to increase negative control nor giving up, might be particularly important. Psychodynamic and interpersonal therapists could explore associations between emotions, negative self-control, and symptoms, while helping patients to understand how relationships inside and outside therapy impact on symptoms.

Our results also suggest that therapists need to be mindful of their own reactions, regardless of psychotherapeutic approach, in order not to maintain problematic regulation processes [7]. For instance, a patient who walls off and increases ED symptoms might trigger expressions of frustration or anger in the therapist, which in turn risks confirming the patient's pathological self-related beliefs and emotion regulation strategies. If therapists instead show interest, acceptance, and validation, while openly acknowledging and discussing challenges to the therapeutic process, patients may find it easier to move from self-hostility toward self-affiliation.

Strengths and limitations

This study had several strengths. Our large, nationally representative clinical sample, including most DSM-5 EDs, strengthened the ecological validity of findings. Additionally, the study concurrently examined both emotional and self-related factors previously shown to be meaningful in EDs, and the analysis of these factors in two clinically relevant sub-samples allowed high specificity. There are, however, also several important limitations.

First, since we only had trait-level cross-sectional data, we cannot infer causality. Although statistical mediation, including contrasting with models stipulating the opposite direction of effect, might indicate the possibility of a causal association, other research designs are needed to support such claims. Second, we had no control over DERS administration, possibly biasing the sample. Although there were no differences in patient related variables (e.g., ED pathology, self-directed behaviors, depression, anxiety, age) depending on if patients were administered the DERS or not, there might be unknown factors that affect the generalizability of the results. Third, the results may only generalize to treatment-seeking females. Fourth, although the DERS variables used in this study are based on Gratz and Roemer's original and clinically relevant conceptualization of emotion dysregulation [6], they are not psychometrically examined and validated in clinical samples. A lower-order correlated traits model including these four as the traits has showed bad fit in university students [59], but no study to our knowledge has examined this solution or alternative second-order or bifactor four-factor solutions in clinical samples (where models showing good fit in control samples often do not fit as well) [46, 49]. However, subscale intercorrelations (Tables S1 and S2), theoretical groundwork [6, 13, 60], and prior findings regarding unique contribution of individual subscales [46, 49, 61] indicate that the combination of Awareness/ Clarity and Goals/Impulse is theoretically relevant and empirically reasonable. Fifth, the patient categorization in this study is not commonly accepted, and we only considered OBE but not purging when dividing participants. However, some prior findings point to relevant differences depending on presence/absence of binge-eating in EDs [39, 62], and stronger unique associations between binge-eating and negative urgency compared to those with purging has been reported in female students [40]. Additionally, there were some relevant differences, and results did differ, between samples which provides some validity to this categorization when considering the constructs under consideration here. Even so, future research needs to examine the potential impact of both binge-eating and purging further. Sixth, in the extended mediation analysis, the use of 99% CI when boot-strapping indirect effects undoubtedly widened the CI:s which, in combination with the inclusion of seven more or less correlated mediators in each model, likely contributed to the observed indirect effects being relatively few and rather weak [54]. Our rationale was due to the exploratory nature of this study and lack of previous findings, although our large samples likely counteracted some uncertainty in the results. Future replication could select the most prominent mediators to refine the mediation models. Lastly, the internal consistency was poor for SASB Cluster 1 and questionable for Cluster 5. We chose to exclude Cluster 1, while all results including Cluster 5 needs to be interpreted with great caution. Internal consistency was acceptable to excellent for all other variables.

Conclusions

We found ED pathology specific association pathways whereby emotion dysregulation was associated with more negative self-directed behaviors, which in turn were associated with greater ED psychopathology. This indicates that addressing patients' self-directed behaviors could be an important way of helping patients deal with their emotions in relation to their ED psychopathology. In participants without loss of control over eating, lower self-love and higher self-attack were influential factors, whereas in participants with loss of control over eating, lower self-affirmation and higher self-blame were influential.

Abbreviations

AN: Anorexia nervosa; AN-R: Anorexia nervosa restricting subtype; AN-BP: Anorexia nervosa binge/purge subtype; BED: Binge eating disorder; BN: Bulimia nervosa; CBT: Cognitive behavioral therapy; CI: Confidence interval; DERS: Difficulties in Emotion Regulation Scale; DSM: Diagnostic and Statistical Manual of mental disorders; ED: Eating disorder; EDE-Q: Eating Disorder Examination Questionnaire; OBE: Objective binge-eating episode; OSFED: Other specified feeding and eating disorders; SASB: Structural Analysis of Social Behavior; SEDI: Structured Eating Disorder; UFED: Unspecified feeding and eating disorders

Authors' contributions

All authors contributed to aims and design. EM completed the analyses and was the major contributor in writing the manuscript. All authors read and approved the final manuscript.

Competing interests

The authors declare that they have no competing interests.

Author details

Centre for Psychiatry Research, Department of Clinical Neuroscience, Karolinska Institute, and Stockholm Health Care Services, Stockholm County Council, Norra Stationsgatan 69, SE-11364 Stockholm, Sweden. [2]Department of Medical Epidemiology and Biostatistics, Karolinska Institutet, Stockholm, Sweden. [3]Institute for Eating Disorders, Oslo, Sweden.

References

1. Schaumberg K, Welch E, Breithaupt L, Hubel C, Baker JH, Munn-Chernoff MA, et al. The science behind the academy for eating disorders' nine truths about eating disorders. Eur Eat Disord Rev. 2017;25(6):432–50.
2. Culbert KM, Racine SE, Klump KL. Research review: what we have learned about the causes of eating disorders – a synthesis of sociocultural, psychological, and biological research. J Child Psychol Psychiatry. 2015; 56(11):1141–64.
3. National Institute for Health and Care Excellence (NICE). Eating Disorders: recognition and treatment: NICE guideline [NG69]. London: NICE; 2017.
4. Forsén Mantilla E, Birgegård A. The enemy within: the association between self-image and eating disorder symptoms in healthy, non help-seeking and clinical young women. J Eat Disord. 2015;3:30.
5. Pearson CM, Wonderlich SA, Smith GT. A risk and maintenance model for bulimia nervosa: from impulsive action to compulsive behavior. Psychol Rev. 2015;122(3):516–35.
6. Gratz KL, Roemer L. Multidimensional assessment of emotion regulation and dysregulation: development, factor structure, and initial validation of the difficulties in emotion regulation scale. J Psychopathol Behav. 2004;26(1):41–54.
7. Benjamin LS. Interpersonal reconstructive therapy for anger, anxiety, and depression: It's about broken hearts, not broken brains. Washington, DC: American Psychological Association; 2018.
8. Monell E, Högdahl L, Forsén Mantilla E, Birgegård A. Emotion dysregulation, self-image and eating disorder symptoms in University Women. J Eat Disord. 2015;3(44).
9. Monell E, Clinton D, Birgegård A. Emotion dysregulation and eating disorders-associations with diagnostic presentation and key symptoms. Int J Eat Disord. 2018;51(8):921–30.
10. Svaldi J, Griepenstroh J, Tuschen-Caffier B, Ehring T. Emotion regulation deficits in eating disorders: a marker of eating pathology or general psychopathology? Psychiatry Res. 2012;197(1–2):103–11.
11. Racine SE, Wildes JE. Dynamic longitudinal relations between emotion regulation difficulties and anorexia nervosa symptoms over the year following intensive treatment. J Consult Clin Psychol. 2015;83(4):785–95..
12. Haedt-Matt AA, Keel PK. Revisiting the affect regulation model of binge eating: a meta-analysis of studies using ecological momentary assessment. Psychol Bull. 2011;137(4):660–81.
13. Preece D, Becerra R, Allan A, Robinson K, Dandy J. Establishing the theoretical components of alexithymia via factor analysis: introduction and validation of the attention-appraisal model of alexithymia. Personal Individ Differ. 2017;119:341–52.
14. Skårderud F. Eating one's words, part II: the embodied mind and reflective function in anorexia nervosa–theory. Eur Eat Disord Rev. 2007;15(4):243–52.
15. Nowakowski ME, McFarlane T, Cassin S. Alexithymia and eating disorders: a critical review of the literature. J Eat Disord. 2013;1:21.
16. Wildes JE, Marcus MD. Development of emotion acceptance behavior therapy for anorexia nervosa: a case series. Int J Eat Disord. 2011;44(5):421–7.
17. Merwin RM, Zucker NL, Lacy JL, Elliott CA. Interoceptive awareness in eating disorders: distinguishing lack of clarity from non-acceptance of internal experience. Cognit Emot. 2010;24(5):892–902.
18. Mallorquí-Bague N, Vintro-Alcaraz C, Sanchez I, Riesco N, Aguera Z, Granero R, et al. Emotion regulation as a Transdiagnostic feature among eating disorders: cross-sectional and longitudinal approach. Eur Eat Disord Rev. 2018;26(1):53–61.
19. Pisetsky EM, Haynos AF, Lavender JM, Crow SJ, Peterson CB. Associations between emotion regulation difficulties, eating disorder symptoms, non-suicidal self-injury, and suicide attempts in a heterogeneous eating disorder sample. Compr Psychiatry. 2017;73:143–50.
20. MacDonald DE, Trottier K, Olmsted MP. Rapid improvements in emotion regulation predict intensive treatment outcome for patients with bulimia nervosa and purging disorder. Int J Eat Disord. 2017;50(10):1152–61.
21. Fairburn CG, Cooper Z, Shafran R. Cognitive behaviour therapy for eating disorders: a "transdiagnostic" theory and treatment. Behav Res Ther. 2003; 41(5):509–28.
22. American Psychiatric Association. Diagnostic and statistical manual of mental disorders. Text Revision, 4th ed. Washington DC: American Psychiatric Association; 2000.
23. Benjamin LS. Structural analysis of social behavior. Psychol Rev. 1974;81(5): 392–425.
24. Godier LR, Park RJ. Compulsivity in anorexia nervosa: a transdiagnostic concept. Front Psychol. 2014;5:778.
25. Bruch H. Anorexia nervosa: therapy and theory. Am J Psychiatry. 1982; 139(12):1531–8.
26. Björck C, Clinton D, Sohlberg S, Hällstrom T, Norring C. Interpersonal profiles in eating disorders: ratings of SASB self-image. Psychol Psychother. 2003; 76(Pt 4):337–49.
27. Patel K, Tchanturia K, Harrison A. An exploration of social functioning in young people with eating disorders: a qualitative study. PLoS One. 2016; 11(7):e0159910.
28. Birgegård A, Björck C, Norring C, Sohlberg S, Clinton D. Anorexic self-control and bulimic self-hate: differential outcome prediction from initial self-image. Int J Eat Disord. 2009;42(6):522–30.
29. Andersen M, Birgegård A. Diagnosis-specific self-image predicts longitudinal suicidal ideation in adult eating disorders. Int J Eat Disord. 2017;50(8):970–8.
30. Haynos AF, Forman EM, Butryn ML, Lillis J. Mindfulness and acceptance for treating eating disorders and weight concerns: evidence-based interventions. Oakland: New Harbinger Publications; 2016.
31. Forsén Mantilla E, Norring C, Birgegård A. Self-image and 12-month outcome in females with eating disorders: extending previous findings. J Eat Disord. 2019;7(15).
32. Pennesi JL, Wade TD. A systematic review of the existing models of disordered eating: do they inform the development of effective interventions? Clin Psychol Rev. 2016;43:175–92.
33. Treasure J, Schmidt U. The cognitive-interpersonal maintenance model of anorexia nervosa revisited: a summary of the evidence for cognitive, socio-emotional and interpersonal predisposing and perpetuating factors. J Eat Disord. 2013;1(13):13.
34. Wonderlich SA, Peterson CB, Smith TL, Klein HM, Mitchell JE, Crow SJ. Integrative cognitive-affective therapy for bulimia nervosa: a treatment manual. New York: Guilford Publications; 2015.
35. Gale C, Gilbert P, Read N, Goss K. An evaluation of the impact of introducing compassion focused therapy to a standard treatment programme for people with eating disorders. Clin Psychol Psychother. 2014; 21(1):1–12.
36. Schaumberg K, Jangmo A, Thornton LM, Birgegård A, Almqvist C, Norring C, et al. Patterns of diagnostic transition in eating disorders: a longitudinal population study in Sweden. Psychol Med. 2019;49(5):819–27.
37. Peat C, Mitchell JE, Hoek HW, Wonderlich SA. Validity and utility of subtyping anorexia nervosa. Int J Eat Disord. 2009;42(7):590–4.
38. Claes L, Vandereyeken W, Vertommen H. Impulsive and compulsive traits in eating disordered patients compared with controls. Personal Individ Differ. 2002;32(4):707–14.
39. Fernandez-Aranda F, Pinheiro AP, Thornton LM, Berrettini WH, Crow S, Fichter MM, et al. Impulse control disorders in women with eating disorders. Psychiatry Res. 2008;157(1–3):147–57.
40. Peterson CM, Fischer S. A prospective study of the influence of the UPPS model of impulsivity on the co-occurrence of bulimic symptoms and non-suicidal self-injury. Eat Behav. 2012;13(4):335–41.
41. Safer DL, Telch CH, Chen EY, Linehan MM. Dialectical behavior therapy for binge eating and bulimia. New York: Guilford Publications; 2009.
42. Hempel R, Vanderbleek E, Lynch TR. Radically open DBT: targeting emotional loneliness in anorexia nervosa. Eat Disord. 2018;26(1):92–104.
43. Birgegård A, Björck C, Clinton D. Quality assurance of specialised treatment of eating disorders using large-scale internet-based collection systems: methods, results and lessons learned from designing the stepwise database. Eur Eat Disord Rev. 2010;18(4):251–9.
44. de Man Lapidoth J, Birgegård A. Validation of the structured eating disorder interview (SEDI) against the eating disorder examination (EDE). Stockholm: Karolinska Institutet; 2010.
45. American Psychiatric Association. Diagnostic and statistical manual of mental disorders. 5th ed. Washington DC: American Psychiatric Association; 2013.

46. Nordgren L, Monell E, Birgegård A, Bjureberg J, Hesser H. Factor structure of the difficulties in emotion regulation scale in treatment seeking adults with eating disorders. J Psychopathol Behav. 2020;42(1):111–26.

47. Medrano LA, Trogolo M. Construct Validity of the Difficulties in Emotion Regulation Scale: Further Evidence Using Confirmatory Factor Analytic Approach. Abnormal Behav Psychol. 2016;2(2).

48. Cho Y, Hong S. The new factor structure of the Korean version of the difficulties in emotion regulation scale (K-DERS) incorporating method factor. Meas Eval Couns Dev. 2017;46(3):192–201.

49. Osborne TL, Michonski J, Sayrs J, Welch SS, Anderson LK. Factor structure of the difficulties in emotion regulation scale (DERS) in adult outpatients receiving dialectical behavior therapy (DBT). J Psychopathol Behav. 2017; 39(2):355–71.

50. Benjamin LS. SASB Intrex user's manual. Utah: University of Utah; 2000.

51. Fairburn CG, Beglin SJ. Assessment of eating disorders: interview or self-report questionnaire? Int J Eat Disord. 1994;16(4):363–70.

52. Luce KH, Crowther JH. The reliability of the eating disorder examination-self-report questionnaire version (EDE-Q). Int J Eat Disord. 1999;25(3):349–51.

53. Welch E, Birgegård A, Parling T, Ghaderi A. Eating disorder examination questionnaire and clinical impairment assessment questionnaire: general population and clinical norms for young adult women in Sweden. Behav Res Ther. 2011;49(2):85–91.

54. Hayes AF. Introduction to mediation, moderation, and conditional process analysis: a regression-based approach. Second ed. New York: The Guolford Press; 2018.

55. Kästner D, Lowe B, Gumz A. The role of self-esteem in the treatment of patients with anorexia nervosa – a systematic review and meta-analysis. Int J Eat Disord. 2019;52(2):101–16.

56. Bowlby J. A secure base: parent-child attachment and healthy human development. New York: Basic Books; 1988.

57. Mikulincer M, Shaver PR. Attachment orientations and emotion regulation. Curr Opin Psychol. 2019;25:6–10.

58. Herman CP, Polivy J. A boundary model for the regulation of eating. Psychiatr Ann. 1983;13(12):918–27.

59. Lee DJ, Witte TK, Bardeen JR, Davis MT, Weathers FW. A factor analytic evaluation of the difficulties in emotion regulation scale. J Clin Psychol. 2016;72(9):933–46.

60. Hayes SC, Wilson KG, Gifford EV, Follette VM, Strosahl K. Experiential avoidance and behavioral disorders: a functional dimensional approach to diagnosis and treatment. J Consult Clin Psychol. 1996;64(6):1152–68.

61. Benfer N, Bardeen JR, Fergus TA, Rogers TA. Factor structure and incremental validity of the original and modified versions of the difficulties in emotion regulation scale. J Pers Assess. 2018;101(6):598–608.

62. Gleaves DH, Brown JD, Warren CS. The continuity/discontinuity models of eating disorders: a review of the literature and implications for assessment, treatment, and prevention. Behav Modif. 2004;28(6):739–62.

12

Dialectical behavior therapy adapted for binge eating compared to cognitive behavior therapy in obese adults with binge eating disorder: A controlled study

Mirjam W. Lammers[1,2]* (iD), Maartje S. Vroling[1,2], Ross D. Crosby[3,4] and Tatjana van Strien[2]

Abstract

Background: Current guidelines recommend cognitive behavior therapy (CBT) as the treatment of choice for binge eating disorder (BED). Although CBT is quite effective, a substantial number of patients do not reach abstinence from binge eating. To tackle this problem, various theoretical conceptualizations and treatment models have been proposed. Dialectical behavior therapy (DBT), focusing on emotion regulation, is one such model. Preliminary evidence comparing DBT adapted for BED (DBT-BED) to CBT is promising but the available data do not favor one treatment over the other. The aim of this study is to evaluate outcome of DBT-BED, compared to a more intensive eating disorders-focused form of cognitive behavior therapy (CBT+), in individuals with BED who are overweight and engage in emotional eating.

Methods: Seventy-four obese patients with BED who reported above average levels of emotional eating were quasi-randomly allocated to one of two manualized 20-session group treatments: DBT-BED ($n = 41$) or CBT+ ($n = 33$). Intention-to-treat outcome was examined at post-treatment and at 6-month follow-up using general or generalized linear models with multiple imputation.

Results: Overall, greater improvements were observed in CBT+. Differences in number of objective binge eating episodes at end of treatment, and eating disorder psychopathology (EDE-Q Global score) and self-esteem (EDI-3 Low Self-Esteem) at follow-up reached statistical significance with medium effect sizes (Cohen's d between .46 and .59). Of the patients in the DBT group, 69.9% reached clinically significant change at end of the treatment vs 65.0% at follow-up. Although higher, this was not significantly different from the patients in the CBT+ group (52.9% vs 45.8%).

(Continued on next page)

* Correspondence: m.lammers@ggnet.nl
[1]Amarum, Expertise Centre for Eating Disorders, GGNet Network for Mental Health Care, Den Elterweg 75, 7207 AE Zutphen, The Netherlands
[2]Radboud University, Behavioural Science Institute, Montessorilaan 3, 6525 HR Nijmegen, The Netherlands
Full list of author information is available at the end of the article

(Continued from previous page)

Conclusions: The results of this study show that CBT+ produces better outcomes than the less intensive DBT-BED on several measures. Yet, regardless of the dose-difference, the data suggest that DBT-BED and CBT+ lead to comparable levels of clinically meaningful change in global eating disorder psychopathology. Future recommendations include the need for dose-matched comparisons in a sufficiently powered randomized controlled trial, and the need to determine mediators and moderators of treatment outcome.

Keywords: Binge eating disorder, Cognitive behavior therapy, Dialectical behavior therapy, Group therapy, Emotion regulation

Plain English summary

Binge eating disorder (BED) is mostly treated with cognitive behavior therapy (CBT). The treatment focusses on reducing efforts to diet. Yet, a substantial number of patients still suffer from binge eating after this treatment. We suggest that patients with BED are better served with a treatment that helps them cope with negative emotions in a healthier way. Dialectical behavior therapy for BED (DBT-BED) is one such treatment. To test this, we compared outcomes of DBT-BED to the intensive CBT program that is common in our treatment center. We did so, in individuals with BED who might especially benefit from DBT-BED: those who are overweight and eat in response to emotions. Greater improvements were observed in the CBT group regarding the number of objective binge eating episodes at the end of treatment, and regarding global eating disorder psychopathology and self-esteem 6 months after treatment. Yet, patients in the CBT group received more therapy hours than in the DBT-BED group, which may have advantaged the CBT treatment. Concurrently, in both groups a comparable percentage of patients showed clinically meaningful changes in global eating disorder psychopathology. In conclusion, our results overall support the intensive CBT program over DBT-BED. Yet, given the fact that DBT-BED is less time-consuming (so cheaper) and presents similar percentages of meaningful change in global eating disorder psychopathology, it is worthwhile to further test the effects of DBT-BED in future studies.

Introduction

Binge eating disorder (BED) is characterized by psychologically distressing, recurrent, brief episodes of uncontrollable overeating [1]. It is associated with psychiatric comorbidity, impaired social functioning and impaired physical well-being [2, 3]. An estimated 70% of BED patients have a body mass index (BMI) between 30 and 40, and about 20% have a BMI of 40 or higher [4]. While aspects of body-image disturbance are part of the diagnostic criteria for anorexia nervosa and bulimia nervosa,

these aspects are not included in the criteria for BED [1]. Nevertheless, several aspects (e.g. body dissatisfaction and the overvaluation of body shape and weight) have shown to be relevant to BED [5]. Current guidelines recommend cognitive behavior therapy (CBT) as the treatment of choice for BED [6, 7]. The most widely supported form of CBT for BED is based on the transdiagnostic model of eating disorders, suggesting that distinctive eating disorders are maintained by similar mechanisms [8]. Clinical perfectionism, interpersonal difficulties, low self-esteem and mood intolerance are acknowledged to act as maintaining factors in many patients. However, the core CBT-protocol focusses on behavior (i.e. dietary restraint) that is related to the overvaluation of body shape and weight [9, 10]. Although CBT is quite effective in BED, about 50% do not fully respond to treatment [11]. This may be related to the fact that overvaluation of body shape and weight is only present in a subset of individuals with BED [12]. In addition, dietary restraint seems to be stronger in bulimia nervosa than in BED [13, 14]. Interventions that focus on other maintaining mechanisms may therefore improve abstinence rates.

One model of interest is the affect regulation model. It assumes that binge eating is triggered by high levels of negative affect and that binge eating reduces negative affect [15, 16]. While mixed empirical support has emerged for the second part of this hypothesis (e.g. [17–20]), the first part has received extensive support from both retrospective studies (e.g. 17, 18, 21]), experimental studies [22] and ecological momentary assessment (EMA) studies [19, 20]. Also, greater elevations of negative affect prior to binge eating were found in BED when compared to bulimia nervosa [20]. Therefore, interventions that specifically target affect-related difficulties may improve outcome in patients with BED.

One treatment that specifically aims to address deficits in affect regulation is dialectical behavior therapy (DBT [23];). DBT, originally developed for patients with borderline personality disorder and ongoing self-harm or suicidal behaviors, has been adapted to treat BED (DBT-BED: e.g. [24]). DBT-BED aims to improve adequate emotion regulation skills in order to replace binge eating as a way of coping with negative affect [16]. To date, two randomized controlled trials have compared DBT-BED in patients with a primary diagnosis of BED to a waitlist control group, showing significantly less eating disordered behavior for DBT-BED at post-treatment and at 6 month follow-up [16, 25]. When compared to an active comparison group treatment (ACGT), post-treatment abstinence rates were favorable for DBT-BED (64% compared to 36% for ACGT), but there were no significant differences between the groups at any time during the 12-month follow-up period [26]. A fourth study [27] compared a more intensive version of DBT-BED to an adjusted, dose-matched, CBT-program in a mixed bulimia nervosa and BED sample of early weak responders to guided self-help cognitive behavior therapy. Although both treatments were helpful in reducing objective binge eating (OBE) episodes, no differences were found between treatments. These data support the idea that DBT can be a viable alternative to CBT in patients with binge eating. However, evidence is scarce and the available data do not favor one treatment over the other.

There are several reasons to assume that a certain subset of patients with BED is more likely to benefit from DBT. All eating disorders are characterized by emotion regulation difficulties, and although some studies suggest that individuals with BED may show these difficulties to a lesser extent than patients with anorexia nervosa or bulimia nervosa, patients with BED show marked emotion regulation difficulties when compared to healthy controls [28, 29]. Individuals who report to eat in response to negative emotions (emotional eating) have been shown to have higher levels of emotion regulation difficulties in comparison to groups without emotional eating [30]. Also, there is evidence suggesting that binge eating in overweight adults with BED is particularly associated with negative affect and not so much with dietary restraint (which is associated with binge eating in *normal weight* adults with BED [31–33]). Therefore, DBT might improve outcome in individuals with BED who are overweight and engage in emotional eating.

This study aimed to add to the current literature by comparing a DBT-BED group treatment to an intensive outpatient CBT-treatment (CBT+) in overweight individuals with BED who report above average levels of emotional eating. Although this CBT 'treatment as usual' comprised significantly more treatment time than the DBT intervention, and as such may have advantaged the CBT group, we hypothesized that DBT would be superior to CBT on measures related to eating disorder pathology and on measures related to emotion regulation.

The reason for this is that we optimized chances for DBT-BED by including only individuals with BED who might be most likely to profit from an emotion regulation intervention.

Method
Study design
This study is an open, quasi-randomized, controlled trial with two arms: CBT+ and DBT-BED. When the study was designed, the CBT+ program had been treatment as usual at our center for 10 years. The program has shown to lead to substantial reductions in eating disorder pathology [34]. For pragmatic reasons we chose to compare DBT-BED with this more intensive program. We reasoned that, given the difference in dosage, we would be able to consider DBT-BED an important alternative to CBT+ if DBT-BED would at least equal the results of CBT+.

All patients that met the inclusion/exclusion criteria (described below) and provided written informed consent to participate in the study were allocated to either CBT+ or DBT-BED. An employee not involved in the clinical trial, randomized eligible patients by flipping a coin. If a treatment group was about to start with only one open slot, the patient to enter the study was assigned to that group rather than randomized. After allocation, participants completed assessments on the first day of treatment (baseline), on the last day of treatment (end of treatment) and 6 months after treatment (follow-up). Enrollment started in October 2011, and was finished by the end of 2016. The design of the study was approved on October 10th 2011 by the Institution of Mental Health Medical Ethics Committee (METiGG: 11.109; CMO Radboud UMC: 2013/226) and was registered retrospectively in the Netherlands Trial Register (NTR4154) on August 28, 2013. Prior to conducting any analyses, given the modest sample size, we made the decision to compare outcome between treatments only on core eating disorder variables.

Participants
Participants were individuals from 18 years upward, who were referred to an expertise center for eating disorders in the Netherlands. If, during a telephone screening, BED seemed plausible, patients were asked to fill out the Dutch Eating Behavior Questionnaire (DEBQ [35];). Subsequently, either a licensed psychologist or psychiatrist conducted a clinical interview, designed a case formulation and determined the presence or absence of BED according to DSM-5 [1]. The case formulation and the DSM-5 classification were then reviewed in a multidisciplinary team. Because individuals with BED who are overweight and engage in emotional eating are arguably most likely to benefit from an emotion regulation

intervention, we only included patients with a BMI ≥ 30 and an above average urge to eat in response to negative emotions (score ≥ 2.38 on the DEBQ subscale Emotional Eating [36];). Exclusion criteria were kept to a minimum to ensure generalization of study results: previous CBT treatment for being overweight or eating disorder; current substance abuse, psychosis, suicidality; severe personality disorder; obesity caused by physical illness; concurrent treatment for being overweight or for eating disorder by medical specialist or dietician. Eligible patients were informed about the study by the clinician who conducted the initial clinical interview. They were given written information together with an informed consent form. All questions were answered. They then were asked to send back a signed form within 2 weeks. During this period a member of the research team was available for additional questions (Fig. 1).

Treatment

Dialectical behavior therapy for binge eating disorder (DBT-BED)

A Dutch prepublication version of the DBT-BED session-to-session protocol (courtesy of C. Telch and D. Safer [24]) was used. DBT-BED teaches skills to help patients regulate emotions in an adaptive way. This is done from a 'dialectical' stance: accept patients as they are and at the same time stimulate them to change in order to help them reach their goals. Treatment included 20 group-sessions of 2 h each, over the course of 20 weeks. In the first two sessions the rational and the goals of therapy were reviewed comprehensively, and an explicit commitment to change was made. The use of diary cards and chain analyses was introduced as well as the concept of therapy interfering behavior. The second phase (sessions 3–18) comprised three modules in which

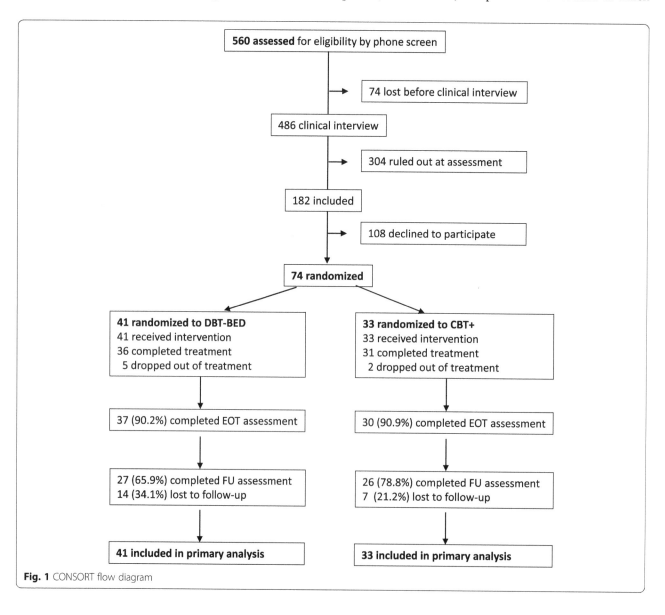

Fig. 1 CONSORT flow diagram

skills in mindfulness, emotion regulation and distress tolerance were taught. The emotion regulation module incorporates lifestyle interventions (i.e. education on a balanced eating pattern and regular physical exercise) to diminish the sensitivity for negative emotions. The third phase focused on the review and enhancement of learned skills, and on plans for the future. During treatment, patients monitored their weight weekly at the treatment center in order to help them face the consequences of (changes in) their eating behavior. A maximum of nine patients could participate in each round, in a closed group format. Six months after the end of treatment, progress was reviewed and skills were refreshed in a single follow-up group session. At that time, further treatment was offered in case this seemed necessary. Each treatment-cycle of 20 weeks was led by two trained psychologists/psychotherapists. Several therapist-pairs were formed as the treatment was provided over a substantial period of time.

Intensive outpatient cognitive behavior therapy (CBT+)

The CBT intervention was an extended version in group format of the manual developed by Fairburn and colleagues [37], addressing binge eating as behavior maintained by dietary restraint and other behavior, like body avoidance, originating from the overvaluation of weight and shape. The session-to-session protocol is available from ML. Treatment included 20 days of group therapy, 1 day per week during 20 consecutive weeks. Each day comprised three modules of 75 min each: 1) discuss daily self-monitoring of eating behavior and related situations, thoughts and feelings, 2) challenge thoughts and conduct behavioral experiments related to food and eating, and 3) challenge thoughts and conduct behavioral experiments related to body image. Over the course of treatment, several topics were covered in all three modules: motivation to change, eating regularly and sufficiently, dealing with triggers for binge eating (including some emotion regulation strategies), body image, body satisfaction, life-style and relapse prevention. In addition, patients monitored their weight weekly at the treatment center in order to diminish the obsession with weight or to break the avoidance of weight, and to monitor the consequences of (changes in) eating behavior. Each treatment-cycle of 20 weeks was led by a team of three: a psychologist, a psychiatric nurse and a psychomotor therapist. Psychomotor therapists addressed maintaining factors like body-avoidance and comparison-making by in-session exercises (e.g. body-exposure) and related homework assignments (see also [38]). Several therapist-combinations were formed as the treatment was provided over a substantial period of time. A maximum of nine patients could participate in each round. New patients entered every 10th week (i.e. a half open group

format). In addition, six group meetings of 90 min each were offered to patients and their partners to enhance mutual understanding and support during the process of change. After treatment, if deemed necessary on clinical grounds, six monthly group sessions were offered to help prevent relapse.

Therapist qualifications/training

All therapists were well trained and experienced in CBT for eating disorders, as this is the treatment as usual at the treatment center. Training in DBT-BED was initially provided by a senior psychologist, independent from this study, and well trained in this specific protocol. Later on, the initially trained therapists trained the co-therapist. Therapists in the DBT-BED-condition were supervised once a month by a leading expert in DBT. Therapists in the CBT-condition did not receive supervision, although peer consultation was ensured. No therapist worked in two treatments at the same time in order to avoid content or procedural overlap. Treatment adherence was assessed (see Supplementary material).

Assessment

Except for demographic information and height (collected at baseline only), all assessment instruments were administered at baseline, at post-treatment and at follow-up. All the assessed psychopathology measures were self-report questionnaires. Staff conducting the assessments was aware of the treatment condition that patients were assigned to.

Eating disorder pathology The Eating Disorder Examination Questionnaire (EDE-Q [39]) was used to assess the number of OBE episodes and global levels of eating disorder psychopathology over the past 28 days. Higher scores indicate greater severity. The EDE-Q is considered reliable for patients with BED [40] and has acceptable to high internal consistency and overall test-retest reliability [41]. However, empirical support for the subscales (restraint, eating concern, shape concern and weight concern) is questionable [42, 43].

Emotion regulation The urge to eat in response to negative emotions was assessed with the 13-item subscale Emotional Eating of the Dutch Eating Behavior Questionnaire (DEBQ [35, 36]). Higher scores indicate higher levels of emotional eating. The reliability and validity of the DEBQ are rated as good (enough) and all subscales have good internal consistency and factorial validity (e.g. [44, 45]).

The subscale Emotional Dysregulation of the Eating Disorder Inventory (EDI-3 [46]) was used to assess the tendency toward poor impulse regulation and mood intolerance. The EDI-3 assesses psychological and behavioral eating disorder symptomatology. Higher scores indicate more psychopathology. The reliability and the validity of the EDI-3 are considered to be good for use in eating disorder patient groups [47].

General psychopathology General psychopathology was measured using the total score of the Symptom Checklist 90 (SCL-90). The SCL-90 consists of 90 items related to the frequency of experienced physical and psychological complaints in the last week. Higher sum scores reflect more general psychopathology. The reliability and validity of the SCL-90 are good [48].

The Beck Depression Inventory-II (BDI-II) consists of 21 questions about the severity of depressive symptoms in the last week. Higher sum scores indicate more depressive symptoms. The reliability and validity of the BDI-II are good [49]. Self-esteem was assessed with the EDI-3 subscale Low Self-Esteem [46].

Weight, body mass index Patients were measured for height and weight, through which we computed their BMI: kg/m^2. Patients were measured for weight on a balanced scale wearing cloths but no shoes.

Dropout Dropout was defined as premature termination of treatment, either patient-initiated or staff-initiated. Patients were allowed to miss a maximum of 2 out of 20 days. If they missed more, they were excluded from treatment and were consequently considered dropout of treatment. When treatment was terminated before the 20-week period ended because staff and patient mutually agreed that treatment goals were achieved, this was considered as completion of treatment instead of dropout.

Power and sample calculation
Initial power analysis suggested that a sample of 34 per group (68 total) would provide a power of .80 to detect a medium effect. A total of 74 participants (33 to CBT+ and 41 to DBT-BED) were randomized. At the conclusion of the trial, it was discovered that the initial power analysis was incorrect. The actual power to detect a medium effect based upon an alpha of .05 is only .58.

Statistical analysis
All analyses were conducted using SPSS Version 25 [50]. Significance tests were based on a two-tailed alpha of 0.05. Primary measures of outcome used to evaluate efficacy included OBE episodes and EDE-Q Global scores. Secondary measures of outcome included DEBQ Emotional Eating, EDI-3 Emotional Dysregulation, SCL-90 total score, BDI-II total score, and EDI-3 Low Self-Esteem. Distribution diagnostics for primary and secondary outcome measures suggested that all outcome measures except OBE episodes were symmetrically

distributed and appropriate for normal assumption models. CBT+ and DBT-BED treatment groups were compared separately at end of treatment and follow-up controlling for baseline assessment using a generalized linear model with a negative binomial distribution for OBE episodes and a general linear model for all other outcome variables. Given that treatment for both CBT and DBT was delivered in group settings, preliminary models were run nesting participants within therapeutic groups. As no significant variation attributable to therapeutic group was found, subsequent analyses were conducted without nesting. Final models included a main effect for treatment group, and a fixed covariate for baseline assessment. Effect sizes between treatments were calculated using both Cohen's [51] d and the *success rate difference* (*SRD* [52]). Cohen's d values were calculated from covariate-adjusted estimated marginal means; Cohen uses values of 0.2, 0.5, and 0.8 to characterize "small", "medium", and "large" differences between groups, respectively. *SRD* values, which can range from − 1 to + 1, represent the probability that a randomly selected case from one treatment will have an outcome preferable to a randomly selected case from another treatment.

Outcome analyses were based upon the intention-to-treat principle [53]. Multiple imputation was used to impute missing data using fully conditional Markov chain Monte Carlo (MCMC [54]) modeling. The final analyses were based upon the pooled results of 20 separate imputation sets. Sensitivity analyses were conducted using both maximum likelihood imputation and available data analyses to evaluate the consistency of results across differing methods for handling missing data.

Clinically meaningful change was operationalized as proposed by Jacobson & Truax [55]. We calculated the percentage of patients on the EDE-Q Global score that shifted from being closer to the mean of the dysfunctional group (current sample: mean = 3.29; SD = .959) to being closer to the mean of a functional group (i.e. a normative non-students sample of males and females from the United Kingdom: mean = 1.92; SD = 1.42 [56]).

Results
Study participants
A total of 74 participants were randomized: 33 to CBT+ and 41 to DBT-BED. Participants included 66 (89.2%) women and 8 (10.8%) men, with an average age of 37.3 (SD = 11.8; range = 18–67) and an average duration of illness of 15.3 years (SD = 10.9; range = 1–45). BMI of participants averaged 39.9 (SD = 5.6; range = 30.5–55.5). The majority of participants ($n = 49$ [66.2%]) lived with a partner/spouse. Treatment groups did not differ significantly on any demographic characteristics, BMI, or outcome measures at baseline.

Study retention

A total of 7 (9.5%) participants dropped out of the treatment and/or study during the course of the trial, including 2 (6.1%) from CBT+ and 5 (12.2%) from DBT-BED (Fisher's Exact p = .451). Of the 74 participants that were randomized, 67 (90.5%) completed end of treatment assessments and 53 (71.6%) completed follow-up assessments. Assessment completion rates for CBT+ and DBT-BED were 90.9% vs. 90.2% (Fisher's Exact p = 1.00) respectively at end of treatment and 78.8% vs. 65.9% (Fisher's Exact p = .301) at follow-up.

Primary outcomes

Mean scores on primary measures of outcome for CBT+ and DBT-BED groups at baseline, end of treatment, and follow-up are presented in Table 1. The CBT+ group experienced greater reductions in EDE-Q Global score that approached significance at end of treatment (p = .060) and reached significance at follow-up (p = .020), with effect sizes ranging from 0.45 at end of treatment to 0.55 at follow-up. Results of sensitivity analyses using maximum likelihood (ML) imputation and available data (AD) analysis produced relatively consistent results at end of treatment (ML: p = .050; AD: p = .052) and follow-up (ML: p = .006; AD: p = .006). Table 2 presents the percentage of participants who completed the EDE-Q that shifted from a dysfunctional level at baseline to a functional level at end-of-treatment and follow-up (cutoff EDE-Q score: 2.47 [55]). Although percentages were higher for CBT+ at both end-of-treatment and follow-up

Table 2 Percentage of Participants that went from above to below the Cutoff of 2.47 on the EDE-Q Global Score

	CBT+	DBT-BED	Fisher's Exact p
End of Treatment	69.6% (16/23)	52.9% (18/34)	.275
Follow-up	65.0% (13/20)	45.8% (11/24)	.238

(69.6 and 65.0% vs 52.9 and 45.8% for DBT-BED), these differences were not significant.

The CBT+ group also showed greater reductions in OBE episodes at end of treatment (p = .035; d = .46), but these differences were no longer significant at follow-up (p = .095). The end of treatment differences between treatment groups in OBE episodes were confirmed in sensitivity analyses (ML: p = .010; AD: p = .010).

Secondary outcomes

Results of secondary outcome analyses are presented in Table 1. *SRD*s show preferable probability of improvement for CBT+ on all secondary measures at both end of treatment and follow-up; however, the only difference in secondary outcome measures that reached significance was for EDI-3 Low Self-Esteem. The CBT+ group experienced greater reductions in EDI-3 Low Self-Esteem that approached significance at end of treatment (p = .072; d = .43) and reached significance at follow-up (p = .014; d = .59). Results of sensitivity analyses confirmed these findings at both end of treatment (ML: p = .053; AD: p = .064) and follow-up (ML: p = .024; AD: p = .018).

Table 1 CBT+ vs. DBT-BED Comparison of Treatment Outcome

Outcome	Group	N	Study Visit (mean, SD)			CBT+ vs. DBT-BED					
						EOT			FU		
			Baseline	EOT	FU	Sig.	d	SRD	Sig.	d	SRD
EDE-Q Global[a]	CBT+	33	3.06 (1.10)	1.64 (1.16)	1.61 (1.11)	.060	.45	.248	.020	.55	.302
	DBT-BED	41	3.48 (0.79)	2.31 (1.09)	2.35 (1.06)						
OBE Episodes[a]	CBT+	33	8.27 (9.65)	0.74 (1.68)	1.85 (5.11)	.035	.46	.253	.095	.37	.204
	DBT-BED	41	7.51 (8.72)	1.64 (3.77)	2.75 (5.58)						
DEBQ Emotional Eating[b]	CBT+	33	3.76 (0.69)	2.55 (0.64)	2.45 (0.86)	.322	.23	.128	.196	.29	.161
	DBT-BED	41	3.77 (0.68)	2.72 (0.64)	2.73 (0.83)						
EDI-3 Emotional Dysregulation[b]	CBT+	33	25.09 (6.80)	21.84 (3.72)	21.23 (4.61)	.392	.21	.117	.253	.27	.150
	DBT-BED	41	27.02 (5.93)	23.81 (6.74)	22.88 (3.76)						
SCL-90[b]	CBT+	33	175.5 (51.9)	136.0 (39.6)	128.8 (37.1)	.257	.27	.150	.152	.34	.188
	DBT-BED	41	185.9 (43.1)	150.7 (45.4)	144.3 (38.4)						
BDI-II[b]	CBT+	33	20.53 (9.89)	7.56 (6.52)	7.21 (6.45)	.193	.31	.172	.098	.39	.215
	DBT-BED	41	21.98 (7.60)	10.69 (8.46)	10.75 (8.20)						
EDI-3 Self-Esteem[b]	CBT+	33	35.44 (9.00)	25.89 (7.96)	24.12 (8.17)	.072	.43	.237	.014	.59	.324
	DBT-BED	41	38.32 (8.47)	30.80 (9.64)	29.75 (8.00)						

EOT End of treatment, *FU* Follow-up, *d* Cohen's *d*, *SRD* Success rate difference
[a]Primary outcome measure
[b]Secondary outcome measure

Treatment adherence

Mean session integrity was 79.1% (SD = 15.0) for DBT-BED and 63.5% (SD = 24.1) for CBT+ with a statistically significant difference in favor of DBT ($p < .001$). To establish interrater reliability, five raters rated four tapes independently. The average kappa coefficient across raters and tapes was .628 ($p < .001$) suggesting good agreement.

Discussion

This controlled study compared an emotion regulation treatment adjusted for BED with an intensive eating disorders-focused form of CBT in obese individuals with BED. Contrary to our expectations, DBT-BED was not superior to and was in fact less efficacious than CBT+ on primary outcome measures, especially on reductions in eating disorder psychopathology at follow-up. The greater reductions in OBE episodes in CBT+ at end of treatment were not retained 6 months after treatment. Reductions on all secondary measures were consistently in favor of the CBT+ group, with self-esteem reaching statistical significance and a medium effect at follow-up.

The failure to support our primary hypothesis may be due to differences in dosage between treatments: CBT+ contained more face-to-face contact time per day (3.75 h versus 2 h per week), offered six group meetings of 90 min to patients with a partner and incorporated six follow-up sessions for some patients (versus one for all patients in DBT-BED). Thus, this latter group received twice-weekly sessions during 6 weeks. Dose-response research in psychotherapy shows that, more than the number of sessions and the total contact time, the frequency of treatment schedules seems to be a relevant factor as more frequent treatment schedules (e.g. twice per week instead of once per week) are found to be more effective [57–59]. Therefore, patients in CBT+, especially those that participated in the 'partner-group', have this advantage.[1] As Chen and colleagues [27] found no superiority of either a more intensive DBT-program or a dose-matched CBT-program, the DBT-BED program in this study may possibly have been as efficacious as CBT if CBT was dose-matched.

Also, again contrary to our expectations, we did not detect any differences between DBT-BED and CBT+ at end of treatment or follow-up on measures related to emotion regulation. This seems remarkable given the theoretical foundation of both therapies with DBT-BED targeting emotion regulation and CBT targeting dietary restraint and other behavior originating from the overvaluation of weight and shape. Possible reasons for

failing to find differences may be related to limited statistical power or to increased treatment time in CBT+. Concurrently, to stay close to clinical practice we did not control for content and therefore conceptual overlap may have occurred. Differential effects of both therapies were possibly compromised because of this. However, it should be noted that findings on the emotion regulation measures in this study are in line with Safer and colleagues [26] who found a consistent lack of differential impact with a broad range of emotion-regulation measures comparing DBT-BED to an active controlled for content comparison. Also, in individuals with bulimia nervosa, CBT has been found to produce decreases in emotion dysregulation [60]. This suggests that decreases in emotion dysregulation might not be attributable to the specific emotion regulation techniques used in DBT-BED, but to therapeutic elements shared across various treatments.

Apart from self-esteem, no significant differences in reduction between the groups were found on measures related to general psychopathology. Depressive features improved considerably in both groups.

Improvements in OBE episodes seemed to diminish slightly between end of treatment and follow-up in both groups but stayed, on average, below the diagnostic threshold (< 4 OBE episodes in 28 days). This is in line with previous findings (e.g. [27]). In addition, a substantial percentage of patients in both groups reached clinically meaningful change in eating disorder psychopathology. Percentages were higher for CBT+ at both end-of-treatment and follow-up, but these differences were not significant.

The study has several limitations. One major limitation of this study is the difference in dosage between DBT and CBT+, which compromises our ability to draw solid conclusions about the observed differences in outcome. A second major limitation is the limited sample size. With higher power we may have found more, and more robust, differences in favor of CBT+, as all nonsignificant differences favored CBT+. However, despite the power issues, we did find significant differences between treatments on both primary measures. Also, treatment adherence was lower in CBT+, possibly due to the fact that therapists received no supervision. Since higher adherence levels are related to better outcome [61, 62], differences in outcome between the two treatments may even have been bigger had the adherence to the CBT+ protocol been higher.

We could have further optimized the assessment of BED pathology by either making use of the Eating Disorder Examination interview (EDE) instead of the EDE-Q [41] or by providing a specific definition of binge eating when administering the EDE-Q (as suggested by Celio and colleagues [63]). In addition, we did not

[1]On the other hand, one could also say that we have advantaged DBT-BED as we selected a sample that we assumed could optimally benefit from the DBT-BED treatment.

control for content which may have compromised differential effects of both therapies. Finally, allocation was strictly not entirely random.

Despite the limitations, the present study has several strengths. To our knowledge, this is the first controlled study in individuals with BED, comparing DBT-BED, previously tested only against a waitlist [16, 25] and an active comparison [26], to a CBT-program. This study is therefore a step forward in evaluating the efficacy of DBT-BED. The selection of a subgroup of BED patients (obese BED patients who report an above average urge to eat in response to negative emotions) optimized the chances of DBT-BED to prove itself as a viable alternative to an intensive outpatient CBT program. Further, although dropout rates in DBT-BED (17.1%) were relatively high when compared to Safer and colleagues [26] (4%), dropout rates in CBT+ (6%) were low when compared to other controlled CBT-treatment studies (e.g. 16.7 to 30% [64, 65]). Besides that, generalizability was optimized by conducting the study in routine clinical practice, with few exclusion criteria, and making use of various therapist-pairs (which enables us to generalize beyond the present therapist sample). Finally, the follow-up period provides insight in the medium-long term effects of both treatments.

In conclusion, the more intensive CBT+ reduced eating disorder related measures and self-esteem more than DBT-BED, even in a population that arguably may be more likely to profit from an emotion regulation intervention. This clearly favors CBT+ above DBT-BED. Yet, when looking at outcome from a different perspective, the data suggest that both groups reached comparable levels of clinically meaningful change in global eating disorder psychopathology. This is particularly interesting given that the DBT-BED program is less time-consuming so less costly than CBT+ as applied in the current study. To be able to fully understand the value of DBT-BED, future research should include dose-matched comparisons of CBT and DBT-BED in a sufficiently powered randomized controlled trial and include longer term follow-up. Furthermore, maybe even more important, future studies should search for mediators and moderators to improve outcome in current efficacious treatments for BED.

Abbreviations
ACGT: Active Comparison Group Therapy; AD: Available Data; BED: Binge Eating Disorder; BDI-II: Beck Depression Inventory-II; BMI: Body Mass Index; CBT: Cognitive Behavioral Therapy; CBT +: Intensive outpatient group CBT-treatment; CMO: Commissie Mensgebonden Onderzoek; COTAN: Commissie Testaangelegenheden Nederland [Dutch committee on tests and testing]; DBT: Dialectical Behavior Therapy; DBT-BED: Dialectical Behavior Therapy adapted for Binge Eating Disorder; DSM-5: Fifth edition of the Diagnostic and Statistical Manual of Mental Disorders; DEBQ: Dutch Eating Behavior Questionnaire; EDE-Q: Eating Disorder Examination Questionnaire; EDI-3: Eating Disorder Inventory-3; MCMC: Markov Chain Monte Carlo; METiGG: Institution of Mental Health Medical Ethics Committee; ML: Maximum Likelihood; NTR: Netherlands Trial Register; SCL-90: Symptom Checklist-90; SD: Standard Deviation; SRD: Success rate difference; UMC: University Medical Center

Acknowledgements
The authors wish to thank all therapists and support staff at Amarum who contributed to collecting the data, Liesbeth Verschoor for her assistance in entering the data, Wies van den Bosch and Thom van den Heuvel for supervising the DBT-arm and Machteld Ouwens for providing feedback on early versions of this paper.

Authors' contributions
TvS initiated the project and provided overall background supervision. ML collected the data and wrote the main part of the manuscript. MV supervised this process. RDC analyzed the data and wrote the statistical analysis and results sections. All authors were involved in interpretation of the data and contributed to writing the manuscript. All authors read and approved the final manuscript.

Competing interests
The authors declare that they have no competing interests other than TvS receiving royalties from the DEBQ and the EDI-3 and RDC being a paid statistical consultant for Health Outcomes Solutions, Winter Park, Florida.

Author details
[1]Amarum, Expertise Centre for Eating Disorders, GGNet Network for Mental Health Care, Den Elterweg 75, 7207 AE Zutphen, The Netherlands. [2]Radboud University, Behavioural Science Institute, Montessorilaan 3, 6525 HR Nijmegen, The Netherlands. [3]Sanford Center for Biobehavioral Research, Fargo, North Dakota, USA. [4]University of North Dakota School of Medicine and Health Sciences, Fargo, North Dakota, USA.

References
1. American Psychiatric Association. Diagnostic and statistical manual of mental disorders. 5th ed. Arlington: American Psychiatric Publishing; 2013.
2. Brownley KA, Berkman ND, Peat CM, Lohr KN, Cullen KE, Bann CM, et al. Binge-eating disorder in adults: a systematic review and meta-analysis. Ann Intern Med. 2016;165(6):409–20.
3. Welch E, Jangmo A, Thornton LM, Norring C, von Hausswolff-Juhlin Y, Herman BK, et al. Treatment-seeking patients with binge-eating disorder in the Swedish national registers: clinical course and psychiatric comorbidity. BMC Psychiat. 2016;16:163.
4. Grucza RA, Przybeck TR, Cloninger CR. Prevalence and correlates of binge eating disorder in a community sample. Compr Psychiatry. 2007;48(2):124–31.
5. Lydecker JA, White MA, Grilo CM. Form and formulation: examining the distinctiveness of body image constructs in treatment-seeking patients with binge-eating disorder. J Consult Clin Psych. 2017;85(11):1095–103.
6. Hay P, Chinn D, Forbes D, Madden S, Newton R, Sugenor L, et al. Royal Australian and new Zealand College of Psychiatrists Clinical practice guidelines for the treatment of eating disorders. Aust NZ J Psychiat. 2014;48(11):977–1008.
7. National Institute for Health and Care Excellence. Eating disorders: Recognition and treatment. 2017. https://www.nice.org.uk/guidance/ng69/chapter/Recommendations#treating-binge-eating-disorder. Accessed 30 May 2019.
8. Fairburn CG, Cooper Z, Shafran R. Cognitive behaviour therapy for eating disorders: a "transdiagnostic" theory and treatment. Behav Res Ther. 2003; 41(5):509–28.

9. Fairburn CG. Cognitive behavior therapy and eating disorders. New York: Guilford Press; 2008.

10. Fairburn CG, Cooper Z, Doll HA, O'Connor ME, Bohn K, Hawker DM, et al. Transdiagnostic cognitive-behavioral therapy for patients with eating disorders: a two-site trial with 60-week follow-up. Am J Psychiat. 2009; 166(3):311–9.

11. Linardon J. Rates of abstinence following psychological or behavioral treatments for binge-eating disorder: meta-analysis. Int J Eat Disord. 2018; 51(8):785–97.

12. Grilo CM. Why no cognitive body image feature such as overvaluation of shape/weight in the binge eating disorder diagnosis? Int J Eat Disord. 2013; 46(3):208–11.

13. Elran-Barak R, Sztainer M, Goldschmidt AB, Crow SJ, Peterson CB, Hill LL, et al. Dietary restriction behaviors and binge eating in anorexia nervosa, bulimia nervosa and binge eating disorder: trans-diagnostic examination of the restraint model. Eat Behav. 2015;18:192–6.

14. Raymond NC, Peterson RE, Bartholome LT, Raatz SK, Jensen MD, Levine JA. Comparisons of energy intake and energy expenditure in overweight and obese women with and without binge eating disorder. Obesity. 2012;20(4):765–72.

15. Hawkins RC, Clement PF. Binge eating: measurement problems and a conceptual model. In: Hawkins RC, Fremouw WJ, Clement PF, editors. The binge purge syndrome: diagnosis, treatment, and research. New York, NY: Springer; 1984. p. 229–51.

16. Telch CF, Agras WS, Linehan MM. Dialectical behavior therapy for binge eating disorder. J Consult Clin Psych. 2001;69(6):1061–5.

17. Abraham SF, Beumont PJV. How patients describe bulimia or binge eating. Psychol Med. 1982;12(3):625–35.

18. Arnow B, Kenardy J, Agras WS. Binge eating among the obese: a descriptive study. J J Behav Med. 1992;15(2):155–70.

19. Berg KC, Crosby RD, Cao L, Crow SJ, Engel SG, Wonderlich SA, et al. Negative affect prior to and following overeating-only, loss of control eating-only, and binge eating episodes in obese adults. Int J Eat Disord. 2015;48(6):641–53.

20. Haedt-Matt AA, Keel PK. Revisiting the affect regulation model of binge eating: a meta-analysis of studies using ecological momentary assessment. Psychol Bull. 2011;137(4):660–81.

21. Vanderlinden J, Grave RD, Fernandez F, Vandereycken W, Pieters G, Noorduin C. Which factors do provoke binge eating? An exploratory study in eating disorder patients. Eat Weight Disord. 2004;9:300–5.

22. Leehr EJ, Krohmer K, Schag K, Dresler T, Zipfel S, Giel KE. Emotion regulation model in binge eating disorder and obesity: a systematic review. Neurosci Biobehav R. 2015;49:125–34.

23. Linehan MM. Cognitive behavioral therapy of borderline personality disorder. New York: Guilford Press; 1993.

24. Safer DL, Telch CF, Chen EY. Dialectical behavior therapy for binge eating and bulimia. New York: Guilford Press; 2009.

25. Masson PC, von Ranson KM, Wallace LM, Safer DL. A randomized wait-list controlled pilot study of dialectical behaviour therapy guided self-help for binge eating disorder. Behav Res Ther. 2013;51(11):723–8.

26. Safer DL, Robinson AH, Jo B. Outcome from a randomized controlled trial of group therapy for binge eating disorder: comparing dialectical behavior therapy adapted for binge eating to an active comparison group therapy. Beh Ther. 2010;41(1):106–20.

27. Chen EY, Cacioppo J, Fettich K, Gallop R, McCloskey MS, Olino T, et al. An adaptive randomized trial of dialectical behavior therapy and cognitive behavior therapy for binge-eating. Psychol Med. 2017;47(4):703–17.

28. Brockmeyer T, Skunde M, Wu M, Bresslein E, Rudofsky G, Herzog W, Friederich HC. Difficulties in emotion regulation across the spectrum of eating disorders. Compr Psychiatry. 2014;55:565–71.

29. Svaldi J, Griepenstroh J, Tuschen-Caffier B, Ehring T. Emotion regulation deficits in eating disorders: a marker of eating pathology or general psychopathology? Psychiatry Res. 2012;197:103–11.

30. Sultson H, Akkermann K. Investigating phenotypes of emotional eating based on weight categories: a latent profile analysis. Int J Eat Disord. 2019; 52(9):1024–34.

31. Carrard I, Van der Linden M, Golay A. Comparison of obese and nonobese individuals with binge eating disorder: delicate boundary between binge eating disorder and non-purging bulimia nervosa. Eur Eat Disord Rev. 2012; 20(5):350–4.

32. Goldschmidt AB, Le Grange D, Powers P, Crow SJ, Hill LL, Peterson CB, et al. Eating disorder symptomatology in normal-weight vs. obese individuals with binge eating disorder. Obesity. 2011;19(7):1515–8.

33. Welsh DM, King RM. Applicability of the dual pathway model in normal and overweight binge eaters. Body Image. 2016;18:162–7.

34. Lammers MW, Vroling MS, Ouwens MA, Engels RCME, Van Strien T. Predictors of outcome for cognitive behaviour therapy in binge eating disorder. Eur Eat Disord Rev. 2015;23(3):219–28.

35. Vanstrien T, Frijters JER, Bergers GPA, Defares PB. The Dutch eating behavior questionnaire (DEBQ) for assessment of restrained, emotional, and external eating behavior. Int J Eat Disord. 1986;5(2):295–315.

36. Van Strien T. Handleiding NVE [Manual DEBQ]. Amsterdam: Hogrefe; 2015.

37. Fairburn CG, Marcus MD, Wilson GT. Cognitive-behavioral therapy for binge eating and bulimia nervosa: a comprehensive treatment manual. In: Fairburn CG, editor. Binge eating: nature, assessment and treatment. New York: Guilford Press; 1993. p. 361–404.

38. Probst M, Knapen J, Poot G, Vancampfort D. Psychomotor therapy and psychiatry: what is in a name. Open Compl Med J. 2010;2:105–13.

39. Fairburn CG, Beglin SJ. Eating disorder examination questionnaire (EDEQ 6. 0). In: Fairburn C, editor. Cognitive behavior therapy and eating disorders. New York: Guilford Press; 2008. p. 309–13.

40. Reas DL, Grilo CM, Masheb RM. Reliability of the eating disorder examination-questionnaire in patients with binge eating disorder. Beh Res Ther. 2006;44(1):43–51.

41. Berg KC, Peterson CB, Frazier P, Crow SJ. Psychometric evaluation of the eating disorder examination and eating disorder examination-questionnaire: a systematic review of the literature. Int J Eat Disord. 2012;45(3):428–38.

42. Aardoom JJ, Dingemans AE, Landt M, Van Furth EF. Norms and discriminative validity of the eating disorder examination questionnaire (EDE-Q). Eat Behav. 2012;13(4):305–9.

43. Carrard I, Rebetez MML, Mobbs O, Van der Linden M. Factor structure of a French version of the eating disorder examination-questionnaire among women with and without binge eating disorder symptoms. Eat Weight Disord. 2015;20(1):137–44.

44. Barrada JR, Van Strien T, Cebolla A. Internal structure and measurement invariance of the Dutch eating behavior questionnaire (DEBQ) in a (nearly) representative Dutch community sample. Eur Eat Disord Rev. 2016;24(6):503–9.

45. COTAN. Beoordeling Nederlandse Vragenlijst voor Eetgedrag, NVE [Review Dutch Eating Behavior Questionnaire, DEBQ]. 2013.

46. Garner DM, Van Strien T. EDI-3. Inventarisatie van eetstoornissymptomen. Handleiding [EDI-3. Inventory of eating disorder symptoms. Manual]. Amsterdam: Hogrefe; 2015.

47. Lehmann V, Ouwens MA, Braeken J, Danner UN, van Elburg AA, Bekker MHJ, et al. Psychometric properties of the Dutch version of the Eating Disorder Inventory-3. SAGE Open. 2013;3(4):2158244013508415.

48. Arrindell WA, Ettema JHM. SCL-90, symptom checklist. Handleiding bij een multidimensionele psychopathology-indicator [manual for a multidimensional psychopathology indicator]. Lisse: Swets Test Publishers; 2003.

49. Beck AT, Steer RA, Brown GK. Beck depression inventory-II (BDI-II). San Antonio: Harcourt Assessment Inc.; 1996.

50. IBM Corp. SPSS statistics for windows, version 25.0. IBM Corp: Armonk; 2017.

51. Cohen J. Statistical power analysis for the behavioral sciences. 2nd ed. Hillsdale New Jersey: Lawrence Erlbaum; 1988.

52. Kraemer HC, Kupfer DJ. Size of treatment effects and their importance to clinical research and practice. Biol Psychiatry. 2006;59(11):990–6.

53. McCoy CE. Understanding the intention-to-treat principle in randomized controlled trials. West J Emerg Med. 2017;18(6):1075–8.

54. Schafer JL. Analysis of incomplete multivariate data. London: Chapman & Hall; 1987.

55. Jacobson NS, Truax P. Clinical-significance: a statistical approach to defining meaningful change in psychotherapy research. J Consult Clin Psych. 1991; 59(1):12–9.

56. Carey M, Kupeli N, Knight R, Troop NA, Jenkinson PM, Preston C. Eating disorder examination questionnaire (EDE-Q): norms and psychometric properties in UK females and males. Psychol Assess. 2019;31(7):839–50.

57. Bell C, Waller G, Shafran R, Delgadillo J. Is there an optimal length of psychological treatment for eating disorder pathology? Int J Eat Disord. 2017;50(6):687–92.

58. Cuijpers P, Huibers M, Ebert DD, Koole SL, Andersson G. How much psychotherapy is needed to treat depression? A metaregression analysis. J Affect Disord. 2013;149(1–3):1–13.

59. Robinson L, Delgadillo J, Kellett S. The dose-response effect in routinely delivered psychological therapies: a systematic review. Psychother Res. 2020; 30(1):79–96.

60. Peterson CB, Berg KC, Crosby RD, Lavender JM, Accurso EC, Ciao AC, et al. The effects of psychotherapy treatment on outcome in bulimia nervosa: examining indirect effects through emotion regulation, self-directed behavior, and self-discrepancy within the mediation model. Int J Eat Disord. 2017;50(6):636–47.

61. Linardon J, Wade TD, Garcia XD, Brennan L. The efficacy of cognitive-behavioral therapy for eating disorders: a systematic review and meta-analysis. J Consult Clin Psych. 2017;85(11):1080–94.

62. Waller G. Evidence-based treatment and therapist drift. Beh Res Ther. 2009; 47(2):119–27.

63. Celio AA, Wilfley DE, Crow SJ, Mitchell J, Walsh BT. A comparison of the binge eating scale, questionnaire for eating and weight patterns-revised, and eating disorder examination questionnaire with instructions with the eating disorder examination in the assessment of binge eating disorder and its symptoms. Int J Eat Disord. 2004;36(4):434–44.

64. Peterson CB, Mitchell JE, Crow SJ, Crosby RD, Wonderlich SA. The efficacy of self-help group treatment and therapist-led group treatment for binge eating disorder. Am J Psychiat. 2009;166(12):1347–54.

65. Wilson GT, Wilfley DE, Agras WS, Bryson SW. Psychological treatments of binge eating disorder. Arch Gen Psychiat. 2010;67(1):94–101.

13

A rational emotive behavior therapy-based intervention for binge eating behavior management among female students: A quasi-experimental study

Jiwon Yang[1] and Kuem Sun Han[2*]

Abstract

Background: Binge eating behavior is highly likely to progress to an eating disorder, with female students particularly at risk.

Objective: This study aimed to verify the effect of a binge eating behavior management program, based on rational emotive behavior therapy (REBT), on binge eating behavior and related cognitive and emotional factors among female college students.

Method: The study, conducted from November 1 to December 2, 2016, involved a pretest-posttest design and nonequivalent control group. The sample included 24 and 22 first- to third-year students, from a college in South Korea, in the experimental and control groups, respectively. Data were collected using self-esteem, covert narcissism, perfectionism, body dissatisfaction, anxiety, depression, and binge eating scales and analyzed via frequency analysis, χ^2 tests, t tests, and analysis of covariance.

Results: The results indicated that the REBT-based binge eating behavior management program exerted positive effects on participants' self-esteem, reducing covert narcissism, body dissatisfaction, anxiety, depression, and binge eating. However, there was no significant difference in perfectionism, although the experimental group's mean score decreased from pretest to posttest.

Conclusions: Based on the results, the program was considered to be effective, and is expected to be useful in preventing the development of eating disorders among female college students by treating binge eating behavior and related cognitive and emotional factors. This intervention could ultimately contribute to the improvement of female college students' health and quality of life.

Keywords: Female, Students, Binge eating disorder, Self-criticism, Narcissism, Perfectionism, Body dissatisfaction, Anxiety, Depression

* Correspondence: hksun@korea.ac.kr
[2]Department of Nursing, Korea University, Seoul, South Korea
Full list of author information is available at the end of the article

Plain English summary

Binge eating behavior results from an individual's distorted body image, dissatisfaction with their physical appearance, and idealization of thin body types, and requires intervention before developing into an eating disorder. The purpose of this study was to address binge eating behavior and related factors among female college students in Korea, ultimately aiming to prevent the development of eating disorders. Our intervention integrated cognitive, emotional, and behavioral techniques used in rational emotive behavior therapy (REBT), aimed at treating binge eating behavior among female college students. The results show that the program was effective, with positive effects on participants' self-esteem, covert narcissism, perfectionism, body dissatisfaction, anxiety, depression, and binge eating.

Background

Over the past two decades, South Korean society has increasingly pursued values based on physical appearance. Consequently, women with normal body weight, particularly college students, have distorted body images, are dissatisfied with their physical appearance, and idealize the thin body type, resulting in inappropriate eating habits and high likelihood of developing eating disorders [1]. According to one study, 37.75% of female college students in South Korea have been shown to be at risk of developing eating disorders, with 38.6% misguidedly considering themselves overweight, leading to problems with their dietary behavior [2]. Moreover, the incidence of bulimia nervosa, an eating disorder, has increased, and women are 15 times more likely than men to develop this disorder. It should also be noted that 44.9% of those treated for bulimia nervosa in South Korea are in their twenties [3].

According to the Health Insurance Review & Assessment (HIRA) Service, the incidence of eating disorders in Korea rose by 18.8% over 5 years from 2008 to 2012, with an annual increase of 4.5%. Of all those diagnosed with eating disorders, 49.2% are between their teens and 30s, highlighting the gravity of the problem among the younger generation. In another study, over 50% of female students attempted to manage their body weight through dieting; more female students are at risk for developing an eating disorder compared to their male counterparts [4]. One study observed that the percentage of female students exhibiting abnormal eating behaviors, such as restrained and binge eating, is consistently on the rise, from 11.3% in 2009 to 21.5% in 2014 [5].

Binge eating behavior is characterized by both the amount of food consumed and loss of control [6]. Binge eating behavior occurs as a central symptom of bulimia nervosa (BN), binge eating disorder (BED), and the binge-purge type of anorexia nervosa (AN-BP) [6]. Binge eating disorder is a mental disorder; binge eating behavior can be seen as a behavioral symptom of and precursor to binge eating disorder [7]. Subjects with an eating disorder often hide their problems and do not ask for expert help, and the disorder seriously impairs the individual's physical and psychosocial functions owing to incorrect eating attitudes [8]. In addition, eating disorders have a high mortality rate among mental disorders, a low recovery rate, and a high risk of recurrence [9]. With such a rapid rise in binge eating behavior—a stage preceding an eating disorder—an intervention for the prevention of eating disorders needs to be developed, as people with eating disorders may develop other physical, mental, and social problems [10]. Particularly, interventions for female students are crucial, as they are at the highest risk for binge eating behaviors [11].

Binge eating behavior is particularly influenced by negative psychological factors [12]. Women who exhibit a binge eating pattern have a stronger desire for recognition, are more sensitive to rejection or criticism, and place greater value on others' opinions relative to women who do not display such behavior [13]. Cognitive factors, including self-esteem, covert narcissism, perfectionism, and body dissatisfaction [14–17], and emotional factors, including anxiety and depression [18], could partially explain binge eating behavior.

In particular, low self-esteem related to body image and outer appearance is reported to be a more potent predictor of binge eating behavior in women than in men [19]. Gordon and Dombeck [20] categorized narcissism as overt and covert narcissism and showed binge eating behavior to be strongly associated with covert narcissism. Covert narcissists have problems in interpersonal relationships, are sensitive toward others' evaluation, and particularly, when they have a negative perception about their body, they demonstrate negative eating attitudes in order to be approved by others [21]. Maples et al. [22] also reported that covert narcissists exhibit abnormal eating behaviors. Perfectionism is a multidimensional construct, and it is characterized by striving to avoid an error or defect and meet the highest standards and expectations [23]. Excessive concerns and worrying about error constitute may induce binge eating behavior, and are reported as major predictors of binge eating behavior over time [24].

Women who exhibit binge eating behavior compare themselves to other women and idealize thin bodies, which is associated with their irrational belief that their value is determined by their weight or appearance. If these women fail to achieve that idealized image, they become dissatisfied with their bodies, which ultimately results in low self-esteem [25]. Anxiety is viewed as a state provoked by a sense of isolation or hostility arising from malfunctioning interpersonal relationships. Particularly, anxiety is an emotion that encompasses emotional aspects such as restlessness and worry as well as physical aspects such as avoidance and dizziness, and it is reported to be closely associated with binge eating [26].

The relationship between depression and eating problems has been consistently discussed [27], and particularly, people who engage in binge eating are reported to undergo more severe stress in their daily living and feel a sense of depression in their lives, which in turn induces binge eating [28]. Another study observed that people who feel more depressed report more binge eating or other mental disorders than those who do not [29].

Ellis [30] developed rational emotive behavior therapy (REBT) to mediate the irrational beliefs that cause emotional and behavioral problems. The cognitive-behavioral perspective holds that individuals who place excessive value on body shape and weight could develop binge eating behavior [31]. In this case, a simple REBT-based intervention with problem-oriented and directional characteristics could be used in the short term because it changes irrational beliefs into rational beliefs, ultimately altering negative emotions/behavior.

REBT has been used in various areas such as clinical psychology, education, and counseling [32], and its effectiveness has been demonstrated in psychotherapy, education, and counseling mediation, regardless of age, manner of delivery, or clinical symptoms [33]. Initially, REBT-based empirical studies largely ignored specific mental disorders and explored the therapy and its effects in pandiagnostic treatments. Therefore, in the early stages of REBT development, there was a lack of research that objectively validated its use with specific diseases [32].

In this study, a binge eating behavior management program based on the REBT theory was developed for female college students, and its effects were tested on self-esteem, covert narcissism, perfectionism, body dissatisfaction, anxiety, depression, and binge eating behavior.

Methods

Ethical approval

The study was approved by the research ethics committee at Sun Moon University prior to data collection (SM-201608-025-2). Prior to their participation, the study's aims and methods were explained to the participants, and they were informed about the voluntary nature of participation, and assured of confidentiality, after which written consent was obtained from each participant.

Experimental design

This was a quasi-experimental study, following a nonequivalent control group pretest-posttest design. The sample size was based on an effect size of 0.5, which was derived from the results of a meta-analysis on the effects of a cognitive-behavioral counseling program [34]; a significance level (α) of .05; and power (1-β) of .80. As per

G*Power 3.1.3, the experimental and control groups required a minimum of 17 participants each. To account for dropout, 48 students (24 in each group) were recruited. However, two students in the control withdrew during the posttest. Accordingly, the final sample included 24 and 22 participants in the experimental and control groups, respectively.

Participants

Current students of S university in C city were recruited through an on-campus recruitment poster. Those who provided informed consent to participate in the study were enrolled. The participant group allocation was determined by flipping a coin (heads: experimental group; tails: control group). Participants were included if they met the following inclusion criteria: tendency to engage in binge eating behavior, as demonstrated by eating attitude scores between 88 and 120 on the Bulimia Test Revised (BULIT-R; see Binge eating section for a discussion of this instrument and its use in the current study); no physical or mental illnesses that could hinder effective communication; and no involvement in any regular binge eating programs or other related educational experiences. The exclusion criteria were as follows: display of improper reward behavior (e.g., self-induced vomiting, diuretics, abuse of prescription drugs or other medications, fasting, or excessive exercise); intellectual disability; substance abuse and/or dependence; diagnosis of any organic mental syndrome; and disabilities that affect education (e.g., hearing and vision impairments).

Procedure

Data collection was conducted from November 1 to December 2, 2016 in the following order: pretest, experimental treatment, and posttest. The data collection methods and procedures are described in the following subsections.

Pretest

The study purpose was explained to all participants prior to participation. All participants provided written informed consent, after which they completed a structured questionnaire regarding general characteristics, and scales on self-esteem, covert narcissism, perfectionism, body dissatisfaction, anxiety, depression, and binge eating. The completed questionnaires were immediately collected.

Experimental treatment

The REBT program was administered to the experimental group. The experimental group attended eight sessions lasting 90–120 min twice per week, with Sessions 4–6 conducted in two groups. The researcher and a graduate student assistant administered the program with the treatment group. The researcher explained the program to the research assistant and trained him in three 1-h sessions regarding the required information, attitudes, and cautionary measures. The control group received education regarding binge eating in one session. During the intervention period, the experimental group was provided with a binge eating-related program, and after termination of the study, the control group was provided with the same intervention program to ensure fairness.

Posttest

Immediately after the eighth session, posttest questionnaires were distributed to both groups. The questionnaire included items regarding self-esteem, inner narcissism, perfectionism, body dissatisfaction, anxiety, depression, and binge eating. Both groups completed the questionnaires and received small gifts for their participation.

During the intervention period, the control group received a binge eating-related intervention program. Upon termination of the study, the control group received the intervention program developed in the current study to ensure fairness.

Measures
Self-esteem

Self-esteem was assessed using Ahn's [35] Korean adaptation of Rosenberg's [36] Self-Esteem Scale. This instrument consists of 10 items, with 5 items for positive self-esteem and 5 items for negative self-esteem. Each item is rated on a 4-point scale from 1 "strongly disagree" to 4 "strongly agree." The total score ranges from 10 to 40, and a higher score indicates higher self-esteem. The reliability of the study as measured with Cronbach's α was .81 in the study by Yoo [37] and .86 in this study.

Covert narcissism

The Covert Narcissism Scale (CNS) developed by Kang and Jeong [38], which was based on Akhtar and Thomson's [39] clinical characteristics of narcissistic personality disorder, was used to measure covert narcissism. Each item is rated on a 5-point scale from 1 "strongly disagree" to 5 "strongly agree." The total score ranges from 45 to 225, and a higher score indicates greater covert narcissism. The reliability of the study as measured with Cronbach's α was .93 in the study by Kang [40] and .89 in this study.

Perfectionism

Perfectionism was measured using a multi-dimensional perfectionism tool, which was first developed by Hewitt and Flett [41] and later adapted into Korean by Kim [42]. This instrument consists of 45 items, with 15 items for self-oriented perfectionism, 15 items for other-oriented perfectionism, and 15 items for socially prescribed perfectionism. Each item is rated on a 7-point scale from 1 "strongly disagree" to 7 "strongly agree." The total score ranges from 45 to 215, and a higher score indicates greater perfectionist tendency.

The Cronbach's α was 0.87 in a study conducted by Jeon [43] and 0.91 in the current study.

Body dissatisfaction

The Body Shape Questionnaire (BSQ), developed by Cooper and colleagues [44] and later adapted into Korean by Noh and Kim [45], was used to determine participants' degree of interest in their body shape. The body dissatisfaction tool consists of 32 items about negative affectivity originating from a feeling of being obese and distortion of the current body weight. Each item is rated on a 6-point scale from 1 "strongly disagree" to 6 "strongly agree." The total score ranges from 32 to 192, and a higher score indicates more frequent feeling of being fat and lower satisfaction with one's body. The Cronbach's α was 0.88 in the original study and 0.94 in the current study.

Anxiety

The State-Trait Anxiety Inventory developed by Spielberger, Gorsuch and Lushene [46], is a commonly used tool to assess anxiety. Kim's Korean adaptation [47], standardized by Hahn, Lee, and Tak [48], was used in the current study. This tool consists of 20 items, and each item is rated on a 4-point scale from 1 "strongly disagree" to 4 "strongly agree." The total score ranges from 20 to 80, and a higher score indicates greater anxiety. The Cronbach's α was 0.92 in a study conducted by Park [49] and 0.93 in the current study.

Depression

Depression was measured using the Korean version of the Center for Epidemiologic Studies Depression Scale (CES-D) developed by Radloff [50] to facilitate epidemiological studies on depression in the general population. Chon and Rhee [51] standardized the CES-D for use in Korean studies. This tool consists of 20 items, and each item is rated on a 4-point scale from 1 "never" to 4 "every day." The total score ranges from 20 to 80, and a higher score indicates increasing severity of depression. The Cronbach's α was 0.91 in a study conducted by Cha [52] and 0.91 in the current study.

Binge eating

In their development of the Bulimia Test, Smith and Thelen [53] relied on DSM-III criteria to diagnose bulimia nervosa. Thelen and colleagues [54] later used the DSM-III-R diagnostic criteria to develop the BULIT-R. The current study used Yoon's [55] version of the tool to measure binge eating. This instrument comprises 36 items assessing five domains: binge eating, emotion, vomiting, food, and body weight. Each item is rated on a five-point scale, and the total score ranges from 36 to 180, where a higher score indicates stronger bulimia nervosa symptoms. In Korean studies, a score of 88 or higher indicates binge eating tendencies, while a score of 121 or higher warrants diagnosis and treatment for eating disorder [55, 56]. The Cronbach's α was 0.90 in a study conducted by Kim [57] and 0.67 in the current study.

Treatment

Table 1 shows the components of the REBT program, which included the following steps: ensuring that participants understood binge eating (first session); identifying participants' belief systems (second session); changing participants' beliefs (third session); forming correct eating habits by achieving cognitive reconstruction (fourth session); focusing on emotional control through emotional confirmation and relaxation (fifth session); focusing on emotional expression (sixth session); attempting behavior modification through

Table 1 Content of the rational emotive behavior therapy-based binge eating behavior management program

Component	Session	Topic	Content	Method
Cognitive Reconstruction	1st	Understanding binge eating	-Introduction to the program's purpose and methods -Creating an alias -Understanding binge eating -Participants share their binging behavior -Discussion and evaluation -Assignment: Dietary diary	Lectures, presentation, discussion, practice, presenting the assignment
	2nd	Identifying belief systems	-Understanding types of beliefs -Distinguishing between rational and irrational beliefs -Self-talking practice -Assignment: Dietary diary -Discussion and evaluation	Lectures, discussion, presentation, practice, discussion
	3rd	Changing beliefs	-Understanding the ABCDE theory -Dispute practice -Applying the ABCDE theory -Discussion and evaluation -Assignment: Applying ABCDE theory to real life	Lectures, practice, role play, discussion, presenting the assignment
	4th	Forming correct eating habits	-Sharing diet experiences -Understanding the advantages and disadvantages of one's diet -Identifying incorrect eating habits -Understanding and planning correct diet habits -Writing to your future self (10 years later) -Discussion and evaluation	Lectures, discussion, presentation, practice
Emotional Control	5th	Emotional confirmation and emotional relaxation	-Identification of positive and negative emotions -Understanding and applying rational emotional imagery -Muscle relaxation training -Discussion and evaluation -Assignment: Applying rational emotional imagery to real life	Lectures, discussion, practice, demonstration, training, presenting the assignment
	6th	Emotional expression	-Understanding and practicing "I-Message" for emotional expression -Discussion and evaluation -Assignment: Applying "I-Message" to real life	Lectures, discussion, practice, role playing, presenting the assignment
Behavior Modification	7th	Problem solving training	-Identifying own problems -Finding ways to troubleshoot -Accepting less than perfect results -Discussion and evaluation -Assignment: Creating a problem-solving paper	Lectures, discussion, practice, role play
	8th	Self-management	-Finding ways to cope with a binging situation -Program evaluation and wrapping up -Share a rolling paper	Discussion, presentation, compensation (presenting gifts)

training on problem-solving skills (seventh session); and ensuring self-management (eighth session). In addition to the REBT program, the researcher conducted weekly private one-to-one interviews with group members by telephone and in person, to prevent a high dropout rate, which might have influenced treatment effects.

A *discussion and evaluation* component was included at the end of each session, to allow participants to present their thoughts and feelings and develop confidence through mutual support and encouragement. This section of the program was designed to reflect participants' opinions regarding each session and improve program quality. Participants were asked to record the times and frequencies of their mealtimes; their thoughts, feelings, and behavior before/after the meal; and whether they were binging, in a *dietary diary,* to measure their eating habits and binging frequency. The participants were asked to write down a list of activities they liked and activities they did not like. Then, they were instructed to reward themselves with activities they liked when they did not binge eat, and engage in activities they did not like after binge eating.

Participants decided to enforce either compensation (e.g., watching movies or shopping for clothes) or punishment (e.g., exercising for 1 h or running for 1 h) based on their own assessments of how well they maintained their dietary records. In the final session, participants presented their dietary diaries, and the researcher used a reinforcement technique involving awarding gifts to participants who had made regular notes and practiced compensation and punishment well.

Statistical analysis

SPSS 20.0 software was used to analyze the data (IBM SPSS Statistics for Windows, Armonk, NY: IBM Corp.). The measurement tools' internal consistency was calculated using the estimated Cronbach's α. A frequency analysis was performed to analyze participants' general characteristics, and χ^2 tests and t tests were performed in crosstabs analysis to assess homogeneity between the control and experimental groups. The Shapiro-Wilk test was used to assess the normality of the general characteristics and dependent variables. The normality of all variables at the baseline for the experimental group and control group was tested with skewness and kurtosis. The absolute skewness was smaller than 3, while the absolute kurtosis was smaller than 10, thereby satisfying the assumption of normality.

A *t*-test was performed to determine whether the self-esteem, covert narcissism, perfectionism, body dissatisfaction, anxiety, depression, and binge eating variables were homogeneous between the control and experimental groups. An analysis of covariance (ANCOVA) was performed to control for the pre-score difference between groups for variables that differed between groups in the pre-homogeneity test. The ANCOVA was also performed to verify the effect of the REBT program.

Results

Homogeneity test for general characteristics

The homogeneity test indicated no significant difference between the groups ($p = .05$); therefore, the two groups were homogeneous with regard to demographic variables (Table 2).

Table 2 Homogeneity of participants' general characteristics ($N = 46$)

Division	Classification	Experimental group ($n = 24$) n (%)	Control group ($n = 22$) n (%)	t	P-value
Age	19–21	22 (91.70)	16 (72.70)	3.168	.205
	22–23	2 (8.30)	6 (27.30)		
	M ± SD	20.52 ± 0.79	20.91 ± 1.16	1.334	.189
Year	1–2	8 (33.30)	9 (40.90)	0.283	.595
	3	16 (66.70)	13 (59.1)		
Major	Nutrition, medical field	10 (41.70)	6 (27.30)	1.049	.306
	Non-nutrition, non-medical field	14 (58.30)	16 (72.70)		
Residence Type	House	10 (41.70)	7 (31.80)	0.406	.780
	Dormitory	9 (37.50)	10 (45.50)		
	Boarding/other	5 (20.80)	5 (22.70)		
Religion	Yes	9 (37.50)	6 (27.30)	0.546	.460
	No	15 (62.50)	16 (72.70)		
Weight (kg)	< 60 kg	14 (58.30)	14 (63.60)	0.136	.713
	> 60 kg	10 (41.70)	8 (36.40)		
	M ± SD	59.05 ± 8.70	58.30 ± 6.66	−0.322	.749

We assumed that certain general characteristics would affect binge eating behavior as religion influences food culture, and the degree of stress depends on an individual's major. We also assumed that type of residence would have an effect on binge eating behavior; for example, a person living alone may have difficulty in forming regular eating habits.

Most participants in the experimental group ($n = 24$) as well as the control group ($n = 22$) were aged 19–21 years, at 91.7 and 72.7%, respectively. Regarding school year, 33.3% in the experimental group and 40.9% in the control group were 1st- or 2nd-year students. The percentage of students majoring in food and medicine was 41.7% and that of students majoring in non-food and non-medicine subjects was 58.3% in the experimental group; the percentages were 27.3 and 72.7%, respectively, in the control group. Regarding living arrangements, 41.7% of participants lived in their homes, 37.5% in the dorm, and 20.8% in a boarding house or other in the experimental group; the percentages were 31.8, 45.5, and 22.7%, respectively, in the control group. Regarding religion, in the experimental group, 37.5% identified themselves as religious, while 62.5% did not; in the control group, 27.3% were religious, while 72.7% were not. In the experimental group, 58.3% of participants weighed under 60 kgs, and 41.7% weighed 60 kgs or more, with a mean body weight of 59.05 kg. In the control group, 63.6% weighed under 60 kgs, and 36.4% weighed 60 kgs or higher, with a mean weight of 58.30 kg.

Homogeneity test for the pre-experimental dependent variables

Table 3 shows the results of the pre-experimental homogeneity test for the dependent variables. The groups were homogeneous in the case of self-esteem, covert narcissism, perfectionism, physical dissatisfaction, anxiety, and depression. The variable of binge eating, however, was not homogenous, as the means (according to a five-point scale) for this item differed significantly (experimental group $M = 93.83$, $SD = 8.42$; control group $M = 99.45$, $SD = 9.94$).

Verifying program effectiveness
Effects on self-esteem
As illustrated in Table 4, the pretest and posttest results for self-esteem indicated that the experimental group's posttest scores ($M = 29.33$, $SD = 4.37$) were higher relative to their pretest scores ($M = 26.79$, $SD = 3.86$), while the control group's scores decreased from the pretest ($M = 26.09$, $SD = 4.85$) to the posttest ($M = 24.77$, $SD = 4.57$).

Effects on covert narcissism
Results for covert narcissism showed that the experimental group exhibited a decrease in scores from pretest ($M = 133.33$, $SD = 19.14$) to posttest ($M = 122.25$, $SD = 23.96$). However, the control group's scores increased from pretest ($M = 135.00$, $SD = 20.39$) to posttest ($M = 138.18$, $SD = 22.23$; Table 4).

Effects on perfectionism
Regarding pretest and posttest perfectionism scores, the change in the experimental group's scores (4.79) was greater relative to that in the control group's scores (1.04), but this difference was nonsignificant. The experimental groups perfectionism scores decreased from pretest ($M = 178.04$, $SD = 29.59$) to posttest ($M = 173.25$, $SD = 30.31$). Further, the control group's scores decreased from pretest ($M = 183.23$, $SD = 26.47$) to posttest ($M = 182.91$, $SD = 25.43$; Table 4).

Effects on body dissatisfaction
The body dissatisfaction results indicated that the experimental group's scores decreased from pretest ($M = 133.04$, $SD = 27.01$) to posttest ($M = 115.17$, $SD = 26.89$). However, the control group's scores increased from pretest ($M = 133.50$, $SD = 26.75$) to posttest ($M = 144.23$, $SD = 17.99$; Table 4).

Effects on anxiety
The experimental group's anxiety scores decreased from pretest ($M = 48.46$, $SD = 10.56$) to posttest ($M = 41.25$, $SD = 9.54$), while the control group's anxiety scores

Table 3 Homogeneity test for pre-experiment dependent variables ($N = 46$)

Variable	Experimental Group ($n = 24$)	Control Group ($n = 22$)	t	P-value
	M ± SD	M ± SD		
Self-Esteem	26.79 ± 3.86	26.09 ± 4.85	−.545	.589
Covert Narcissism	133.33 ± 19.14	135.00 ± 20.39	0.286	.776
Perfectionism	178.04 ± 29.59	183.23 ± 26.47	0.624	.536
Body Dissatisfaction	4.16 ± 0.84	133.50 ± 26.75	0.058	.954
Anxiety	48.46 ± 10.56	50.64 ± 11.93	0.657	.515
Depression	41.54 ± 10.56	44.45 ± 10.11	0.974	.336
Binge Eating	93.83 ± 8.42	99.45 ± 9.94	2.075	.044*

Table 4 Differences in dependent variables between groups

Variable	Group	Pretest M ± SD	Posttest M ± SD	F^a	P-value
Self-esteem	Exp.	26.79 ± 3.86	29.33 ± 4.37	9.144	.004**
	Cont.	26.09 ± 4.85	24.77 ± 4.57		
Covert narcissism	Exp.	133.33 ± 19.14	122.25 ± 23.96	4.424	.041*
	Cont.	135.00 ± 20.39	138.18 ± 22.23		
Perfectionism	Exp.	178.04 ± 29.59	173.25 ± 30.31	1.52	.225
	Cont.	183.23 ± 26.47	182.91 ± 25.43		
Body dissatisfaction	Exp.	133.04 ± 27.01	115.17 ± 26.89	12.441	.001***
	Cont.	133.50 ± 26.75	144.23 ± 17.99		
Anxiety	Exp.	48.46 ± 10.56	41.25 ± 9.54	10.544	.002**
	Cont.	50.64 ± 11.93	50.91 ± 10.41		
Depression	Exp.	41.54 ± 10.16	37.21 ± 8.90	13.245	.001**
	Cont.	44.45 ± 10.11	47.32 ± 9.01		
Binge eating	Exp.	93.83 ± 8.42	69.67 ± 14.73	20.538	< .001***
	Cont.	99.45 ± 9.94	93.36 ± 16.13		

* $p < .05$, ** $p < .01$, *** $p < .001$
a Measured by an analysis of covariance, *Exp.* Experimental group, *Cont.* Control group

increased from the pretest (M = 50.64, SD = 11.93) to the posttest (M = 50.91, SD = 10.41; Table 4).

Effects on depression

The experimental group's depression scores decreased from pretest (M = 41.54, SD = 10.16) to posttest (M = 37.21, SD = 8.90). However, the control group's scores increased from the pretest (M = 44.45, SD = 10.11) to the posttest (M = 47.32, SD = 9.01; Table 4).

Effects on binge eating

The difference between the pretest and posttest scores in the experimental group (24.16) were greater relative to those in the control group (6.09). Scores decreased from pretest (M = 93.83, SD = 8.42) to posttest (M = 69.67, SD = 14.73) in the experimental group. In addition, the control group's score on binge eating decreased from pretest (M = 99.45, SD = 9.94) to posttest (M = 93.36, SD = 16.13; Table 4).

Discussion

The REBT-based binge eating behavior management program developed in this study reduced participants' irrational beliefs, that is, the cognitive factors of covert narcissism, perfectionism, and body dissatisfaction, and the emotional factors of anxiety and depression, as well as the behavioral factor of binge eating, while positively impacting participants' self-esteem. We discuss these results below.

First, after completing the REBT-based binge eating behavior management program, the experimental group had a significantly higher self-esteem score than the control group, thereby providing evidence for effectiveness of this program. Previous findings of Saelid and Nordahl [58], who applied a short three-session program using the ABC model of REBT, support our findings. However, our results are in contrast with the result of a previous study, where a cognitive behavioral program did not effectively increase self-esteem in female undergraduates [59], although that program's effectiveness may have been impacted by its inclusion of a cognitive restructuring intervention in only one out of the eight sessions (specific methods were not included in the report of the earlier study). On the other hand, our program significantly increased self-esteem by converting irrational beliefs to rational ones by specifically using a technique known as refutation based on the ABCDE model. Further, checking the restructured cognition through role play and presenting a task in each session to help participants to practice it in their daily living seemed to have contributed to their increased self-esteem.

Second, after the REBT-based binge eating management program, the experimental group had a significantly lower covert narcissism score than the control group, thereby providing evidence for the effectiveness of this program. This is similar to previous results of reduction in social media addiction tendencies through cognitive therapy with a focus on maladaptive cognitive emotional control strategies [60]. Further, Jeon [61] also reported that mindfulness intervention, a type of cognitive behavioral therapy, for participants with high covert narcissism significantly lowered covert narcissism, which supports our findings. As people with high covert narcissism fear criticism and rejection and feel embarrassment, we believe that encouraging the expression of their emotions through the "expressing negative emotions" activity in session 6, and helping them forgive and accept themselves through the "accepting less perfect results" activity in session 7, would have facilitated the positive outcome.

Third, after the REBT-based binge eating management program, while the posttest mean perfectionism score was low in the experimental group, there were no statistically significant differences in perfectionism between the experimental group and control group. We assume that the participants' experience of psychological pressure to see positive changes after the study could have contributed to lowering perfectionism, albeit nonsignificantly. In addition, considering that perfectionism is a continuous character trait that is difficult to be significantly altered even with therapeutic interventions [62], we can surmise that a significant difference could not be observed owing to the short intervention period. Subsequent studies should utilize more diverse intervention methods and periods to alter perfectionism and compare them.

Fourth, after the REBT-based binge eating behavior management program, the experimental group had a significantly lower body dissatisfaction score than the control group, thereby providing evidence for the effectiveness of this program. Previous studies on the effect of cognitive behavioral therapy on body satisfaction of female college students with a negative body image [63] and the effect of cognitive behavioral program and meditation on body image in female middle school students [64] support our results. The participants of our program exhibited abnormal eating behaviors due to their body dissatisfaction, such as going on a diet to attain a thin and beautiful body figure. The program taught them of the risk of binge eating and diet and attempted to convert their irrational belief favoring a slim body shape into a rational belief through refutations of notions such as "do you really have to be skinny?" "Is everyone skinny in the real world?" and "what are the benefits of being skinny?" Further, the "accepting less perfect results" activity attempted to lower participants' dissatisfaction with their bodies. We believe these intervention techniques would have led to the positive outcome of lowering body dissatisfaction.

Fifth, after the REBT-based binge eating management program, the experimental group had a significantly lower anxiety score than the control group, thereby providing evidence for the effectiveness of this program. Previous results that REBT-based group counseling program was effective in lowering test anxiety in elementary school students [65] and high school students [66] support our findings. In this study, the addition of emotional control and behavioral correction interventions for cognitive restructuring rendered the program more effective in lowering anxiety. We also believe that

directly intervening with emotional control would have contributed to significant improvement.

Sixth, after the REBT-based binge eating behavior management program, the experimental group had a significantly lower depression score than the control group, thereby providing evidence for the effectiveness of this program. As described in our review of previous studies, depression, in addition to anxiety, was an important predictor of binge eating. Our results are supported by a previous study in which cognitive behavioral therapy was found to be superior to supportive expressive therapy in lowering depression in patients with binge eating [67]. The study that observed that correcting irrational beliefs through a REBT-based group counseling program led to a significant reduction of depression Stice [68] also supports our findings. Fischer et al. [69] reported that the intervention group that underwent a cognitive behavioral group therapy showed significantly greater reduction in depression compared to the control group among binge eaters [70], and a study on the effects of cognitive behavioral therapy on depression in female college students with a negative body image Park and Son [63] also confirmed that the therapy is effective for female college students showing binge eating behaviors, which are in line with our study. Through this program, the participants examined negative thinking, and explored and honestly expressed their depressive emotions about themselves. Further, by using a rational emotive imagery technique as an intervention, the participants were capacitated to experience positive and healthy emotions instead of negative and inappropriate emotions that are provoked when thinking about a negative event. This intervention for emotional control seems to have contributed to the effectiveness of the program.

Seventh, the experimental group had a significantly reduced binge eating score than the control group in the posttest evaluation, thereby providing evidence for the effectiveness of this program. The participants noted in their evaluations that writing a diet journal to monitor their binge eating behaviors and their thoughts and emotions and rewarding and punishing themselves accordingly substantially helped them reduce binge eating behaviors. They also reported that the assignment that required them to continue practicing to refute their irrational beliefs after the end of the session was beneficial for altering their irrational beliefs, regulating negative emotions, and lowering binge eating. In this study, the emotional relaxation training in session 5 and expression of negative emotions and conversing with others without hurting their own or others' feelings by using "I-message" in session 6 seem to have contributed to emotional control and ultimately to lowering binge eating.

Ultimately, these results provide evidence that the integrative cognitive, emotional, and behavioral techniques of REBT are appropriate and useful for intervention in binge eating behavior and bringing about positive changes in the factors involved. However, a few limitations need consideration. First, this study was conducted with female college students attending one university; therefore, the findings cannot be generalized. Second, as this program is an intervention for binge eating behavior and related factors, its ultimate goal is the prevention of eating disorders. In order to verify the effectiveness of the intervention in the long run, a long-term follow-up is needed, as the current study did not examine its long-term effects. Third, because the Cronbach's α (=.67) for binge eating behavioral measures was low, other measures should be considered in future studies. Fourth, although we considered participants' weight, more restrictive selection criteria (e.g., body mass index) should be considered in future. Finally, because the study was conducted using the nonequivalent control group design, the results have limited generalizability. Despite these limitations, this study is significant in that it is the first to apply REBT in a binge eating behavior intervention for young female students. Furthermore, by examining the risk factors of binge eating, it informs the direction subsequent studies may take to develop binge eating behavior intervention programs.

Conclusions

In summary, the REBT-based binge eating management program for female college students positively altered their self-esteem, and led to reduction in covert narcissism, body dissatisfaction, anxiety, depression, and binge eating. This program was applied to female students, but we suggest that subsequent studies expand the target population according to age, sex, and degree of symptoms based on the intervention components of the program. Since the ultimate aim of this program is to prevent eating disorders, we suggest future researchers to conduct long-term follow-ups to examine whether the effects of the program persist after its completion. In addition, while a group counseling technique was used in this study, subsequent studies may develop and assess interventions using social media or mobile phone applications to enable ease of participation for those who cannot participate in person.

Abbreviations
BULIT-R: Bulimia Test Revised; BSQ: Body Shape Questionnaire; CES-D: Center for Epidemiologic Studies Depression Scale; CNS: Covert Narcissism Scale; REBT: Rational emotive behavior therapy

Acknowledgements
This study was supported by Korea Nursing Research Center. We thank the families who participated in the study and the researchers who shared their research instruments.

Authors' contributions
KSH developed the research concept and supervised the data collection. JWY collected and analyzed the data, and was responsible for the writing of the manuscript. All authors read, provided feedback, and approved the final manuscript.

Competing interests
The authors declare that they have no competing interests.

Author details
Department of Nursing, Kyungil University, Gyeongsan-si, South Korea.
Department of Nursing, Korea University, Seoul, South Korea.

References
1. Izydorczyk B. A psychological typology of females diagnosed with anorexia nervosa, bulimia nervosa or binge eating disorder. Health Psychol Rep. 2015;3(4):312–25. https://doi.org/10.5114/hpr.2015.55169.
2. Woo J. A survey of overweight, body shape perception and eating attitude of Korean female university students. J Exerc Nutrition Biochem. 2014;18(3):287–92. https://doi.org/10.5717/jenb.2014.18.3.287.
3. National Health Insurance Service. "Bulimia" in women is 15 times more than men. In: NHIS press release: Ministry of Health and Welfare; 2015. https://129.go.kr/news/news02_view.jsp?n=8357. Accessed 20 Jan 2018.
4. Lee IH, Hwang HK. Anxiety, body checking, and eating disorder related symptoms in non-clinical group: the mediated moderating effect of body checking cognition and behavior. Kor J Psychol Health. 2015;20(2):405–68.
5. Byun YS, Lee NH, Lee KH. Factors influencing eating problems among Korean university women. J Korean Acad Fundam Nurs. 2014;21(4):362–9. https://doi.org/10.7739/JKAFN.2014.21.4.362.
6. American Psychiatric Association. Diagnostic and statistical manual of mental disorders (DSM-V). 5th ed. Washington, DC: American Psychiatric Association; 2013.
7. Stephen EM, Rose JS, Kenney L, Rosselli-Navarra F, Weissman RS. Prevalence and correlates of unhealthy weight control behaviors: findings from the national longitudinal study of adolescent health. J Eat Disord. 2014;2:16. https://doi.org/10.1186/2050-2974-2-16.
8. Nakai Y, Nin K, Noma S. Eating disorder symptoms among Japanese female students in 1982, 1992 and 2002. Psychiatry Res. 2014;219(1):151–6. https://doi.org/10.1016/j.psychres.2014.05.0189.
9. Lindberg L, Hjern A. Risk factors for anorexia nervosa: a national cohort study. Int J Eat Disord. 2003;34(4):397–408. https://doi.org/10.1002/eat.10221.
10. Burton AL, Abbott MJ. Processes and pathways to binge eating: development of an integrated cognitive and behavioural model of binge eating. J Eat Disord. 2019;7:18. https://doi.org/10.1186/s40337-019-0248-0 Published 2019 Jun 7.
11. Stice E, Marti CN, Durant S. Risk factors for onset of eating disorders: evidence of multiple risk pathways from an 8-year prospective study. Behav Res Ther. 2011;49(10):622–7. https://doi.org/10.1016/j.brat.2011.06.009.
12. Russell SL, Haynos AF, Crow SJ, Fruzzetti AE. An experimental analysis of the affect regulation model of binge eating. Appetite. 2017;110:44–50. https://doi.org/10.1016/j.appet.2016.12.007.
13. Short MM, Mushquash AR, Sherry SB. Perseveration moderates the relationship between perfectionism and binge eating: a multi-method daily diary study. Eat Behav. 2013;14(3):394–6. https://doi.org/10.1016/j.eatbeh.2013.06.001.
14. Herman CP, Polivy J. Causes of eating disorders. Annu Rev Psychol. 2002;53:187–213. https://doi.org/10.1146/annurev.psych.53.100901.135103.
15. Stein D, Kaye WH, Matsunage H, Orbach I, Har-Even D, Frank G, et al. Eating related concerns, mood, and personality traits in recovered bulimia nervosa subjects: a replication study. Int J Eat Disord. 2002;32(2):225–9. https://doi.org/10.1002/eat.10025.
16. Tomori M, Rus-Makovec M. Eating behavior, depression, and self-esteem in high school students. J Adolesc Health. 2000;26(5):361–7. https://doi.org/10.1016/S1054-139X(98)00042-1.

17. Kim HJ. Effects of covert narcissism, shame, and depression on binge-eating among university students [master's thesis]. Jinju: Gyeongsang National University; 2014. Korean.

18. Rosenbaum DL, White KS. The relation of anxiety, depression, and stress to binge eating behavior. J Health Psychol. 2015;20(6):887–98. https://doi.org/10.1177/1359105315580212.

19. Dorairaj K, Thompson K, Wilksch S, Wade T, Paxton S, Austin S, Byrne S. Risk factors for eating disorders: investigating the relationships between global self-esteem, body-specific self-esteem and dietary restraint. J Eat Disord. 2013;1(S1):O31. https://doi.org/10.1186/2050-2974-1-S1-O31.

20. Gordon KH, Dombeck JJ. The associations between two facets of narcissism and eating disorder symptoms. Eat Behav. 2010;11:288–92. https://doi.org/10.1016/j.eatbeh.2010.08.004.

21. Back MD, Schmukle SC, Egloff B. Why are narcissists so charming at first sight: decoding the narcissism-popularity link at zero acquaintance. J Pers Soc Psychol. 2010;98(1):132–45. https://doi.org/10.1037/a0016338.

22. Maples J, Collins B, Miller JD, Fischer S, Seibert A. Differences between grandiose and vulnerable narcissism and bulimic symptoms in young women. Eat Behav. 2011;12(1):83–5. https://doi.org/10.1016/j.eatbeh.2010.10.001.

23. Frost RO, Marten P, Lahart C, Rosenblate R. The dimensions of perfectionism. Cognit Ther Res. 1990;14:449–68. https://doi.org/10.1007/BF01172967.

24. Mackinnon SP, Sherry SB, Graham AR, Stewart SH, Sherry DL, Allen SL, et al. Reformulating and testing the perfectionism model of binge eating among undergraduate women: a short-term, three-wave longitudinal study. J Couns Psychol. 2011;58:630–46. https://doi.org/10.1037/a0025068.

25. Luppino FS, de Wit LM, Bouvy PF, Stijnen T, Cuijpers P, Penninx BW, et al. Overweight, obesity, and depression: a systematic review and meta-analysis of longitudinal studies. Arch Gen Psychiatry. 2010;67(3):220–9. https://doi.org/10.1001/archgenpsychiatry.2010.2.

26. Ostrovsky NW, Swencionis C, Wylie-Rosett J, Isasi CR. Social anxiety and disordered overeating: an association among overweight and obese individuals. Eat Behav. 2013;14:145–8. https://doi.org/10.1016/j.eatbeh.2013.01.009.

27. Araujo DMR, Santos GFDS, Nardi AE. Binge eating disorder and depression: a systematic review. World J Biol Psychiatry. 2010;11(2–2):199–207. https://doi.org/10.3109/15622970802563171.

28. Wolff GE, Crosby RD, Roberts JA, Wittrock DA. Differences in daily stress, mood, coping, and eating behavior in binge eating and nonbinge eating women. Addict Behav. 2000;25(2):205–16. https://doi.org/10.1016/S0306-4603(99)00049-0.

29. Goldschmidt AB, Wall MM, Zhang J, Loth KA, Neumark-Sztainer D. Overeating and binge eating in emerging adulthood:10-year stability and risk factors. Dev Psychol. 2016;52:475–83. https://doi.org/10.1037/Fdev0000086.

30. Ellis A. Reason and emotion in psychotherapy. New York: Birch Lane Press; 1994.

31. Allen KL, Byrne SM, McLean NJ. The dual-pathway and cognitive-behavioural models of binge eating: prospective evaluation and comparison. Eur Child Adolesc Psychiatry. 2012;21(1):51–62. https://doi.org/10.1007/s00787-011-0231-z.

32. David D. Rational emotive behavior therapy. New York: Oxford University Press; 2014.

33. David D, Cotet C, Matu S, Mogoase C, Stefan S. 50 years of rational-emotive and cognitive-behavioral therapy: a systematic review and meta-analysis. J Clin Psychol. 2018;74(3):304–18. https://doi.org/10.1002/jclp.22514.

34. Kim NJ. The meta-analysis for effectiveness of cognitive behavior therapy program: focusing on the references of 2005 to 2015 [master's thesis]. Seoul: Dankook University; 2015. Korean.

35. Ahn SY. Effect of body dissatisfaction on self-esteem and depression in binge eater group [master's thesis]. Seoul: Yonsei University, Seoul, South Korea; 1994. Korean.

36. Rosenberg M. Self-esteem scale. In: Robinson JP, Shaver PR, Wrightsam LS, editors. Measure of personality and social psychological attitudes, vol. 1. Cambridge: Academic; 1965. p. 80–2.

37. Yoo SA. A study on factors affecting eating disorders in female college students [master's thesis]. Gwangju: Nambu University Graduate School; 2014. Korean.

38. Gang SH, Chung NW. A study on the development and validation of the covert narcissism scale. Korean J Counsel Psychotherapy. 2002;14(4):969–90.

39. Akhtar S, Thomson A. Overview: narcissistic personality disorder. Am J Psychiatry. 1982;139(1):12–20. https://doi.org/10.1176/ajp.139.1.12.

40. Kang MS. The effect of female college students' covert narcissism and self-silencing on eating attitude [master's thesis]. Seoul: Myongji University; 2014. Korean.

41. Hewitt PL, Flett GL. Perfectionism in the self and social contexts: conceptualization, assessment and association with psychopathology. J Pers Soc Psychol. 1991;60(3):456–70. https://doi.org/10.1037/0022-3514.60.3.456.

42. Kim YS. The effects of perfectionism and self-esteem on immediate depressive reaction and enduring depressive reaction after experiencing achievement-related stress [master's thesis]. Seoul: Catholic University; 1998. Korean.

43. Jeon MJ. The mediating effect of self-efficacy on the relationship between perfectionism and disordered eating behavior of the adolescent [master's thesis]. Seoul: Sungkyunkwan University; 2015. Korean.

44. Cooper PJ, Taylor MJ, Cooper Z, Fairburn CG. The development and validation of the body shape questionnaire. Int J Eat Disord. 1987;6(4):485–94. https://doi.org/10.1002/1098-108X(198707)6:4<485::AID-EAT2260060405>3.0.CO;2-O.

45. Noh YK, Kim BW. The validation study of the body shape questionnaire (BSQ): in female university students. Korean J Counsel. 2005;6(4):1163–74.

46. Spielberger CD, Gorsuch RL, Lushene RE. Manual for the state-trait anxiety inventory. Palo Alto: Consulting Psychologists Press; 1970.

47. Kim JT. The relationship between trait anxiety and sociality: focusing on Spielberger's STAI [master's thesis]. Seoul: Korea University Seoul; 1978. Korean.

48. Hahn DW, Lee CH, Tak JK. Standardization of Spielberger state-trait anxiety inventory. Korean Psychol Assoc Annu Conf. 1993;1993(0):505–12.

49. Park HR. The effect of female college student's self-compassion, depression and anxiety on eating attitude [master's thesis]. Seoul: Myongji University; 2014. Korean.

50. Radloff LS. The CES-D scale: a self-report depression scale for research in the general population. Appl Psychol Meas. 1977;1(3):385–401. https://doi.org/10.1177/014662167700100306.

51. Chon JK, Rhee MK. Preliminary development of Korean version of CES-D. Korean J Clin Psychol. 1992;11(1):437–55.

52. Cha YJ. A study on construction of suicidal ideation prediction model in adolescents [dissertation]. Seoul: Korea University; 2008. Korean.

53. Smith MC, Thelen MH. Development and validation of a test for bulimia nervosa. J Consult Clin Psychol. 1984;52(5):863–72. https://doi.org/10.1037/0022-006X.52.5.863.

54. Thelen MH, Farmer J, Wonderlich J, Smith MC. A revision of the bulimia test: BULIT-R. Psychol Assess. 1991;3(1):119–24. https://doi.org/10.1037/1040-3590.3.1.119.

55. Yoon HY. The relationship between female college students' binge eating behavior, depression, and attribution style [master's thesis]. Seoul: Catholic University; 1996. Korean.

56. Lee JA. Cognitive traits of binge eating behavior groups [master's thesis]. Seoul: Korea University; 1998. Korean.

57. Kim SJ. The effects of a cognitive-behavioral group counseling program on body dissatisfaction, self-esteem and depression of high school girl students with binge eating [master's thesis]. Daegu: Keimyung University; 2005. Korean.

58. Sælid GA, Nordahl HM. Rational emotive behaviour therapy in high schools to educate in mental health and empower youth health. A randomized controlled study of a brief intervention. Behav Cogn Psychother. 2016;46(3):196–210. https://doi.org/10.1080/16506073.2016.1233453.

59. Han JH. Effects of cognitive behavioral group treatment of bulimia neuroticism [master's thesis]. Seoul: Deoksung University University; 2003. Korean.

60. Lee EJ. The relationship between university students' inner self-love and SNS addiction tendency [master's thesis]. ChunAn: Soonchunhyang University Graduate School; 2015. Korean.

61. Jeon AR. The influence of the counselor's implicit narcissism and mindfulness on behavior of reversal [master's thesis]. Seoul: Graduate School of Education, Sogang University; 2011. Korean.

62. Flett GL, Hewitt PL. Treatment interventions for perfectionism-a cognitive perspective: introduction to the special issue. J Ration Emot Cogn Behav Ther. 2008;26:127–31. https://doi.org/10.1007/s10942-007-0063-4

63. Park SJ, Son CN. The effects of cognitive behavioral therapy on body image

satisfaction, self-esteem, and depression of female college students with negative body images. Kor J Psychol Health. 2002;7(3):335–51.

64. Hwang HJ, Kim KH. The effects of cognitive-behavioral programs and meditation training programs on improvement of body dissatisfaction and binge eating and weight loss of middle school girls. Kor J Psychol Health. 1999;4(1):140–54.

65. Jeong DH. The effect of the REBT Group counseling program on exam anxiety in elementary school students [master's thesis]. Busan: Graduate School of Education, Pusan National University of Education; 2006. Korean.

66. Lee EY. Comparison of the effects of MBSR and REBT on test anxiety reduction [master's thesis]. Seoul: Graduate School, Chung-Ang University; 2008. Korean.

67. Garner DM. Pathogenesis of anorexia nervosa. Lancet. 1993;341:1631–5. https://doi.org/10.1016/0140-6736(93)90768-c.

68. Stice E. Clinical implications of psychosocial research on bulimia nervosa and binge-eating disorder. Clin Psychol. 1999;55:675–84. https://doi.org/10.1002/(SICI)1097-4679(199906)55:6%3C675::AID-JCLP2%3E3.0.CO;2-3.

69. Fischer S, Meyer AH, Dremmel D, Schlup B, Munsch S. Short-term cognitive-behavioral therapy for binge eating disorder: long-term efficacy and predictors of long-term treatment success. Behav Res Ther. 2014;14:36–42. https://doi.org/10.1016/j.brat.2014.04.007.

70. Telch CF, Agras WS, Rossister EM. Group cognitive-behavioral treatment for the nonpurging bulimia: an initial evaluation. J Consult Clin Psychol. 1990;58(5):629–35. https://doi.org/10.1037//0022-006x.58.5.629.

14

Can we change binge eating behaviour by interventions addressing food-related impulsivity?

Başak İnce[1], Johanna Schlatter[2], Sebastian Max[3], Christian Plewnia[3], Stephan Zipfel[2,4], Katrin Elisabeth Giel[2,4] and Kathrin Schag[2,4*] (iD)

Abstract

Background: An extensive amount of research has underlined the potential role of impulsivity in the development and maintenance of binge eating behaviour. Food-related impulsivity has particularly received attention given its close relationship with overeating and binge eating episodes. Besides the available evidence, our understanding regarding the effectiveness of treatment modalities for binge eating targeting impulsivity and related constructs (e.g., food craving, inhibitory control, and reward sensitivity) is limited. Thus, this systematic review aimed to investigate whether binge eating behaviour is changeable by interventions that are impulsivity-focused and food-related and whether one of these interventions is superior to the others.

Method: A search on PubMed and PsycINFO was performed for relevant articles published up to September 2020. Studies delivering food-related impulsivity treatment to individuals suffering from binge eating episodes and including a control condition without this treatment were investigated. Following the search, 15 studies meeting the eligibility criteria were analysed.

Results: Analyses revealed that available impulsivity-focused approaches can be categorised as psychotherapy, pharmacotherapy, computer-assisted cognitive training, and direct neuromodulation interventions. Regarding their effectiveness, it appeared that all of these approaches might be promising to change food-related impulsivity in individuals with binge eating episodes, particularly to decrease binge eating symptoms. However, a superior intervention approach in this early state of evidence could not be determined, although food-related cue exposure, transcranial direct current stimulation, and the combination of several interventions seem fruitful.

Conclusion: Efforts to treat binge eating behaviour with interventions focusing on food-related impulsivity appear to be promising, particularly concerning binge eating frequency, and also for food craving and inhibitory control. Given limited research and varying methods, it was not possible to conclude whether one impulsivity-focused intervention can be considered superior to others.

Keywords: Binge eating, Eating behaviour, Food, Impulsivity, Treatment, Training, Psychotherapy, Pharmacotherapy, Neurostimulation

* Correspondence: kathrin.schag@med.uni-tuebingen.de
[2]Department of Psychosomatic Medicine and Psychotherapy, University Hospital Tübingen, Osianderstraße 5, 72076 Tübingen, Germany
[4]Competence Center of Eating Disorders Tübingen (KOMET), Tübingen, Germany
Full list of author information is available at the end of the article

Plain English summary

As one of the core symptoms of bulimia nervosa and binge eating disorder, binge eating behaviour negatively influences the physical and psychosocial well-being of a significant number of people. Current first-line treatments for bulimia nervosa and binge eating disorder are effective, but often do not result in sustainable remission for a substantial number of patients. Existing treatments targeting binge eating might benefit from interventions directly targeting impulsivity, particularly food-related impulsivity, which can be a potential etiological and/or maintaining factor for binge eating behaviour. With this systematic review investigating novel impulsivity-focused treatments for individuals with binge eating behaviour, promising approaches to change food-related impulsivity are described. The included studies use several impulsivity-focused treatments, ranging from specific psychotherapy that includes so-called cue exposure treatment, as well as computer training, pharmacotherapy, or direct stimulation of the brain with special equipment. Despite the limited number of studies and lack of data available to conclude the superiority of one of these approaches, the reviewed treatments seem promising to improve treatment outcomes.

Background

Binge eating behaviour refers to the consumption of a large amount of food in a short period of time accompanied by feelings of loss of control over eating [1]. Even though binge eating behaviour can be observed in many individuals irrespective of an eating disorder (ED) diagnosis (e.g., people with obesity or emotional eating), it is considered to be the core feature of bulimia nervosa (BN) and binge eating disorder (BED). BN and BED are frequently presenting EDs affecting people worldwide. According to the data collected from 14 countries for the World Mental Health Survey of the World Health Organization, lifetime prevalence estimates were 1.0% for BN and 1.9% for BED [2]. Since binge eating behaviour causes weight gain, medical complications, and psychosocial impairments [3], it is important to explore and further understand the underlying and maintaining mechanisms behind this dysfunctional behaviour.

According to systematic reviews and meta-analyses, a great number of studies have identified the personality trait impulsivity as a potential aetiological and/or maintaining factor for binge eating behaviour [4–6]. Impulsivity is not only a personality trait, but also a significant construct for the understanding and diagnosis of a variety of psychological illnesses (e.g., attention-deficit/hyperactivity disorder, borderline personality disorder, and substance use disorder) [7]. Moeller and colleagues [8] defined impulsivity as "a predisposition toward rapid, unplanned reactions to internal or external stimuli without regard to the negative consequences of these reactions to the impulsive individual or others" (p. 1784). More recently, Gullo and colleagues [9] investigated the facets of impulsivity by considering different models and summarised that reward sensitivity and disinhibition are the aspects of impulsivity that play the main role in addictive-like behaviour. Negative urgency, i.e. the tendency to show impulsive behaviour particularly in negative mood is currently accepted as a factor of impulsivity, following reward sensitivity and disinhibition [9].

In particular, food-related impulsivity has received attention given its close relationship with binge eating behaviour [5]. Dawe and Loxton [10] initially proposed a relationship between food-related impulsive tendencies and binge eating. According to the authors, individuals who binge eat suffer from increased food craving, i.e. an intense desire to eat particular foods as they perceive food and related stimuli highly rewarding [11]. Having a high level of reward sensitivity towards food-related stimuli could increase the likelihood of binge eating and decrease the ability to inhibit or control eating [10]. Similarly, Treasure and colleagues [12] propose that individuals with binge eating behaviour have a hyper-responsive reward system and impaired inhibitory control towards food-related cues. Regardless of the type of instrument used, namely self-report measures, behavioural tasks, and electroencephalography (EEG), the evidence supports a positive association between increased impulsivity and binge eating behaviour in both healthy and clinical samples [5, 8]. For example, electrocortical process analyses in EEG studies have shown alterations regarding conflict processing, inhibitory control deficits, and higher levels of frontal beta activity which has been positively associated with disinhibited eating [13, 14]. Studies investigating the neurobiological basis of binge eating behaviour report an enhanced attentional bias towards food stimuli, alterations in the reward system, and impairments in cognitive functions like poor inhibitory control skills towards food [15, 16]. Moreover, evidence suggests that individuals with high levels of negative urgency are more likely to consider food as a way of coping with negative emotions, thus engaging in binge eating behaviour [17, 18]. Taken together, this bio-psychological model of food-related impulsivity including increased reward sensitivity, disinhibition, and negative urgency strongly resembles the three-pathway model of alcohol craving [19] and hints that substance addictions and impulsive eating behaviours might share similar psychobiological processes.

Moreover, evidence suggests that impulsivity predicts the development of binge eating behaviour [20–22]. For example, negative urgency together with negative affect predicts binge eating onset in a longitudinal study examining school children over a time span of 1 year [22].

Impulsivity seems also to increase the risk for other mental disorders like substance use disorders and additional psychological problems like self-harming behaviours and negative affect [23]. Lastly, impulsivity also predicts treatment outcomes, with higher levels of impulsivity interfering with treatment success by making it difficult to implement newly acquired skills or resulting in possible relapse [24].

Cognitive-behavioural therapy (CBT), interpersonal therapy (IPT), and dialectical behaviour therapy (DBT) are considered first-line treatments for individuals with BN and BED [25–27]. However, meta-analyses and review studies indicate that available conventional treatments have difficulties in decreasing binge eating behaviour, with up to 50% of patients not benefiting from these treatments and remaining symptomatic [27, 28]. One reason for this might be that although theoretical models and research concerning binge eating behaviour emphasize impulsivity, the translation of this evidence into treatment is still limited. Impulsivity and related constructs are hardly targeted in treatment approaches for binge eating [29]. Thus, integrating impulsivity into treatment for binge eating behaviour could be a fruitful approach to improve treatment outcomes and decrease relapse rates.

In this regard, this study aims to systematically review existing impulsivity treatment approaches for individuals with binge eating behaviour, in order to discuss their effectiveness and provide recommendations for future research and clinical work. In particular, we investigated interventions which use food stimuli as they directly target impulsive eating behaviour, i.e. binge eating. Such impulsive eating behaviours might also be more easily modifiable and measurable than the underlying trait. We define treatment in this article as any form of intervention targeting binge eating behaviour, i.e. in forms of psychotherapeutic, computer-assisted cognitive training, neuromodulation or pharmacological approaches.

Taken together, we aim to answer the following research questions:

(1) Is there any evidence that food-related impulsivity can be changed by impulsivity-focused interventions in individuals with binge eating behaviour?
(2) If so, is there any evidence to conclude that one of these interventions is superior to the others?

Materials and methods

This systematic review was conducted based on the PRISMA-Statement [30, 31].

Search strategy

A search on the scientific databases PubMed and PsycINFO and additional hand search was performed for relevant articles published up to September 2020 with no starting date. For the PubMed search, the following search terms were used:

(binge-eating disorder [MeSH Terms] OR "binge eating"[Title/Abstract] OR „binge-eating"[Title/Abstract] OR "BED"[Title/Abstract] OR bulimia [MeSH Terms] OR bulimia [Title/Abstract] OR Hyperphagia [MeSH Terms] OR Hyperphagia [Title/Abstract] OR overeating [Title/Abstract] OR overeating [MeSh Terms]) AND (impulsive behavior [MeSH Terms] OR impulsiv*[Title/Abstract] OR impulsivity [MeSH Terms] OR reward [MeSH Terms] OR reward [Title/Abstract] OR disinhibit*[Title/Abstract] OR "loss of control"[Title/Abstract] OR "inhibition psychology"[MeSH Terms]) AND (therapy [MeSH Terms] OR therapy [Title/Abstract] OR "behavioural change "[MeSH Terms] OR behavioural change [Title/Abstract] OR Intervention [Title/Abstract] OR Intervention [MeSH Terms] OR "Stop Signal "[Title/Abstract] OR "Stop Signal "[MeSH Terms] OR Training [Title/Abstract] OR "training support"[MeSH Terms] OR behavioural modification [MeSH Terms] OR behavioural modification [Title/Abstract] OR "transcranial magnetic stimulation "[Title/Abstract] OR "transcranial direct current stimulation "[Title/Abstract] OR "vagus nerve stimulation "[Title/Abstract] OR "deep brain stimulation "[Title/Abstract]).

For the PsycINFO search, the following search terms were used with a filter for academic journals:

(TI (binge eating OR binge-eating OR BED OR Bulimia OR Hyperphagia OR overeating) OR AB (binge eating OR binge-eating OR BED OR Bulimia OR Hyperphagia OR overeating)) AND (TI (impulsiv* OR reward OR disinhibit* OR "loss of control") OR AB (impulsive behavior OR impulsiv* OR reward OR disinhibit* OR "loss of control")) AND (TI (therapy OR behavioural change OR behavioral change OR intervention OR training OR behavioural modification OR transcranial magnetic stimulation OR transcranial direct current stimulation OR vagus nerve stimulation OR deep brain stimulation) OR AB (therapy OR behavioural change OR behavioral change OR intervention OR training OR behavioural modification OR transcranial magnetic stimulation OR transcranial direct current stimulation OR vagus nerve stimulation OR deep brain stimulation)).

Eligibility criteria

As recommended in the PRISMA statement, eligibility was based on the PICOS criteria: participants, interventions, comparators, outcome and study design [31].

Participants

Studies including individuals of any age or gender who suffer from binge eating episodes with a diagnosis of BED, BN, EDNOS, OSFED or subclinical binge eating behaviour. Studies were excluded if the subjects suffer from neurological disorders (e.g., Parkinson's disease).

Interventions

In order to be included, studies must offer some form of impulsivity-focused intervention that targets food-related impulsivity (e.g., group therapy, neuromodulation, or computer-assisted cognitive training). The term "impulsivity-focused intervention" requires at least one factor of impulsivity to be targeted in the treatment, e.g. reward sensitivity, inhibitory control, and/or negative urgency.

Comparators

As a comparison group, studies with a control group in which participants did not receive a food-related impulsivity-focused treatment were included. Another intervention in the control group (e.g. treatment as usual) was possible, though it was not a necessary inclusion criterion. Studies with within-subject comparisons, i.e. where sessions with the food-related impulsivity-focused treatment were compared with sessions without this treatment in the same subjects, were also included.

Outcome

Studies were considered to be eligible if they included at least one measure related to food-related impulsivity. For example, this could be the assessment of binge eating episodes by standardised interviews or questionnaires (EDE, EDEQ), or by experimental paradigms, e.g. Stop Signal task or Go/No Go task with the presentation of food stimuli. Changes of trait impulsivity by interviews, self-reports or experimental paradigms were also reported though this was not a necessary inclusion criterion.

Study design

Clinical studies, experimental studies, and observational studies were included. Case studies were excluded.

Study selection and data collection

Three authors of the present article independently assessed the eligibility of the articles that were identified following the database search based on the eligibility criteria. The first and the second author independently screened the articles by scanning their titles and abstracts and removed duplicated articles. These two authors and the last author performed the evaluation of the full texts of studies that were potentially relevant to the eligibility criteria. In the case of contrary opinions, the single studies were discussed with the last author.

Extracted data for the included articles are displayed in Table 1 and contain: (i) characteristics of the study participants (diagnosis, number of participants and type of control group); (ii) characteristics of the interventions (session numbers, format); (iii) type of impulsivity and related measures; and (iv) summary of main findings.

Results

The detailed information regarding the selection procedure is presented in the flowchart in Fig. 1. 972 articles from the systematic search in PubMed and PsycINFO and 13 additional articles through hand search were identified. After the title/abstract screening, 66 studies remained for full-text investigation. Finally, 15 studies were analysed in this systematic review after excluding studies that did not fulfil one or more of the eligibility criteria. Participants were adults in all studies and included patients with an eating disorder diagnosis, with the exception of one study which included patients with subjective binge eating episodes [44]. Studies were categorised based on the treatment approach used: psychotherapy, pharmacotherapy, computer-assisted cognitive training, or direct neuromodulation interventions (i.e. neurostimulation and neurofeedback) (see Table 1).

Interventions using a psychotherapy approach

Three studies were identified as including psychotherapy approaches [3, 32, 33]. One study investigated cue exposure therapy in virtual reality (VR-CET) as second-level treatment after CBT in patients with BN or BED, in comparison to additional cognitive behavioural therapy (A-CBT). The VR-CET was developed based on the classical conditioning model of binge eating to reduce food cravings by breaking the connection between the craved food(s) and binge eating behaviour. To achieve this, a virtual environment is simulated which depicts the usual location of binge eating episodes and includes exposures of their frequently consumed foods during binge eating episodes [3]. Even though participants in both treatment groups had improvements, participants in the VR-CET showed significantly greater abstinence rates from binge eating episodes and lower binge eating and purging frequency, as well as lower food craving, in comparison to the participants who received A-CBT. In the study by Preuss and colleagues [32], a novel treatment called ImpulsE, which strengthens emotion-based and food-related inhibitory control abilities, was compared with CBT as treatment as usual (TAU) for patients with obesity and a subgroup of patients with BED. The ImpulsE treatment included motivational techniques for change, emotion regulation skills and a food-specific, computer-assisted, Stop Signal inhibition training. Findings revealed a significant reduction in the frequency of overeating, perceived lack of perseverance and urgency in both conditions. However, significant binge eating reduction in patients with BED at post-treatment and 3-month follow up was found only in the ImpulsE group. The ImpulsE group also

Table 1 Summary of the studies investigating impulsivity focused interventions to reduce binge eating behaviour

Study	Sample	Intervention	Dose	Impulsivity and Related Measures	Summary of Findings
Psychotherapy approach					
Ferrer-Garcia et al. (2017) [3]	N = 64 adults with BED or BN after CBT fails	Virtual Reality & Cue Exposure Therapy (VR-CET) vs. Additional CBT (A-CBT)	6 individual sessions twice a week	1. EDE (binge eating episodes)	1. Both groups reduced binge eating, VR - CET was significantly superior compared to A-CBT regarding the reduction of binge eating frequency and achievement in abstinence from binge eating episodes (53% vs. 25%).
				2. EDE (purging episodes)	2. Both groups reduced purging behaviour, VR-CET was also significantly superior to A-CBT for achievement in abstinence from purging episodes (75% vs. 31.5%).
				3. EDI - Bulimia subscale (self-reported binge eating tendency)	3. Both groups improved self-reported binge eating tendency, but VR-CET was significantly superior to A-CBT.
				4. FCQ (state and trait version)	4. Both groups reduced both state and trait food craving, but VR-CET was significantly superior to A-CBT.
Preuss et al. (2017) [32]	N = 69 treatment seeking obesity patients (40.6% OSFED, 33.3% BED)	ImpulsE (psychotherapeutic treatment to increase inhibitory control and emotion regulation) + food-specific stop-signal inhibition training vs. TAU (CBT for obesity and BED)	10, 100-min sessions in group format	1. EDEQ (frequency of episodes of overeating and objective binge eating)	1. Frequency of disinhibited overeating decreased in both conditions. Significant binge eating reduction in patients with BED at post-treatment and 3-month FU in ImpulsE group, no change in TAU.
				2. SST with food stimuli (inhibitory control)	2. Significantly greater reduction in inhibitory control in ImpulsE group compared with TAU.
				3. UPPS Impulsive Behaviour Scale (urgency, lack of premeditation, lack of perseverance and sensation seeking)	3. Perceived lack of perseverance and urgency significantly decreased in both groups.
Schag et al. (2019) [33]	N = 80 adults with BED	IMPULS (impulsivity focused group intervention) vs. Control group without intervention	8, 90-min sessions in group format	1. EDE (binge eating episodes)	1. Binge eating episodes in the past 4 weeks were significantly reduced in both groups at the end of treatment. Binge eating was reduced more in the IMPULS group vs. control group at 3 months follow up.
				2. DEBQ (external eating subscale)	2. External eating was reduced more in IMPULS group at the end of treatment and follow up. Control group showed reduction only at follow up.
				3. BIS-15 & BIS/BAS (trait impulsivity)	3. Trait impulsivity was not significantly reduced in any group.

Table 1 Summary of the studies investigating impulsivity focused interventions to reduce binge eating behaviour (Continued)

Study	Sample	Intervention	Dose	Impulsivity and Related Measures	Summary of Findings
Pharmacotherapy approach					
Chao et al. (2019) [34]	N = 150 obese adults with binge eating	IBT-alone vs. IBT-liraglutide vs. Multicomponent (IBT + liraglutide + portion-controlled diet)	21 sessions of IBT vs. 21 sessions of IBT + 3.0 mg/d as a once-daily vs. 21 sessions of IBT + 3.0 mg/d as a once-daily + 12-week, 1000- to 1200-kcal/d diet	1. EDEQ (binge eating episodes) 2. FCI (frequency of food cravings) 3. EDI (dietary disinhibition)	1. At week 24, the IBT-liraglutide and multicomponent groups showed a significant within-group mean decline. The multicomponent group had a greater decrease compared to the IBT-alone group at week 24. All groups had significant within-group declines in binge eating at week 52, with a greater decline in the multicomponent group. 2. All groups had significant and similar declines in total food cravings at both 24 and 52 weeks. 3. All groups had a significant within-group decline at week 24 and 52. At week 24, the IBT-alone and IBT-liraglutide groups did not differ, but the decline was significantly less in the IBT-alone group compared to the multicomponent group. At week 52, there was no significant group difference.
Da Porto et al. (2020) [35]	N = 60 type 2 diabetic outpatients with BED	dulaglutide vs. gliclazide modified release +metformin	dulaglutide 150 mg/week vs. gliclazide modified release 60 mg/day + metformin (dosage 2–3 g/day)	1. BES (binge eating)	1. Binge eating behaviour was only significantly reduced in the dulaglutide group.
Quilty et al. (2019) [36]	N = 49 women with BED	Psychostimulant medication (Methylphenidate) vs. CBT TAU	12 weeks of medication usage (initial dosage: 18 mg; final dosage 72 mg) vs. 12 weekly individual sessions for CBT	1. EDE (objective binge eating) 2. BES (subjective binge eating) 3. The UPPS Impulsive Behaviour Scale (urgency, lack of premeditation, lack of perseverance and sensation seeking)	1. Objective binge episodes decreased in both groups, with no treatment effect. 2. Subjective binge episodes decreased in both conditions, with no treatment effect. 3. Perseverance and negative urgency scores decreased in both conditions over time with no treatment effect. Higher levels of UPPS perseverance and negative urgency scores were associated with a better treatment outcome in both conditions.
Computer-assisted cognitive training approach					
Brockmeyer et al. 2019 [37]	N = 50 with BN or BED	Real ABM to avoid food cues vs. Sham ABM	10 sessions within 4 weeks	1. EDE (binge eating episodes) 2. FCQ (trait food craving, food cue reactivity) 3. Bogus Taste Test (food intake) 4. AAT (approach and attention bias towards food)	1. Both groups had significantly fewer binge eating episodes after the training. 2. Both groups reported significantly lower trait food craving and reduced food cue reactivity after the training. 3. There was no significant change in food intake in any group. 4. There was no significant change in approach and attention bias towards food in any group.

Table 1 Summary of the studies investigating impulsivity focused interventions to reduce binge eating behaviour (*Continued*)

Study	Sample	Intervention	Dose	Impulsivity and Related Measures	Summary of Findings
Giel et al. (2017) [38]	N = 22 women with BED	Food specific inhibition training based on antisaccade paradigm vs. Control group with free vision instruction	3 individual sessions within 2 weeks	1. EDEQ (number of binge eating episodes in the last 4 weeks) 2. FCQ (state version) 3. YFAS (food addiction total score)	1. There were significantly lower numbers of binge eating episodes in both groups. 2. Reduced error rates and increase in food related inhibitory control in both groups. 3. No effect on food craving or food addiction were found in any group.
Turton et al. (2018) [39]	n = 27 women with BN and n = 17 with BED vs. lean and overweight controls	Food specific Go/No-Go training vs. General Go/No-Go training (within-subject-design)	1 individual session	1. Taste test for food consumption following the training 2. 24-h post food diary including a sense of 'loss of control' and purging episodes 3. FCQ (food craving)	1. Small non-significant reductions in high-calorie food consumption in the food specific vs. the general training. 2. No treatment effect on binge eating or purging symptoms in the 24-h post diary. 3. No treatment effect on food craving.
Direct neuromodulation approach (neurostimulation and neurofeedback)					
Burgess et al. (2016) [40]	N = 30 adults with BED or sub-BED	Real tDCS on DLPFC (anode right, cathode left) vs. sham tDCS on DLPFC (within-subject-design)	2 individual sessions	1. FPCT (Food craving) 2. In-lab food intake test 3. 5-day at-home binge eating survey (urge to binge eat and binge eating frequency 5 days)	1. & 2. Food craving and food intake were reduced after tDCS compared to sham stimulation. 3. Urge to binge eat in men was reduced after tDCS vs. sham; no reduction concerning binge eating frequency in both conditions.
Gay et al. (2016) [41]	N = 47 women with BN	High frequency rTMS on left DLPFC vs. sham rTMS on left DLPFC	10 individual sessions over 2 consecutive weeks	1. Number of binge episodes in the last 15 days after stimulation 2. Number of vomiting episodes in the last 15 days after stimulation	1. No significant reduction was found in any groups, and there was no difference between groups. 2. No significant reduction was found in any groups, and there was no difference between groups.
Kekic et al. (2017) [42]	N = 39 adults with BN	tDCS on DLPFC (anode right/cathode left) vs. tDCS on DLPFC (anode left/cathode right) vs. sham tDCS on DLPFC (within-subject-design)	2 individual sessions	1. Urge to binge eat on visual analogue scale 2. FCT (food craving) 3. Temporal Discounting (general reward processing) 4. Self-reported binge eating and purging frequency 24 h after stimulation	1. Both active conditions vs. sham show significant reduction in urge to bingeeat. 2. There was no group difference for food craving. 3. Increased discounting in both active conditions vs. sham condition 4. No differences between conditions were found.
Max et al. (2020) [43]	N = 27 with BED	anodal 1 mA tDCS on DLPFC vs. sham tDCS (within-subject) vs. anodal2 mA tDCS on DLPFC vs. sham tDCS (within-subject design)	2 individual sessions	1. food-related antisaccade task (latency, error rate)	1. Significant reduction of error rate over time in all conditions; Latencies were decreased in the 2 mA vs. sham and vs. 1 mA condition.

Table 1 Summary of the studies investigating impulsivity focused interventions to reduce binge eating behaviour (*Continued*)

Study	Sample	Intervention	Dose	Impulsivity and Related Measures	Summary of Findings
				2. Frequency of binge eating episodes in the past seven days	2. Compared to sham stimulation, the frequency of binge eating episodes decreased at the 2 mA condition over time whereas it did not change significantly at the 1 mA condition.
Schmidt & Martin (2016) [44]	N = 75 healthy women with subjective binge eating episodes	EEG-neurofeedback with cue exposure vs. mental imagery with cue exposure vs. waitlist	10 individual sessions	1. EDEQ (binge eating episodes)	1. EEG-neurofeedback and MI groups showed decreased binge eating frequency, but this decrease was significant only at EEG-neurofeedback group at post test and 3-months follow up.
				2. FCQ (trait version)	2. Food craving was reduced in both EEG-neurofeedback (large effect) and MI groups (medium effect).
Van den Eynde et al. (2010) [45]	N = 38 adults with BN or EDNOS-bulimic type	High frequency rTMS on the left DLPFC vs. sham rTMS on the left DLPFC	1 individual session	1. Urge to eat, urge to binge eat, hunger on visual analogue scale immediately after stimulation	1. Urge to eat was significantly reduced in real rTMS group vs. sham stimulation. Urge to binge eat and hunger were reduced in both real rTMS and sham conditions.
				2. Binge eating frequency 24 h after stimulation	2. Significantly fewer binge-eating episodes over the 24 h following were reported in real rTMS compared to sham.
				3. FCQ (state version)	3. Both groups reduced food craving, and there was no group difference.

Note. AAT Approach–Avoidance Task. *ABM* Approach Bias Modification, *BED* Binge Eating Disorder, *BES* Binge Eating Scale, *BIS/BAS* Behavioral Inhibition System/Behavioral Activation System Questionnaire, *BIS-15* Barrat Impulsiveness Scale-short version, *BN* Bulimia Nervosa; *CBT,* Cognitive Behavioural Therapy, *DEBQ* Dutch Eating Behaviour Questionnaire, *DLPFC* Dorsolateral Prefrontal Cortex, *EDE* Eating Disorders Examination Interview, *EDEQ* Eating Disorder Examination Questionnaire, *EDI* Eating Disorders Inventory, *EDNOS* Eating Disorder Not Otherwise Specified, *FCI* Food Craving Inventory, *FCQ* Food Craving Questionnaire, *FCT* Food Challenge Task, *FPCT* Food Photo Craving Test, *IBT* Intensive Behavioral Therapy, *MI* Mental Imagery, *OSFED* Other Specified Feeding or Eating Disorder, *rTMS* Repetitive Transcranial Magnetic Stimulation, *SST* Stop Signal Task, *sub-BED* sample with subthreshold BED, *TAU* Treatment as Usual, *tDCS* Transcranial Direct Current Stimulation, *TFEQ* Three-factor Eating Questionnaire, *YFAS* Yale Food Addiction Scale

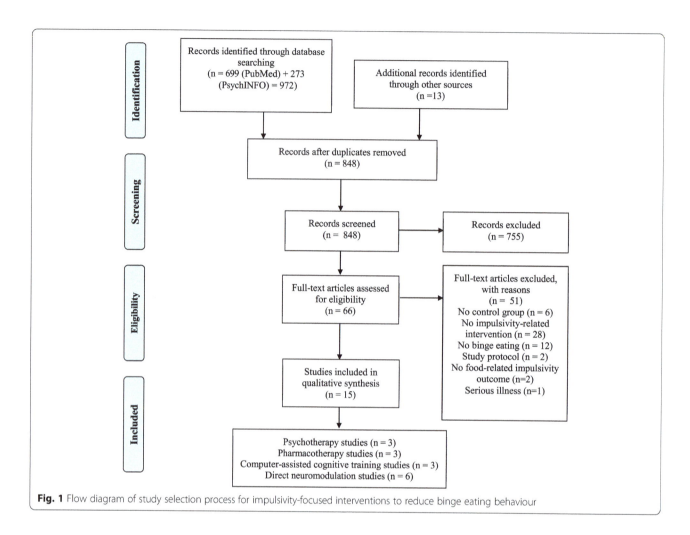

Fig. 1 Flow diagram of study selection process for impulsivity-focused interventions to reduce binge eating behaviour

resulted in significantly greater reduction in inhibitory control compared with TAU, but no differences in trait-like impulsivity.

Schag and colleagues [33] investigated the efficacy of a newly developed cognitive-behavioural group treatment for impulsive eating in patients with BED called IMPULS. This treatment program mainly focusses on reducing impulsive eating behaviour and consists of several techniques such as food cue exposure, stimulus and response control. The IMPULS group was not superior to the control group receiving no intervention in terms of reducing binge eating episodes directly after treatment. However, the improvement in binge eating frequency at 3-month follow up continued only in the IMPULS group, reporting that binge eating frequency was more reduced compared to the control group at follow up. In terms of external eating, the IMPULS group showed improvement both at the end of treatment and follow up, whereas the control group showed an improvement only at follow up. Trait impulsivity was not reduced in either group. Taken together, these studies suggest that psychotherapy treatments that focus on

impulsivity are fruitful in targeting food-related impulsive behaviour, but seem not to be able to change the impulsivity trait per se.

Interventions using a pharmacotherapy approach

Three studies were identified investigating the efficacy of pharmacotherapy for binge eating [34–36]. The first study investigated whether liraglutide would be helpful to reduce reward sensitivity towards food and meal intake among people with obesity and binge eating behaviour [34]. Liraglutide is a glucagon-like peptide-1 (GLP-1) agonist reducing activation of brain areas associated with appetite and reward, and is used in the treatment of type 2 diabetes and obesity. For this purpose, participants were randomised to intensive behaviour therapy (IBT) alone, IBT-liraglutide, or multicomponent therapy including IBT, liraglutide, and portion-controlled diet. Binge eating episodes were significantly decreased in the IBT-liraglutide and multicomponent groups, and the multicomponent group was superior to the IBT-alone group at week 24. Although binge eating episodes were significantly decreased in all groups at week 52, the multicomponent group showed a greater reduction. In terms of food cravings and dietary disinhibition, all groups had significant within-group declines at both 24 and 52 weeks. However, the IBT-alone group showed significantly less decline in dietary disinhibition compared to the multicomponent group at week 24. Furthermore, a recent study also administered medications for the treatment of type 2 diabetes to treat binge eating behaviour [35]. The efficacy of dulaglutide, a GLP-1 receptor agonist that modulates appetite and reward-related brain areas, was compared to gliclazide, an antidiabetic medication, in a sample of outpatients with type 2 diabetes and BED. Binge eating behaviour was only significantly reduced in in the dulaglutide group. In another study, Quilty and colleagues [36] tested the efficacy of methylphenidate, which is usually prescribed to treat ADHD, known to reduce impulsivity, and influence appetite and weight. They compared this medication with CBT as TAU. Findings revealed that both treatments, i.e. methylphenidate and CBT resulted in decreased binge eating. Furthermore, it was found that perseverance and negative urgency scores were decreased over time in both conditions. Higher levels of these scores at baseline assessment were associated with better treatment outcomes. The possible reasoning behind this finding is that the subjects with higher negative urgency and perseverance might have had experienced higher levels of stress. Thus, they might have had higher levels of treatment motivation and adherence. Since all these studies differed in methodology and participants had comorbidities, it is hard to comment on the efficacy of impulsivity-focused pharmacotherapy approaches. Findings of two studies comparing medication with psychotherapy [34, 36] did not provide evidence for a superiority of impulsivity-focused medication, although the coupling with psychotherapy seems promising and effective.

Interventions using a computer-assisted cognitive training approach

There were three studies that included computer-assisted cognitive trainings for decreasing impulsivity symptoms among individuals with binge eating behaviour [37–39]. Two studies were based on decreased inhibitory control tendencies and therefore utilised food-related inhibitory control computer trainings for the treatment. Giel and colleagues [38] developed a food-specific inhibition training in an eye tracking antisaccade paradigm, i.e. looking at the opposite direction of the given stimulus as quickly as possible, for individuals with BED. The training was compared to a free vision condition in the control group. In their study, they found that both conditions resulted in a reduction of binge eating episodes and an increase in inhibitory control. However, the participants in the control condition looked at high-

caloric food stimuli more often than the participants in the training group over all sessions. In another study, a food-specific and a non-food Go/no-go inhibition training with one session for each training condition was administered in a within-subjects design in women with BN or BED [39]. In the Go/no-go training, the patients are instructed to press a specific button when a go cue is shown and to withhold this response when a no-go cue is shown. In this study, neither the food-specific nor the general inhibition training led to a statistically significant decrease in food intake and both conditions did not differ concerning binge eating and purging symptoms. A more recent study [37] examined the efficacy of an approach bias modification (ABM) in which patients with BN or BED are trained to avoid visual cues of high-calorie foods. Participants receiving real ABM did not show significantly greater reductions in the number of objective binge eating episodes, trait food craving, and food cue reactivity than participants receiving sham ABM who were not trained to avoid food cues. Furthermore, no change in food intake, approach bias, and attention bias toward food was found in any group. Based on the available studies, there is hardly evidence that such computer-assisted cognitive trainings are effective for decreasing binge eating behaviour. This might be due to the low dose [39], due to the chosen paradigm in the control group which might also be effective [38], or due to not targeting the necessary underlying mechanisms of action [37].

Interventions using a direct neuromodulation approach

Six studies were identified as directly targeting the brain for the treatment of impulsivity symptoms in people with binge eating behaviour. More specifically, one study used neurofeedback [44] whereas five studies investigated the effectiveness of non-invasive brain stimulation methods comparing verum with sham stimulation [40–43, 45].

Schmidt and Martin [44] tested the efficacy of EEG-neurofeedback combined with cue exposure against two comparison groups including mental imagery with cue exposure and a wait-list control group in healthy women with subjective binge eating episodes. They found that binge eating frequency decreased in both intervention groups. However, this decrease was only significant in the EEG-neurofeedback group. Furthermore, food craving was significantly reduced in the EEG-neurofeedback group (with a large effect) and the mental imagery with cue exposure group (with a medium effect) compared to the control group.

The neurostimulation studies targeted the dorsolateral prefrontal cortex (DLPFC) given its relationship with impulsivity and cognitive control. Among these neurostimulation studies, two tested the efficacy of repetitive transcranial magnetic stimulation (rTMS) [41, 45]. Van den Eynde and colleagues [45] compared verum rTMS (10 Hz) over the left DLPFC to sham in patients with bulimic disorders and reported less urge to eat immediately after stimulation and fewer binge eating episodes 24h after stimulation in the verum condition. However, Gay and colleagues [41] did not find a reduction after verum or sham rTMS (10 Hz) over the left DLPFC even after 10 stimulation sessions in terms of binging and purging episodes.

Furthermore, there were three studies administering transcranial direct current stimulation (tDCS) [40, 42, 43]. Burgess and colleagues [40] showed decreased in-lab food intake and food craving in patients with BED, and decreased urge to binge eat, particularly in men, following anodal verum tDCS administration (2 mA) over the right DLPFC in comparison to sham stimulation. However, no effect on binge eating frequency was found in any condition. Similarly, in the study of Kekic and colleagues [42], patients with BN received two stimulation conditions (anode right DLPFC/cathode left DLPFC; 2 mA, and anode left DLPFC/cathode right DLPFC; 2 mA) compared with sham condition in a counterbalanced order. In the two verum conditions, a suppressed urge to binge eat and increased self-regulatory control were demonstrated. A recent randomised proof-of-concept-study investigated the efficacy of anodal tDCS over the right DLPFC (1 mA vs. 2 mA vs. sham) combined with a food-modified antisaccade task to increase response inhibition skills in BED patients [43]. In the food-modified antisaccade task, participants were instructed to look as fast as possible on the opposite side of the screen when they saw a food picture. Significant improvement concerning the latency in the antisaccade task and reduced binge eating frequency was reported only for the 2 mA condition. The authors also report a learning effect concerning error rate over time in all three conditions suggesting that patients with BED can benefit from the repeated execution of a computer-assisted cognitive task addressing the underlying cognitive impairments, particularly response inhibition. To summarise, findings regarding the efficacy of rTMS concerning a reduction of binge eating episodes are mixed. However, there is slightly more consistent evidence that tDCS and EEG-neurofeedback combined with cue exposure appear to decrease binge eating and food craving.

Discussion

The aim of this systematic review was to investigate the available interventions addressing impulsivity, particularly concerning impulsive eating behaviour among patients with binge eating behaviour. Following the database search, 15 studies were investigated under four categories based on the delivered treatment approaches: psychotherapy, pharmacotherapy, computer-assisted cognitive

training, and direct neuromodulation interventions (i.e. neurostimulation and neurofeedback).

Summary and interpretation of findings

Trials concerning impulsivity-focused psychotherapeutic treatments are surprisingly really scarce. The treatments included in this review appeared to decrease binge eating and impulsive eating behaviour among individuals who suffer from BED and BN significantly more in comparison to psychotherapeutic approaches without a specific focus on food-related impulsivity [3, 32]. However, studies did not add evidence for the efficacy of these treatment approaches on improvements of impulsivity as a trait.

The studies investigating the efficacy of pharmacotherapy to decrease binge eating episodes have different methodologies making it hard to draw a conclusion. Though Glucagon-like peptide-1 [34, 35] and methylphenidate [36] seem helpful to reduce food cravings, administration of these medications appears not to result in a greater improvement when compared to psychotherapeutic approaches [34, 36]. Moreover, review studies on pharmacological approaches for the treatment of binge eating suggest that topiramate as an antagonist of kainate/AMPA glutamate receptor is able to reduce binge eating frequency by suppressing appetite [46, 47]. Further, Lisdexamfetamine dimesylate (LDX) has been suggested to regulate the dopamine and noradrenaline neurotransmitter systems that are involved in eating behaviour and reward regulation, and thus decrease binge eating [48]. LDX is also the only approved medication for adults with BED by the US Food and Drug Administration (FDA) [49, 50]. Thus, both these drugs can also be considered to address food-related impulsivity, even though the impulsivity concept was not explicitly included in the articles as a supposed working mechanism.

There were three studies that used a computer-assisted cognitive training approach. Although studies administering a food-specific inhibition training to address food-related impulsivity among patients with binge eating seemed to increase inhibitory control, no evidence was found for the superiority of these approaches in decreasing binge eating episodes or food craving in comparison with control conditions [37–39]. It might be that the presentation of food stimuli itself – independent from the used training task - induces habituation effects likely regarded as one underlying mechanism for food cue exposure interventions (see below).

Most of the food-related impulsivity treatment studies identified in the current review were direct neuromodulation interventions. However, it is important to state here that neither the methodologies of the studies nor the findings were identical. The findings of the two studies with rTMS were mixed, showing no significant or superior effect in one study [41], but a significant effect in the 24 h following the treatment for the decrease in binge eating episodes in the other [45]. This makes it hard to draw any conclusions about the efficacy of rTMS. On the other hand, tDCS as another non-invasive neuromodulation approach seemed to be a more fruitful approach to decrease binge eating and food craving because the related studies delivered more consistent findings (significantly greater reduction in real conditions compared to sham conditions) [40, 42, 43]. However, it is important to note that all neuromodulation studies did not use an active intervention in the control condition, but only a sham stimulation which lowers the impact of these results. In contrast, when compared to an active control condition, a combination of EEG-neurofeedback and cue exposure [44] resulted in decreased binge eating frequency with significantly greater outcomes compared to control. The inclusion of an active control condition can be considered as particular strength for this study.

Regarding our first research question, it is plausible to conclude that impulsive eating behaviour might be changed through impulsivity-related interventions in individuals with binge eating episodes. Available approaches appear to be especially promising for decreasing binge eating symptoms. Although there is less evidence, there are supportive findings for improvements in food craving and inhibitory control following food-related impulsivity treatments. One major issue concerning the first research question is the lack of active interventions in the control conditions. Only six out of the 15 studies included in this systematic review had an active treatment group as a comparator. Nevertheless, in these six studies with active control conditions, the results suggest that impulsivity-focused treatment is at least not inferior to treatment as usual.

Moreover, it is difficult to make a comment about our second research question regarding whether one impulsivity-focused intervention is superior to the others to decrease binge eating episodes for several reasons. First, the detailed systematic search in two scientific databases revealed only 15 studies meeting the eligibility criteria. Second, although separated into four categories, the studies were heterogeneous regarding the treatment paradigms, the intensity of treatments (e.g, session numbers, delivery format etc.), and research methodology. Furthermore, none of the treatment approaches in these studies resulted in improvements in all the features of food-related impulsivity (e.g., binge eating episodes, impulsivity trait, food craving etc.).

Besides not having enough evidence to draw a distinct conclusion, food-related cue exposure can be considered as a promising approach as some studies that used this intervention technique, either in psychotherapy [33], virtual reality or neurofeedback [3, 44] found improvement in binge eating behaviour. The proposed mechanisms of cue exposure concerning impulsivity are multifaceted: cue reactivity and conditioning (e.g. [51]), habituation processes, increased self-efficacy, and self-control (e.g. [52]). Contextual cues related to food and eating might also lead appetitive conditioned responses [53], thus integrating virtual reality tools into cue exposure focused treatment modalities for binge eating might also be beneficial. However, further research is necessary to answer this question. Furthermore, investigating the efficacy of impulsivity-focusing medications would be valuable given their supposed mechanisms of suppressing appetite and regulating the reward pathway. Another fruitful approach that is worthy to be mentioned are neuromodulation techniques, in particular tDCS [40, 42, 43]. Moreover, combinations of several interventions seem to be very promising, either the combination of psychotherapy with computer-assisted cognitive trainings [32], pharmacotherapy with behavioural interventions [34], or neuromodulation with computer-assisted cognitive trainings [43]. For example, such neuromodulation interventions combined with well-elaborated, food-related computer training paradigms might target binge eating behaviour more directly and thus, enhance its effectivity (e.g. [54]).

Overall, it is quite surprising that such few studies have been published concerning this topic, especially such few psychotherapy studies. This might be due to the fact that psychotherapeutic trials are very time-consuming and complex. Studies concerning interventions specifically focusing on negative urgency are also lacking. It could be that some earlier conducted studies were labelled differently, for example negative urgency is a fairly new accepted impulsivity factor and studies might have been done before under the umbrella of emotion regulation strategies.

Concerning the addressed mechanisms, it could be that the efficacy of the intervention depends on the specific maintaining factor for the binge eating behaviour that is targeted (i.e., reward sensitivity, disinhibition or negative urgency). A patient engaging in binge eating behaviour which is mainly due to having high levels of reward sensitivity might not benefit from a treatment if it only focuses on inhibitory control. Moreover, people with subclinical binge eating, BED or BN might benefit differently from the impulsivity interventions, as demonstrated with the identified studies using rTMS for patients with BN or EDNOS-bulimic type. Thus, rTMS might provide a better treatment outcome in individuals who do not engage in purging behaviours, like in patients with BED. Otherwise, impulsivity-focused treatments could be helpful in specific patient subgroups, for example if first-line CBT fails [3] or in patients with increased trait impulsivity or comorbid mental disorders like addictive behaviours or ADHD that are related to impulsivity.

Taking together, it is reasonable to say that the findings for treating binge eating behaviour with a focus on food-related impulsivity are promising. However, it is important to bear in mind that research in this field is still in its infancy. The reported evidence is really heterogeneous and scarce, and publication bias cannot be ruled out, although some studies report negative findings that do not favour impulsivity-focused treatments. Thus, there are still many more studies needed to draw a concise conclusion concerning our research questions.

Considerations for future research and clinical work

Findings of the present systematic review reveal that studies targeting food-related impulsivity are heterogeneous in many aspects. In this regard, future research may benefit from combining successful aspects of the available interventions as well as including active treatment control conditions rather than wait-list or sham control conditions only (see above).

Food-related impulsivity among patients with binge eating behaviour is suggested to have multiple components rather than being a single construct. More specifically, evidence underlines reward sensitivity, inhibitory control, and attentional bias towards food-related cues that can account for food-related impulsivity features [12]. Given that the studies included in this review focused on different aspects of impulsivity and provided mixed findings, it is possible to argue that identifying the underlying impulsivity aspect in each individual and then providing a more targeted intervention might increase treatment success. Another option would be to develop an impulsivity-focused treatment program that addresses all main components of impulsivity as these components often interact with each other. For example, high reward sensitivity towards food stimuli in combination with low inhibitory control skills may trigger a binge eating episode especially when also combined with negative mood in terms of negative urgency. Thus, an impulsivity-focused treatment might be most beneficial if it addresses these interrelations as well.

Moreover, future research is needed to compare impulsivity focused treatments with other active treatments, in particular concerning neurostimulation studies (see above). Last, it is of high importance to choose an adequate control condition [55] and this might also explain the negative findings in the computer-assisted cognitive training programmes.

Conclusion

Even though first-line treatment modalities (e.g., CBT, IPT, and DBT) are available for binge eating behaviour, recovery is only achieved by 50% of treated patients as the treatments do not generally address important underlying and maintaining mechanism of binge eating behaviour, i.e. food-related impulsivity. With this systematic review, available novel approaches based on food-related impulsivity for binge eating behaviour were presented. In conclusion, although more research is needed, these interventions appear to be fruitful for future research and clinical attempts for the treatment of binge eating behaviour and related impulsive factors.

Abbreviations
ABM: Approach Bias Modification; ADHD: Attention Deficit Hyperactivity Disorder; BED: Binge Eating Disorder; BN: Bulimia Nervosa; CBT: Cognitive-Behavioral Therapy; DBT: Dialectical Behaviour Therapy; DLPFC: Dorsolateral Prefrontal Cortex; ED: Eating Disorder; EDE: Eating Disorders Examination; EDEQ: Eating Disorders Examination Questionnaire; EDNOS: Eating Disorder Not Otherwise Specified; EEG: Electroencephalography; GLP-1: Glucagon-like peptide-1; IBT: Intensive Behaviour Therapy; IPT: Interpersonal Therapy; LDX: Lisdexamfetamine Dimesylate; OFSED: Other Specified Feeding or Eating Disorders; RCT: Randomised Controlled Trial; rTMS: Repetitive Transcranial Magnetic Stimulation; TAU: Treatment as Usual; tDCS: Transcranial Direct Current Stimulation; VR-CET: Cue Exposure Therapy in Virtual Reality

Acknowledgements
We would like to thank Jessica Cook (Department of Psychosomatic Medicine and Psychotherapy, Tübingen, Germany) for her revision concerning English spelling and grammar.

Authors' contributions
KS, KEG and SZ drafted the review topic and research question. KS and JS developed the search terms and eligibility criteria. Bl, JS and KS screened, reviewed, selected and analysed studies included in the review. CP and SM gave imported intellectual content concerning the interpretation of the neuromodulation studies. Bl and KS drafted the manuscript. All authors critically revised the manuscript.

Competing interests
All authors declared that they have no competing interest.

Author details
[1]Department of Psychology, Haliç University, Istanbul, Turkey. [2]Department of Psychosomatic Medicine and Psychotherapy, University Hospital Tübingen, Osianderstraße 5, 72076 Tübingen, Germany. [3]Department of Psychiatry and Psychotherapy, Neurophysiology & Interventional Neuropsychiatry, University of Tübingen, Tübingen, Germany. [4]Competence Center of Eating Disorders Tübingen (KOMET), Tübingen, Germany.

References
1. American Psychiatric Association. Diagnostic and statistical manual of mental disorders. 5th ed. Arlington: American Psychiatric Association; 2013.
2. Kessler RC, Berglund PA, Chiu WT, Deitz AC, Hudson JI, Shahly V, et al. The prevalence and correlates of binge eating disorder in the World Health Organization world mental health surveys. Biol Psychiatry. 2013;73(9):904–14.
3. Ferrer-Garcia M, Gutierrez-Maldonado J, Pla-Sanjuanelo J, Vilalta-Abella F, Riva G, Clerici M, et al. A randomised controlled comparison of second-level treatment approaches for treatment-resistant adults with bulimia nervosa and binge eating disorder: assessing the benefits of virtual reality Cue exposure therapy. Eur Eat Disord Rev. 2017;25(6):479–90.

4. Fischer S, Smith GT, Cyders MA. Another look at impulsivity: a meta-analytic review comparing specific dispositions to rash action in their relationship to bulimic symptoms. Clin Psychol Rev. 2008;28(8):1413–25.

5. Giel KE, Teufel M, Junne F, Zipfel S, Schag K. Food-related impulsivity in obesity and binge eating disorder-a systematic update of the evidence. Nutrients. 2017;9(11):1170.

6. Wu M, Hartmann M, Skunde M, Herzog W, Friederich HC. Inhibitory control in bulimic-type eating disorders: a systematic review and meta-analysis. PLoS One. 2013;8(12):e83412.

7. Whiteside SP, Lynam DR. The five factor model and impulsivity: using a structural model of personality to understand impulsivity. Personal Individ Differ. 2001;30(4):669–89.

8. Moeller FG, Barratt ES, Dougherty DM, Schmitz JM, Swann AC. Psychiatric aspects of impulsivity. Am J Psychiatry. 2001;158(11):1783–93.

9. Gullo MJ, Loxton NJ, Dawe S. Impulsivity: four ways five factors are not basic to addiction. Addict Behav. 2014;39(11):1547–56.

10. Dawe S, Loxton NJ. The role of impulsivity in the development of substance use and eating disorders. Neurosci Biobehav Rev. 2004;28(3):343–51.

11. Ng L, Davis C. Cravings and food consumption in binge eating disorder. Eat Behav. 2013;14(4):472–5.

12. Treasure J, Cardi V, Leppanen J, Turton R. New treatment approaches for severe and enduring eating disorders. Physiol Behav. 2015; 152(Pt B):456–465.

13. Leehr EJ, Schag K, Dresler T, Grosse-Wentrup M, Hautzinger M, Fallgatter AJ, et al. Food specific inhibitory control under negative mood in binge-eating disorder: evidence from a multimethod approach. Int J Eat Disord. 2018; 51(2):112–23.

14. Tammela LI, Pääkkönen A, Karhunen LJ, Karhu J, Uusitupa MIJ, Kuikka JT. Brain electrical activity during food presentation in obese binge-eating women. Clin Physiol Funct Imaging. 2010;30(2):135–40.

15. Kessler RM, Hutson PH, Herman BK, Potenza MN. The neurobiological basis of binge-eating disorder. Neurosci Biobehav Rev. 2016;63:223–38.

16. Smith KE, Mason TB, Schaefer LM, Juarascio A, Dvorak R, Weinbach N, et al. Examining intra-individual variability in food-related inhibitory control and negative affect as predictors of binge eating using ecological momentary assessment. J Psychiatr Res. 2020;120:137–43.

17. Racine SE, Burt SA, Keel PK, Sisk CL, Neale MC, Boker S, et al. Examining associations between negative urgency and key components of objective binge episodes. Int J Eat Disord. 2015;48(5):527–31.

18. Wolz I, Hilker I, Granero R, Jiménez-Murcia S, Gearhardt AN, Dieguez C, et al. Food addiction in patients with eating disorders is associated with negative urgency and difficulties to focus on long-term goals. Front Psychol. 2016;7:61.

19. Verheul R, van den Brink W, Geerlings P. A three-pathway psychobiological model of craving for alcohol. Alcohol Alcohol. 1999;34(2):197–222.

20. Meule A, Platte P. Facets of impulsivity interactively predict body fat and binge eating in young women. Appetite. 2015;87:352–7.

21. Oliva R, Morys F, Horstmann A, Castiello U, Begliomini C. The impulsive brain: neural underpinnings of binge eating behavior in normal-weight adults. Appetite. 2019;136:33–49.

22. Pearson CM, Zapolski TC, Smith GT. A longitudinal test of impulsivity and depression pathways to early binge eating onset. Int J Eat Disord. 2015; 48(2):230–7.

23. Waxman SE. A systematic review of impulsivity in eating disorders. Eur Eat Disord Rev. 2009;17(6):408–25.

24. Manasse SM, Espel HM, Schumacher LM, Kerrigan SG, Zhang F, Forman EM, et al. Does impulsivity predict outcome in treatment for binge eating disorder? A multimodal investigation. Appetite. 2016;105:172–9.

25. Excellence NIfHaC. Eating disorders: recognition and treatment - NICE guideline 2017 [23.05.2017]. Available from: https://www.nice.org.uk/guidance/ng69.

26. Hilbert A, Petroff D, Herpertz S, Pietrowsky R, Tuschen-Caffier B, Vocks S, et al. Meta-analysis of the efficacy of psychological and medical treatments for binge-eating disorder. J Consult Clin Psychol. 2019;87(1): 91–105.

27. Slade E, Keeney E, Mavranezouli I, Dias S, Fou L, Stockton S, et al. Treatments for bulimia nervosa: a network meta-analysis. Psychol Med. 2018;48(16):2629–36.

28. Citrome L. Binge eating disorder revisited: what's new, what's different, what's next. CNS Spectr. 2019;24(S1):4–13.

29. Lavender JM, Mitchell JE. Eating disorders and their relationship to impulsivity. Curr Treat Opt Psychiatr. 2015;2(4):394–401.

30. Liberati A, Altman DG, Tetzlaff J, Mulrow C, Gotzsche PC, Ioannidis JP, et al. The PRISMA statement for reporting systematic reviews and meta-analyses of studies that evaluate health care interventions: explanation and elaboration. J Clin Epidemiol. 2009;62(10):e1 34.

31. Moher D, Liberati A, Tetzlaff J, Altman DG. Preferred reporting items for systematic reviews and meta-analyses: the PRISMA statement. PLoS Med. 2009;6(7):e1000097.

32. Preuss H, Pinnow M, Schnicker K, Legenbauer T. Improving inhibitory control abilities (ImpulsE)-a promising approach to treat impulsive eating? Eur Eat Disord Rev. 2017;25(6):533–43.

33. Schag K, Rennhak SK, Leehr EJ, Skoda EM, Becker S, Bethge W, et al. IMPULS: impulsivity-focused group intervention to reduce binge eating episodes in patients with binge eating disorder - a randomised controlled trial. Psychother Psychosom. 2019;88(3):141–53.

34. Chao AM, Wadden TA, Walsh OA, Gruber KA, Alamuddin N, Berkowitz RI, et al. Effects of liraglutide and behavioral weight loss on food cravings, eating behaviors, and eating disorder psychopathology. Obesity. 2019; 27(12):2005–10.

35. Da Porto A, Casarsa V, Colussi G, Catena C, Cavarape A, Sechi L. Dulaglutide reduces binge episodes in type 2 diabetic patients with binge eating disorder: a pilot study. Diab Metab Synd. 2020;14(4):289–92.

36. Quilty LC, Allen TA, Davis C, Knyahnytska Y, Kaplan AS. A randomized comparison of long acting methylphenidate and cognitive behavioral therapy in the treatment of binge eating disorder. Psychiatry Res. 2019;273: 467–74.

37. Brockmeyer T, Friederich HC, Küppers C, Chowdhury S, Harms L, Simmonds J, et al. Approach bias modification training in bulimia nervosa and binge-eating disorder: a pilot randomized controlled trial. Int J Eat Disord. 2019; 52(5):520–9.

38. Giel KE, Speer E, Schag K, Leehr EJ, Zipfel S. Effects of a food-specific inhibition training in individuals with binge eating disorder-findings from a randomized controlled proof-of-concept study. Eat Weight Disord. 2017; 22(2):345–51.

39. Turton R, Nazar BP, Burgess EE, Lawrence NS, Cardi V, Treasure J, et al. To go or not to go: a proof of concept study testing food-specific inhibition training for women with eating and weight disorders. Eur Eat Disord Rev. 2018;26(1):11–21.

40. Burgess EE, Sylvester MD, Morse KE, Amthor FR, Mrug S, Lokken KL, et al. Effects of transcranial direct current stimulation (tDCS) on binge eating disorder. Int J Eat Disord. 2016;49(10):930–6.

41. Gay A, Jaussent I, Sigaud T, Billard S, Attal J, Seneque M, et al. A lack of clinical effect of high-frequency rTMS to dorsolateral prefrontal cortex on bulimic symptoms: a randomised, double-blind trial. Eur Eat Disord Rev. 2016;24(6):474–81.

42. Kekic M, McClelland J, Bartholdy S, Boysen E, Musiat P, Dalton B, et al. Single-session transcranial direct current stimulation temporarily improves symptoms, mood, and self-regulatory control in bulimia nervosa: a randomised controlled trial. PLoS One. 2017;12(1):e0167606.

43. Max SM, Plewnia C, Zipfel S, Giel KE, Schag K. Combined antisaccade task and transcranial direct current stimulation to increase response inhibition in binge eating disorder. Eur Arch Psychiatry Clin Neurosci. 2020.

44. Schmidt J, Martin A. Neurofeedback against binge eating: a randomized controlled trial in a female subclinical threshold sample. Eur Eat Disord Rev. 2016;24(5):406–16.

45. Van den Eynde F, Claudino AM, Mogg A, Horrell L, Stahl D, Ribeiro W, et al. Repetitive transcranial magnetic stimulation reduces cue-induced food craving in bulimic disorders. Biol Psychiatry. 2010;67(8):793–5.

46. Leombruni P, Lavagnino L, Fassino S. Treatment of obese patients with binge eating disorder using topiramate: a review. Neuropsychiatr Dis Treat. 2009;5:385 92.

47. Marazziti D, Corsi M, Baroni S, Consoli G, Catena-Dell'Osso M. Latest advancements in the pharmacological treatment of binge eating disorder. Eur Rev Med Pharmacol Sci. 2012;16(15):2102–7.

48. Guerdjikova AI, Mori N, Casuto LS, McElroy SL. Novel pharmacologic treatment in acute binge eating disorder - role of lisdexamfetamine. Neuropsychiatr Dis Treat. 2016;12:833–41.

49. Griffiths KR, Yang J, Touyz SW, Hay PJ, Clarke SD, Korgaonkar MS, et al. Understanding the neural mechanisms of lisdexamfetamine dimesylate (LDX) pharmacotherapy in binge eating disorder (BED): a study protocol. J Eat Disord. 2019;7(1):23.

50. Food and Drug Administration. FDA expands uses of Vyvanse to treat binge-eating disorder. Press Release. 2015:30.

51. Jansen A. A learning model of binge eating: cue reactivity and cue exposure. Behav Res Ther. 1998;36(3):257–72.

52. Loeber S, Croissant B, Heinz A, Mann K, Flor H. Cue exposure in the treatment of alcohol dependence: effects on drinking outcome, craving and self-efficacy. Br J Clin Psychol. 2006;45(Pt 4):515–29.

53. van den Akker K, Jansen A, Frentz F, Havermans RC. Impulsivity makes more susceptible to overeating after contextual appetitive conditioning. Appetite. 2013;70:73–80.

54. Plewnia C. T023 Targeting the biased brain. Non-invasive brain stimulation to ameliorate cognitive control. Clin Neurophysiol. 2017;128(3):e7.

55. Zipfel S, Junne F, Giel KE. Measuring success in psychotherapy trials: the challenge of choosing the adequate control condition. Psychother Psychosom. 2020;89(4):195–9.

15

Impact of an oral health education intervention among a group of patients with eating disorders (anorexia nervosa and bulimia nervosa)

Laura S. Silverstein[1], Carol Haggerty[2], Lattice Sams[1], Ceib Phillips[3] and Michael W. Roberts[4*] (iD)

Abstract

Background: It is recognized that eating disorders are serious psychosocial illnesses that affect many adolescents and adults. A pre and post survey study was developed to assess demographics, oral health knowledge and self-image of patients with eating disorders participating in a hospital-based eating disorder clinic using an original oral health education program. The program's aim is to change the self-image and oral health practices of patients with anorexia-binge eating/purging (AN-BP) and bulimia nervosa (BN) disorders.

Methods: A pre-survey was completed by each study participant prior to attending the three educational sessions over a six-week period. A post survey questionnaire was completed after participation in all the educational presentations. Forty-six patients attended all three educational sessions and completed the pre and post-questionnaires.

Results: Most patients knew in advance that AN-BP and BN behavior can cause erosion of the teeth but only 30% knew the most likely location for the erosion to occur. But, following completion of the educational interventions, 73% answered the location correctly. Patients who reported going to the dentist regularly were significantly more likely to respond that their teeth/mouth had a positive effect on how they looked to themselves and to others, their general health, and their general happiness. Positive responses to the effect of the teeth/mouth on kissing and romantic relationships were also significantly higher for those who go to the dentist regularly compared to those who do not.

Conclusions: There is a need to further understand AN-BP and BP patients' oral health knowledge and self-image perceptions as it relates to their smile (teeth, mouth) to assist in developing a standardized oral health program for eating disorder centers to implement into their daily curricula. A dental team member in an interdisciplinary eating disorder treatment team is important. Including an oral health education program improves patients' oral hygiene and oral health knowledge, as well as provides a supportive environment to empower the patients to take control of their overall oral health.

Keywords: Oral health education, Eating disorders, Anorexia nervosa and bulimia nervosa

* Correspondence: mike_roberts16@unc.edu
[4]Division of Pediatric and Public Health, University of North Carolina Adams School of Dentistry, 228 Brauer Hall CB #7450, Chapel Hill, NC 27599-7450, USA
Full list of author information is available at the end of the article

Plain English summary

Using a pre and post survey, this study examined the demographics, oral health knowledge and self-image among a group of patients diagnosed with AN-BP or BN. The study participants completed a survey instrument before attending three educational presentations. A post survey questionnaire was completed after the final educational presentation. After participating in the educational presentations, 95% knew that tooth erosion was the most common oral effect of eating disorders (pre education = 78%) and 73% knew where the erosion most commonly occurred (pre education = 30%). Patients who went to a dentist regularly were significantly more likely to report that their teeth/mouth had a positive effect on how they looked to themselves and others, romantic relationships, general health, and their level of happiness. Providing an oral health education program improves the patients' oral health knowledge and empowers them to be proactive in caring for their teeth.

Introduction

Eating disorders are psycho-social illnesses that affect many adolescents and adults [1]. Individuals with eating disorders can also have additional health issues [2]. Some of these include diabetes, loss of menses in females, heart failure, very low self- esteem, metabolic, cardiovascular and endocrine disturbances [2], and distorted perception of body image [3]. In addition to these systemic problems, oral/dental trauma and dental caries, increase in xerostomia and parotid salivary gland swelling, dental erosion, and periodontal disease have been cited in the literature and are most associated with anorexia-binge eating/purging (AN-BP and bulimia nervosa (BN) [4]. Roberts and Li stated that the very negative self-perception and self-esteem that many individuals with anorexia nervosa and bulimia nervosa reported could be, in part, a cause for their lack of oral hygiene and increase in dental disease [3].

Often there are general health education programs in eating disorder clinics. However, we are unaware of any established oral health education programs to change and improve patients' oral health behaviors and self-perception as it relates to their smile [5, 6]. According to the Academy of Eating Disorders, the American Psychological Association, and the American Dental Association, proper oral health care for patients with eating disorders is fragmented. Johnson et al. reported "In addition to patient's lack of knowledge, there is very little evidence, if any, documenting the collaborative interaction between oral health and eating disorder professionals. Individuals who receive treatment for an eating disorder are typically not viewed as needing specialized, preventive oral care and commonly fail to receive appropriate oral health care, or recommendations

from the eating disorder treatment team" [7]. There is no indication that these patients have access to the proper oral health education and information. Without adequate oral health education for patients with eating disorders, oral disease can become severe and impact the patient's ability to eat, speak, and socialize [7].

The extent of oral/dental education in curricula within eating disorder treatment centers is unexplored to date [5, 6, 8]. Evidence of patients' self-image as it relates to their smile is also unexplored. The limited studies evaluating perception of oral health knowledge in eating disorder treatment programs suggest the need to further explore provider and client/patient barriers and perception towards oral care [7]. Integrating an oral health program focusing on improving self-image through dental education is essential in providing patients an interdisciplinary approach to care for the entire person. Understanding eating disorder patients' oral health knowledge and perceptions of self-image as it relates to their smile will assist in developing a standardized oral health program for eating disorder treatment centers to implement into their daily curricula.

Methods

The authors designed a pre and post survey study to assess demographics, oral health knowledge, and self-image of patients diagnosed with AN-BP and BN participating in a hospital-based eating disorder clinic. The authors consulted and collaborated with eating disorder specialists, dentists, dental hygienists, and psychiatrists in designing the surveys and the education program. An original oral health education program, called Smiles Matter, was created consisting of three different presentations/discussions. Each Smiles Matter session consisted of 15–20 min of didactic learning, 10 min of a group/personal exercise, and 10 min of questions that the patients had about their oral health or the topic of the day (Fig. 1).

Patients were consented prior to participating in the study and educational program. A pre-survey was completed by each participant prior to attending the three educational sessions. The presentations were given weekly and addressed general oral health education, esthetics, effects of eating disorders and oral pain, and nutrition for oral health. A post survey questionnaire was completed after the patient had participated in all three educational presentations. A respondent could choose not to answer all questions and some did so. Therefore, the denominator for some questions is different depending upon the number of responses.

The pre-survey consisted of 37 questions and the post survey consisted of 17 questions. Copies of the survey instruments are available from the author. The pre-survey asked questions on the following topics: demographics, oral health knowledge, oral habits and oral health

Smiles Matter Presentations and Discussions: Oral Health Education Program Topics

Session 1:
General Oral Health Education

- A. Oral hygiene
  - a. Demonstrate brushing and flossing techniques, discuss toothpastes and what they contain and purpose. Use large models with tooth brushes to demonstrate correct technique.
  - b. The best tooth brushes to use, electric vs. manual tooth brush.
- B. Educational and interactive activity.
  - a. Review intent of oral hygiene practices.
  - b. Distribute calendars for the patient to place sticker on at end of day if they did well.

Session 2:
Esthetics, Effects of Eating Disorders, and Pain

- A. Impact on the teeth
  - a. What eating disorders can do to your smile, erosion of teeth, pain in mouth and what may be the causes?
  - b. Discuss what happens to your teeth when you brush immediately after purging (vomiting) and sharing how you can minimize the damage to the teeth.
- B. Educational and reflective activity
  - a. Have patients draw a picture of their smile and then draw an ideal smile. Discuss the differences in the two drawings.
  - b. Write down educational and future goals. Talk about how smiles and success are related.

Session 3:
Nutrition for Oral Health

- A. Nutrition
  - a. Discuss how good nutrition affects overall health including oral manifestations, healthy diets for the oral cavity, problems with acidic foods, sugar containing foods, sodas, diet drinks.
  - b. End on a positive note. Discuss what negative issues can be reversed by maintaining good oral health and focusing on their smile.
  - c. Loss of tooth structure cannot be reversed. But an improvement in the smile can be achieved. It may require restorative dental care too help undue damage but much is possible.
    - i. First step is getting purging habit under control.
    - ii. Reduce ingestion of acidic or acid encouraging foods.
- B. Educational Activity
  - a. Nutrition exercise
    - i. Discuss what foods stimulate saliva, cognitive level.
    - ii. Plan a meal day. What foods will stick to your teeth, what will stimulate saliva and raise the pH of the mouth versus lowering the pH?
  - b. Address any questions from the patients.

Fig. 1 Smiles Matter Presentations and Discussions: Oral Health Education Program Topics

behaviors prior to diagnosis, oral health and habits since diagnosis with AN-BP or BN and current self-perceptions. The post-survey addressed similar issues after the patients participated in the education program. Chi-square analyses were performed to compare those who completed only the pre-survey questionnaire and those who completed both surveys and to assess the effect of age (< 23 vs > =23) and dental visit frequency (regularly vs occasionally/if a problem) on the pre-survey self-perception items. Discordance between pre and post survey responses were analyzed using the McNemar Test or its extension, the Bowken's Test of Symmetry. All analyses were conducted using SAS®v9.4software. Level of significance was set at 0.05 for all analyses. Statistical results were not corrected for multiplicity of comparisons because of the nature of the study.

The study design and all questionnaires, presentations, consents to participate and hand-outs were reviewed and approved by the Institutional Review Boards (IRB) at the University of North Carolina at Chapel Hill (IRB #15–3295). All study sites ceded review responsibility to the UNC-Chapel Hill IRB for management. The study is registered with ClinicalTrials.gov

(Identifier: NCT03921632). Funding for this study was provided by the Department of Pediatric Dentistry.

Study population
Patients enrolled in three in-patient treatment programs participated in the study; Center of Excellence for Eating Disorders at the University of North Carolina School of Medicine, Carolina House Eating Disorder Treatment Center, and Veritas Collaborative. Patients between the ages of 13 years old and 50 years old were eligible to participate in the study. While there are now eight recognized classifications of eating disorders in the DSM V [9], this study was limited to patients with anorexia nervosa and bulimia nervosa. Most of the patients who participated in the study did classify themselves as having anorexia nervosa.

Results
Sixty-seven patients were initially screened (92% Caucasian/100% females) and completed the pre-survey questionnaire but only 46 completed both pre- and post-questionnaires and attended all three of the educational module presentations. This was due to the patient being

released from the clinic or problems with scheduling return visits. There were no statistically significant differences between those who completed the protocol and those who did not (Table 1).

Of those who completed the protocol, the mean age at the time of diagnosis was 21.4 years (SD = 10.3) and at the beginning of the study 25.2 years old (SD = 10.8). The majority (69%) of the patients had AN-BP. Fifty-nine percent reported seeing a dentist regularly but 20% reported seeing a dentist only when they had a dental problem. Only 15% of the patients reported being referred to a dentist since their eating disorder was diagnosed. While most patients knew in advance eating disorders behavior can cause erosion of the teeth ($N = 35$; 76%) only 30% ($N = 14$) knew the most likely location in the mouth for erosion to occur. Eight-8 % also reported tooth sensitivity as an oral effect of an eating disorder; 78% reported dry mouth as an effect while 57% thought salivary gland enlargement and 38% oral cancer were possible oral effects (Table 2).

Before the intervention, there were no statistically significant differences ($p > 0.06$) in the proportion of positive responses for those less than 23 years of age (54%) compared to those 23 or older (46%) with respect to the effect that the teeth / mouth have on self-perception. Patients who reported going to the dentist regularly were significantly more likely to respond that their teeth/mouth had a positive effect on how they looked to themselves ($p = 0.03$), how they looked to others ($p = 0.03$), their general health ($p = 0.01$), and their general happiness ($p < 0.001$) than those who only reported going occasionally, or if they had a problem. Positive responses to the effect of the teeth/mouth on kissing and romantic relationships were also significantly higher for those who go to the dentist regularly compared to those who don't ($p = 0.04$ and 0.002 respectively). Table 2. Sixty-three percent ($N = 27$) of the patients said they had a plan to use the Smiles Matter material. Only 11% ($N = 5$) did not plan to see a dentist or would go only if they had a problem while 67% ($N = 30$) planned to see a dentist within 6 months. After participating in the program, 95 % of the patients ($N = 41$) correctly identified dental erosion as the most common dental finding of eating disorders. Similarly, 73% ($N = 32$) after the program answered correctly where erosion is most likely to occur in the mouth (Table 3).

Discussion

Evidence-based communication programs are critical for health professionals managing the prevention, treatment, and post treatment of patients of patients with AN-BP and BN eating disorders. It is important that oral health education programs be included to assist eating disorder patients improve their self-image and shift their focus to the importance of their smile and oral health. The results of this study suggests improved communication and providing appropriate information to AN-BP and BN eating disorder patients will help change behaviors

Table 1 Comparison of those who participated in both the pre and the post survey ($N = 46$) and those who only participated in the pre-survey ($N = 21$)

Variable	Participated in Both Surveys		Completed Only Pre-Survey		P Value
	Mean	SD	Mean	SD	
Age at Entry	25.2	10.8	26.9	10.7	0.55
Age at Diagnosis	21.4	10.3	20.6	8.2	0.77
	N	%	N	%	
Eating Disorder					0.77
Anorexia nervosa	31	69	13	62	
Bulimia Nervosa	10	22	5	24	
Other	4	9	3	14	
Ever Seen a Dentist					0.79
No	1	2	0	0	
Within last year	27	59	15	71	
Last 2 years	10	22	3	14	
More than 2 years	8	17	3	14	
Frequency of Dental Visit					0.93
Regularly	27	59	13	65	
Occasionally	10	22	4	20	
Only if problem	9	20	3	15	

Table 2 Effect of dental visit frequency on correct identification of possible oral effects of eating disorders and positive self-perception before the intervention

Possible effects of eating disorders	Regularly		Occasionally/only if problem		P value
	N	%	N	%	
Tooth erosion	22 of 26	84	13 of 20	65	0.45
Probable erosion sites	10 of 26	38	4 of 20	20	0.33
Tooth sensitivity	24 of 26	92	14 of 20	70	0.37
Dry mouth	20 of 26	81	13 of 20	66	0.99
Enlarged saliva glands	16 of 26	62	8 of 20	40	0.53
Oral cancer	12 of 26	46	4 of 20	20	0.21
No pain	14 of 26	54	7 of 20	35	0.02
Positive self-perception responses					
Confidence	15 of 26	58	5 of 20	25	0.15
Look to others	15of 26	58	3 of 20	15	0.03
Kissing	12 of 26	46	2 of 20	10	0.04
General health	17 of 26	65	5 of 20	25	0.01
Attendance	7 of 26	27	2 of 20	10	0.54
Success	7 of 26	27	4 of 20	20	0.60
Smiling/laughing	19 of 26	73	7 of 20	35	0.12
Looks to themselves	15 of 26	58	4 of 20	20	0.03
Social life	10 of 26	37	3 of 20	15	0.18
Enjoy eating	14 of 26	54	6 of 20	30	0.27
Speech	14 of 26	54	5 of 20	25	0.10
Choice of foods	8 of 26	30	4 of 20	20	0.17
Enjoy Life	14 of 26	54	3 of 20	15	0.08
Romantic relationship	10 of 26	37	1 of 20	5	0.002
General happiness	11 of 26	42	0 of 20	0	< 0.001
Weight	4 of 26	15	2 of 20	10	0.37

and improve their oral health. The intent of this study was to survey the effectiveness of an original oral health education program, "Smiles Matter", which aimed to improve patient's oral hygiene practices and oral health knowledge, and provide a supportive environment to empower them to take control of their oral health as well as their general health. Throughout the study, participating patients verbally shared that they had not previously had specialized, preventive oral care or recommendations from their eating disorder treatment team targeted to oral health.

It is important that eating disorder patients have access to a dental home to help provide a supportive environment for their oral health, their self-image as it relates to their smile, and their general health. The study found that patients who went to the dentist more frequently had a more positive response to how their teeth affected their lives. It is important for eating disorder treatment centers to provide an oral health educational program and to include an oral health educational program in their treatment protocol.

The primary limitation of this study was the small sample size. It was a challenge to identify patients who were available to complete all components of the study due to the intensity, length, and location of the eating disorder treatment programs. The dropout rate (patients not completing the entire program) was another limiting factor. While additional history was probably recorded in the patient's clinical record (e.g. duration of illness, psychiatric comorbidity) this information was not recorded/analyzed in the present study.

Conclusions

While statistical significance were shown in this study, the need to further understand eating disorder patients' oral health knowledge and perceptions of self-image as it relates to their smile (teeth, mouth) is important to assist in developing a standardized oral health program

Table 3 Impact of "Smiles Matter" program

Plan to See a Dentist	N	%				
No	2	4				
Within 6 months	30	67				
Within 1 year	10	22				
Only if a problem	3	7				
Have a Plan to Use Smiles Matter						
No	16	37				
Yes	27	63				
Change in Knowledge						
Dental Erosion						
	Post "Smiles Matter"					
	Correct		Incorrect			
Pre "Smiles Matter"	N	%	N	%		P value
Correct	34	79	1	2.3	(N = 35)	0.03
Incorrect	7	16	1	2.3		
	(N = 41)					
Erosion Location						
Correct	12	27	2	4.6	(N = 14)	0.001
Incorrect	20	45	10	22.7		
	(N = 32					

for eating disorder treatment centers to implement into their daily curricula/protocol. Including an oral health education program in eating disorder treatment centers appears to improve patients' oral hygiene and oral health knowledge, as well as provides a supportive environment to empower the patients to take control of their overall oral health. Whether the initial improvement in oral habits and awareness will be maintained over time could not be determined by this study.

Abbreviations
AN_BP: Anorexia-binge eating/purging; BN: Bulimia nervosa; IRB: Institutional Review Board; UNC: University of North Carolina-Chapel Hill

Acknowledgements
The authors acknowledge the assistance of Abigail Callahan, Helen May and Samantha Glover in conducting this study.
Dr. Silverstein was a dental student at the University of North Carolina Adams School of Dentistry when this study was conducted.

Authors' contributions
LSS assisted in developing the study protocol and the educational interventions, recruited the study participants and drafting the manuscript. CH assisted in developing the study protocol and the educational interventions. LS assisted in developing the study protocol and the educational interventions. CP was the biostatistician who completed the statistical analysis of the collected data. MWR assisted in developing the study protocol, edited the educational interventions and drafting the manuscript. All authors read and approved the final manuscript.

Competing interests
The authors declare that they have no competing interests.

Author details
[1]Department of Pediatric Dentistry, Children's Hospital Colorado, 1575 N Wheeling Street, Aurora, CO 80045, USA. [2]Division of Comprehensive Oral Health, University of North Carolina Adams School of Dentistry, Chapel Hill, NC 27599-7450, USA. [3]Division of Craniofacial and Surgical Sciences, University of North Carolina Adams School of Dentistry, Chapel Hill, NC 27599-7450, USA. [4]Division of Pediatric and Public Health, University of North Carolina Adams School of Dentistry, 228 Brauer Hall CB #7450, Chapel Hill, NC 27599-7450, USA.

References
1. Grilo CM, White MA, Masheb RM. DSM-IV psychiatric disorder comorbidity and its correlates in binge eating disorder. Int J Eat Disord. 2009;42(3):228–34.
2. Hicks TM, Lee J, Nguyen T, La Via M, Roberts M. Knowledge and practice of eating disorders among a group of adolescent dental patients. J Clin Pediatr Dent. 2013;38(1):39–43.
3. Roberts MW, Li S-H. Oral findings in anorexia nervosa and bulimia nervosa: a study of 47 cases. J Am Dent Assoc. 1987;115(3):407–10.
4. Romanos GE, Javed F, Romanos EB, Williams RC. Oro-facial manifestations in patients with eating disorders. Appetite. 2012;59(2):499–504.
5. Kisely S, Quek L-H, Pais J, Lalloo R, Johnson NW, Lawrence D. Advanced dental disease in people with severe mental illness: systematic review and meta-analysis. Br J Psychiatry. 2011;199(3):187–93.
6. DeBate RD, Plichta SB, Tedesco LA, Kerschbaum WE. Integration of oral health care and mental health services: dental hygienists' readiness and capacity for secondary prevention of eating disorders. J Behav Health Serv Res. 2006;33(1):113–25.
7. Johnson L, Boyd L, Rainchuso L, Rothman A, Mayer B. Eating disorder professionals' perceptions of oral health knowledge. Int J Dent Hyg. 2017;15(3):164–71.
8. Mental Health. A Report of the Surgeon General. Rockville: US Department of Health and Human Services, Substance Abuse and Mental Health Services Administration, Center for Mental Health Services, National Institutes of Health, National Institute of Mental Health; 1999.
9. Feeding and Eating Disorders. American Psychiatric Association. In: Diagnostic and statistical manual of mental disorders. 5th ed. Arlington: American Psychiatric Publishing; 2013.

16

Eating disorders and oral health: a scoping review on the role of dietitians

Tiffany Patterson-Norrie[1*] , Lucie Ramjan[2], Mariana S. Sousa[3], Lindy Sank[4] and Ajesh George[5]

Abstract

Background: Compromised nutritional intake due to eating disorder related behaviors, such as binge eating and purging, can lead to multi-system medical complications, including an irreversible impact on oral health. However, dental anxiety, fear or embarrassment may hinder individuals with an eating disorder from seeking assistance for their oral health concerns. As key health professionals in eating disorder treatment, dietitians are well positioned to provide basic dental screening, however, their capacity to perform this role in practice has not been established. The aim of this review was to identify current evidence on the role of dietitians in promoting oral health among individuals with eating disorders.

Methods: A comprehensive search of eight electronic databases and the grey literature was conducted to address the following three focus areas: 1) guidelines and recommendations on the role of dietitians in oral health 2) knowledge, attitudes and practices of dietitians regarding oral health promotion and; 3) current models of oral health care and resources for dietitians.

Results: Twelve articles were included. The review indicated that current national and international position statements encourage dietitians to conduct basic oral health screening and promote oral health in high risk populations, such as those with an eating disorder. However, no evidence was found to indicate dietitians performed oral health screening or education in populations with an eating disorder. In other population settings, dietitians were found to play a role in oral health promotion, however, were noted to have mixed knowledge on oral health risk factors, prevention and treatment and generally were not providing referrals. Some oral health promotion resources existed for dietitians working in pediatric, HIV and geriatric clinical areas however no resources were identified for dietitians working in eating disorder settings.

Conclusion: Despite current evidence showing that dietitians can play a role in oral health care, no models of care exist where dietitians promote oral health among individuals with an eating disorder. There are also no training resources and screening tools for dietitians in this area. Further research is required to develop this model of care and assess its feasibility and acceptability.

Keywords: Dietitians, Early intervention, Oral health, Feeding and eating disorders, Health personnel

* Correspondence: 17802808@student.westernsydney.edu.au
[1]Centre for Oral Health Outcomes & Research Translation (COHORT), School of Nursing and Midwifery , Western Sydney University/South Western Sydney Local Health District/ Ingham Institute for Applied Medical Research, Liverpool BC, Locked Bag 7103, Sydney, NSW 1871, Australia
Full list of author information is available at the end of the article

Plain English summary

Eating disorder related behaviors including binge eating and purging are known to lead to significant medical and dental complications. Barriers including dental anxiety or embarrassment may hinder individuals with an eating disorder from seeking assistance for their oral health concerns. Dietitians form part of the primary care team for eating disorders and therefore are well positioned to provide basic dental screening and education, however, their capacity to perform this role in practice has not been established. A review of the literature was conducted and focused on guidelines for oral health promotion, dietitian knowledge, attitudes and practices towards oral health promotion, and the availability of resources in this area. Recommendations that supported the role of the dietitian in oral health promotion were identified. Additionally, dietitians were found to be aware of the importance of oral health, however were not providing referrals. Overall, there was limited evidence of adequate oral health resources to assist dietitians. Despite the limited evidence, it highlights their capability to provide pre-emptive oral health promotion in other clinical settings. Further research is needed to explore how to support dietitians to promote oral health among populations with an ED.

Background

The prevalence, incidence and magnitude of eating disorders (ED) is increasing worldwide [1–3]. Around 1.2 million people in the United Kingdom [4], and approximately 30 million individuals in the United States are thought to currently have an eating disorder [5–7]. In Australia, ED are estimated to affect 4–9% of the population [8–10] and are the second leading cause of mental disorder disability among females [5, 8, 10, 11]. Eating disorders affect an individual's social and functional roles, and increase overall risk of morbidity and mortality [5, 12]. From an economic standpoint, ED can also place significant financial strain on the individual and health system with the total burden of disease in Australia estimated to be $52.6 billion per year [13], with the impact on productivity reaching $15 billion [10].

Compromised nutritional intake as a result of restrictive or obsessive dieting and purging.

behaviors among people with ED can lead to multi-system medical complications such as bradycardia, electrolyte imbalance and renal failure [1, 12, 14]. Somewhat less well known, these behaviors can also have an irreversible impact on oral health [15, 16]. The results from two systematic reviews and meta-analyses confirmed an association between tooth erosion, poor oral health and ED. Individuals with an ED were five times more likely to have tooth erosion and

overall higher decay, regardless of ED subtype [17, 18]. Furthermore, ED related dental complications can perpetuate body dissatisfaction leading to a decline in self-esteem, quality of life and psychosocial functioning [19–21]. When combined with the psychological and emotional stress of managing an ED, the impact of having an oral health complication can exacerbate ED signs and symptoms such as limited oral intake or food avoidance and inhibit treatment goals [20].

It is well known that good oral health is integral to general health, yet there are a number of barriers that may deter individuals from prioritizing their oral health care practices and seeking treatment for their oral health concerns. In vulnerable low income populations, individuals reported oral health behaviors such as living with chronic dental issues including dental pain or decaying teeth without seeking intervention, and accessing dental services only when dental concerns became unbearable [22, 23]. Significant relationships between poorer self-reported oral health outcomes, lower socioeconomic status and mental health vulnerabilities were also noted [22–24]. Specifically for individuals with a mental health condition, barriers to maintaining oral health included a reduced awareness of the presence/risk of oral health problems, the affect of medications such as antidepressants resulting in manifestations such as dry mouth, lower self-esteem and body image, poor diet and fear and distrust of dental providers [24–26]. Although individuals with ED were generally found to be concerned about their teeth especially the long term impact of dental issues such as enamel erosion [27, 28], their perceived barriers for not seeking dental intervention included reduced energy levels, anxiety, uncertainty about oral hygiene and distrust of dental providers [27, 28]. If left untreated, oral health complications can impede dietary intervention and ongoing ED treatment due to dental pain or discomfort [29–31].

Given the risk of dental problems among individuals with ED and their risk of poorer oral health outcomes, it is important to consider the promotion of oral health in this population. Previous research has supported the role of non-dental health professionals in raising awareness of dental problems and performing screening assessments in vulnerable or at-risk populations [30, 31]. Dietitians form an integral part of the multidisciplinary primary care team often working towards the stabilization of acutely unwell patients and helping to safely assist the client towards re-nourishment, relapse prevention and recovery [32–34]; this places them in a unique position to promote oral health in an ED clinical setting. However, to date, the potential role of the dietitian in promoting oral health among people with ED has received little attention and has not been clearly defined.

The aim of this scoping review was to identify current evidence supporting the role and scope of dietitians in this area. Specifically, this review was guided by the following focus areas:

- Guidelines and recommendations on the role of dietitians in oral health
- Knowledge, attitudes and practices (KAP) of dietitians in oral health promotion
- Current models of oral health care and resources for dietitians

Terminology
Dietitian/ registered dietitian
A dietitian has tertiary qualifications in nutrition and dietetics which specifically involves the study of medical nutrition therapy, dietary counselling and food service management in addition to qualifications of a nutritionist. To obtain these qualifications, a dietitian must have "undertaken a course of study that included substantial theory and supervised and assessed clinical practice" [35].

Nutritionist
A nutritionist is a tertiary qualified professional who has the expertise to provide a range of nutrition services related to public health nutrition and community health [35].

Non-dental professional
An individual that is not recognized as a dentist, dental hygienist, dental therapist or other qualified oral health professional. Therefore, a non-dental professional can include, but is not limited to, nutritionists, dietitians, medical doctors, nurses, midwives and other allied health professionals.

Methods
Design
Utilizing the framework as described by Arksey and O'Malley, a scoping review was undertaken to investigate and summarize the nature and breadth of the role and scope of dietitians in providing oral health promotion (OHP) for individuals with ED, as well as to identify current gaps in the literature [36]. A scoping review was chosen as it allows for the researcher to follow an iterative search approach enabling the focus areas to be re-modeled and re-defined especially given the paucity of research on this topic, which would increase the complexity of conducting a review.

Search strategy
A preliminary search was undertaken by author TPN using Google Scholar to identify keywords based on published abstracts and articles. A total of eight databases were then searched including: MEDLINE (Ovid), Embase, EBSCO, PubMed, Cochrane, SCOPUS, Web of Science and ProQuest. Search strategies were enabled by Boolean operators (AND, OR, NOT), Truncations e.g. (diet*), medical subject headings (MESH) and descriptive key-terms where appropriate. In addition, a grey literature search was conducted to source government or non-government related material to assist in answering the aims of this review. Keywords used included: dietitian, oral health assessment, oral health screening, eating disorder, bulimia nervosa, anorexia nervosa, guidelines, training, resources, knowledge, attitudes, perceptions, practices, behaviors.

Inclusion and exclusion criteria
All studies published up until October 2019 that addressed at least one of the focus areas were included in this review. There were no restrictions placed on database searches in terms of year of publication, study design or study quality for all focus areas. Only articles published in English were eligible for inclusion.

Articles and resources found on the world wide web were eligible for inclusion if the sources originated from a reputable research foundation, network, association, organization or government source. There was no restriction placed on year of publication for grey literature. Depending on the country of registration, dietitians can be identified by different titles such as dietitian, registered dietitian, registered dietitian nutritionist and so on. Therefore, due to the paucity of research in this area, studies that included dietitians or nutritionists were included in this study.

Data screening, selection and extraction
The screening and selection were carried out by two authors (TPN, MSS). The process can be viewed in Fig. 1. Articles that met at least one of the inclusion requirements were included. All included articles were then categorized into the three focus areas. Initial results indicated that more expansive searching was required in all focus areas based on the meagre results acquired. The focus areas were revised from specifically investigating the ED population to other settings where dietitians were playing a role in oral health promotion. Data were extracted by one reviewer (TPN) and verified by three reviewers (MSS, LR, AG). Information extracted from the articles included: location of study, article type, study aims, study design,

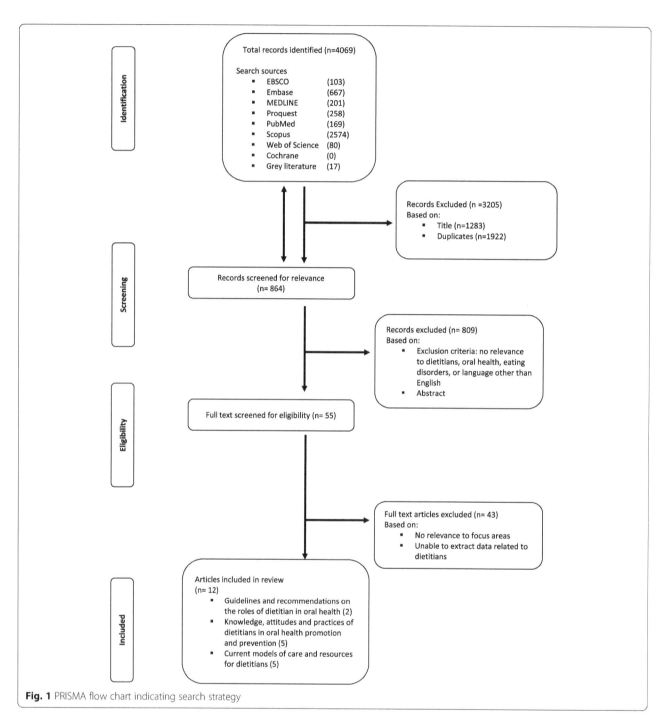

Fig. 1 PRISMA flow chart indicating search strategy

details of the study including participant demographics, study findings and conclusions.

Results

A search of the literature yielded a total of 4069 records. Of these, 3205 were excluded based on title ($n = 1283$) and duplicates ($n = 1922$), resulting in 864 abstracts which were screened for relevance. From this, 55 articles were identified for full text review and a total of 12 articles were included in this scoping review. The articles were categorized under the following focus areas: i) Guidelines and recommendations on the role of dietitians in oral health ($n = 2$) ii) Knowledge, attitudes and practices (KAP) of dietitians in oral health promotion ($n = 5$) and; iii) current models of oral health care and resources for dietitians ($n = 5$) (Table 1). Literature and resources identified in the focus areas originated from Australia ($n = 3$ [38, 46, 49]), United States ($n = 8$ [37, 39–44, 48]), and Israel ($n = 1$ [45]).

Table 1 Included articles that identify available guidelines for dietitians, KAP of dietitians regarding oral health promotion and current models of oral health care and resources for dietitians

Author (Year)/ Location	Article Type	Aims	Study Design	Details of Study	Conclusion	Focus area
Decker, R.T. (2013) USA [37]	Position statement	To provide the position of The Academy of Nutrition and Dietetics regarding oral health and nutrition as well as describe the roles and responsibilities of dietetics practitioners in oral health education, practice and research.	N/A	Position statement on the role of the dietitians in oral health promotion	• The Academy supports the collaboration and integration of oral health with nutrition services, education and research. • Skills of screening oral health and making referrals is essential for dietitians. • Supports education that reinforces and illustrates the role of nutrition in oral health. • Collaboration between oral health practitioners and dietitians is recommended. • Eating disorders is highlighted as an at-risk group and some oral health manifestations typical to this population, such as xerostomia are specified. However, no specific information exists to detail the support dietitians should provide to this population. • A general table is provided where dietitians can identify oral related manifestations of nutrition deficits.	Guidelines and recommendations
Dietitians Australia and Dental Health Services Victoria (2015) Australia [38]	Joint Position statement	To provide evidence based oral health information to dietitians; to guide how oral health can be incorporated into the various roles of dietitians and to provide a framework for workforce capacity building workforce.	N/A	Joint position statement on the role of the dietitian in oral health promotion	• There is consensus that the dietitian's role, dependent on setting, should: incorporate oral health screening, especially in priority at risk groups; recognize risk factors; provide nutritional management and/or provide guidance/ referral to oral health professionals; develop and deliver health promotion and education messages. • Specific oral health advice for dietitians is provided for medically compromised/special needs patients including individuals with an eating disorder. • Specific oral health advice for dietitians is provided for medically compromised/special needs patients including individuals with an eating disorder. Key advice includes encouraging good oral hygiene and providing advice on oral care after vomiting.	Guidelines and recommendations

Table 1 Included articles that identify available guidelines for dietitians, KAP of dietitians regarding oral health promotion and current models of oral health care and resources for dietitians *(Continued)*

Author (Year)/ Location	Article Type	Aims	Study Design	Details of Study	Conclusion	Focus area
Faine, M.P. (1995) USA [39]	Peer reviewed journal article	Assess the knowledge of the role of diet in dental caries aetiology in nutritionists and dental hygienists.	Cross-sectional	136 registered dietitians and 37 registered dental hygienists	• Awareness varied across different topics related to caries-preventative measures. While 95% of nutritionists recognised fluoride uptake into developing teeth makes dental enamel more resistant to dental caries, only 16% understood that fluoride may hinder bacterial activity. • Most nutritionists (53%) demonstrated awareness of the infectious nature of dental caries but only 38% recognised mothers can transmit bacteria to their children. • Nearly all nutritionists correctly identified high vs. low cariogenic snack foods. Nearly all (97%) of nutritionists were aware of and discussed childhood caries with clients. • Two thirds of nutritionists surveyed incorrectly linked the severity of dental decay to concentration of sugars in food. • Most nutritionists were knowledgeable on recommendations including limiting nighttime bottle feeding to reduce childhood caries risk	Knowledge attitudes and practices
Fuller, L.A. (2014) USA [40]	Peer reviewed journal article	To assess the oral health knowledge, confidence and practices of Virginia personnel in the special supplemental food program for Women, Infants and Children (WIC).	Cross-sectional 22-item investigator-designed questionnaire (content validity and reliability established). Some questions sourced from previously tested questionnaires.	159 WIC personnel including –registered dietitians (20%) –nutritionists (33%), –dietetic technicians (5%), –licensed practical nurses (~ 4%) and registered nurses (~ 1%).	• WIC respondents who were over 40 years of age and with 10+ years' experience were more knowledgeable about caries transmission and the dental decay process than younger and less experienced WIC respondents. • More than half (64%) of respondents were not confident in performing oral screening. • Respondents with higher academic qualifications were more confident (90%) in oral health counselling. • One third of respondents were performing oral screenings for decay. • Most (87%) respondents who were older and more experienced were providing oral health counselling to parents on toothbrushing and were	Knowledge, attitudes and practices

Table 1 Included articles that identify available guidelines for dietitians, KAP of dietitians regarding oral health promotion and current models of oral health care and resources for dietitians (*Continued*)

Author (Year)/ Location	Article Type	Aims	Study Design	Details of Study	Conclusion	Focus area
					also more likely to provide referrals to dentists.	
Gold, J.T. (2016) USA [41]	Peer reviewed journal article	Assess the oral health knowledge, practices and attitudes of staff in the Special Supplemental Nutrition Program for Women, Infant and Children (WIC) in north central Florida.	Cross-sectional 28 item questionnaire-developed and validated from previously validated questionnaires.	39 WIC staff including, 9 nutritionists/dietitians.	• Majority of nutritionists (> 78%) were knowledgeable about the importance of maintaining good oral health in children, risk factors and the role of caregivers. • Poor knowledge (33%) around the use of fluoridated toothpaste in children under the age of 2 and nighttime on demand breastfeeding as a risk factor. • All nutritionists were confident in providing oral health counselling for women and children and dental referral if required. • All nutritionists discussed the relationship between dietary choices and caries with parents. • More than two thirds (67%) of nutritionists regularly provided counselling on the importance of tooth brushing and dental visits. • None of the nutritionists were undertaking oral health risk screenings of children and less than half (44%) were referring women and children to dentists.	Knowledge attitudes and practices
Koerber, A. (2006) USA [42]	Peer reviewed journal article	Explore the attitudes and practices of health professionals in a Latino community regarding the association between diabetes and periodontitis to guide interventions for oral health promotion.	Qualitative	Participants (N = 14) - 50% Nurses (n = 7) - 36% Dentists (n = 5) - 14% Nutritionist (n = 2) Nutritionist years of experience: ~ 13-20 yrs.	• Knowledge on the relationship between diabetes and its associated symptoms and caries risk was adequate but lacked depth. • All nutritionists considered oral health and diabetes to be important. • Nutritionists were eager to provide oral health education. • None of available resources used by nutritionists discussed the need for oral health and self-care prevention measures with diabetic patients. • Nutritionists were not referring to dentists but demonstrated willingness to do so. • Nutritionists requested more training and suggested development of guidelines and new protocols on the diabetes-periodontitis	Knowledge attitudes and practices

Table 1 Included articles that identify available guidelines for dietitians, KAP of dietitians regarding oral health promotion and current models of oral health care and resources for dietitians (*Continued*)

Author (Year)/ Location	Article Type	Aims	Study Design	Details of Study	Conclusion	Focus area
Shick EA. (2005) USA [43]	Peer reviewed journal article	Examine the effects of knowledge and confidence on dental referral practices among WIC nutritionists in North Carolina.	Cross-sectional 118 item questionnaire-developed from previously tested questionnaires and pilot tested	324 nutritionists	association as well as patient information handouts and videotapes. • Most nutritionists were knowledgeable about basic oral hygiene and caries related diet recommendations. • Nutritionists were less aware (33%) of potential caries transmission from carers and importance of fluoride for children. • Nutritionists were very confident about providing oral health counselling and dental referrals (90–96%). They were Less confident (39.3%) about undertaking oral health risk screenings of children. • Confidence in undertaking oral health risk screenings (OR.2.12), and making dental referrals (OR 3.02) was associated with more frequent referrals.	Models of care and resources
Karmally W. (2014) USA [44]	Webinar	Provide education on the association between nutrition and oral health conditions and discuss practical strategies for dietitians to integrate oral health information with nutrition counselling.	N/A	Webinar approved for continued professional education	• Webinar discusses the relationship between nutrition, disease and oral health and provides strategies on how dietitians can incorporate oral health into the nutrition assessment (including oral health screening).	Models of care and resources
Brody R.A. (2014) Israel [45]	Peer reviewed journal article	To assess the changes in knowledge and practice of dietitians, working in geriatric care in Israel, following a training program in nutrition focused physical assessment of the oral cavity.	Prospective pilot study using a pre- posttest design. Investigator designed 29 item knowledge pre-test (face and content validity established) and patient data collection forms (practices)	30 dietitians completed the pre-and post-test questionnaires. Testing conducted pre-training, immediately post-training and 12 months post-training (3 timepoints) Training was provided to dietitians which included oral related anatomy, performing extra-oral and intra-oral examination and screening for dysphagia and vitamin deficiencies	• Pretesting suggests that dietitians had limited nutrition focused physical assessment oral health knowledge. At each timepoint following training, knowledge had increased. • Three months post training, dietitians were more likely to perform oral health screenings rather than not assessing or obtaining history from the medical record. • Dietitians were 5.7 x more likely to refer to other allied health professionals 3 months post-training.	Models of care and resources
Jeganathan, S. (2010) Australia [46]	Peer reviewed journal article	Develop and validate a 3-item oral health assessment questionnaire (OHQ) for use by dietitians to screen individuals with HIV at risk of dental	Cross-sectional	Tool to be validated: 3 item oral health assessment questionnaire (OHQ) and the Oral health Impact profile 14 (OHIP-14) was administered	• Questionnaire completed by 273 participants. • The OHQ was found to be a valid and sensitive screening tool for	Models of care and resources

Table 1 Included articles that identify available guidelines for dietitians, KAP of dietitians regarding oral health promotion and current models of oral health care and resources for dietitians (Continued)

Author (Year)/ Location	Article Type	Aims	Study Design	Details of Study	Conclusion	Focus area
		complications for referral to dental health services.		to 273 clients	dietitians to initiate further investigation for oral health screening and referral to dental professionals. • The sensitivity for the OHQ was 84% and the specificity was 55%. • Compared to the 'Gold Standard' Oral health Impact profile-14 (OHIP), the OHQ demonstrated adequate validity (rho = 0.617 (95% CI 0.54, 0.69), $P < 0.0001$).	
The Albion Centre, oral health promotion working group - NSW Health (2015) Australia [47]	Oral health resource	Oral health screening and referral tool for health professionals (including dietitians) working with individuals with HIV.	N/A	Oral health resource includes three item oral health assessment tool, take home advice for clients, referral pathways and information about common dental problems encountered by individuals with HIV	N/A	Models of care and resources
Pac West MCH distance Learning Network, University of Washington (2005) USA [48]	Oral health education and screening resource	Provides actions that non-dental and dental health professionals can take to identify individuals at risk of oral health complications and provides guidelines for action.	N/A	Module 5 of an online resource for actions that non-dental health professionals can consider when addressing oral health complications which includes: potential oral health screening and prevention activities, suggestions for screening tools for nutrition related oral health problems, mechanisms for referral and further resources and initiatives	N/A	Models of care and resources
Author (Year)/ Location	Article Type	Aims	Study Design	Details of Study	Conclusion	Focus area
Decker, R.T. (2013) USA [37]	Position statement	To provide the position of The Academy of Nutrition and Dietetics regarding oral health and nutrition as well as describe the roles and responsibilities of dietetics practitioners in oral health education, practice and research.	N/A	Position statement on the role of the dietitians in oral health promotion	• The Academy supports the collaboration and integration of oral health with nutrition services, education and research. • Skills of screening oral health and making referrals is essential for dietitians. • Supports education that reinforces and illustrates the role of nutrition in oral health. • Collaboration between oral health practitioners and dietitians is recommended. • Eating disorders is highlighted as an at-risk group and some oral health	Guidelines and recommendations

Table 1 Included articles that identify available guidelines for dietitians, KAP of dietitians regarding oral health promotion and current models of oral health care and resources for dietitians *(Continued)*

Author (Year)/ Location	Article Type	Aims	Study Design	Details of Study	Conclusion	Focus area
					manifestations typical to this population, such as xerostomia are specified. However, no specific information exists to detail the support dietitians should provide to this population. • A general table is provided where dietitians can identify oral related manifestations of nutrition deficits.	
Dietitians Australia and Dental Health Services Victoria (2015) Australia [38]	Joint Position statement	To provide evidence based oral health information to dietitians; to guide how oral health can be incorporated into the various roles of dietitians and to provide a framework for workforce capacity building workforce.	N/A	Joint position statement on the role of the dietitian in oral health promotion	• There is consensus that the dietitian's role, dependent on setting, should: incorporate oral health screening, especially in priority at risk groups; recognize risk factors; provide nutritional management and/or provide guidance/ referral to oral health professionals; develop and deliver health promotion and education messages. • Specific oral health advice for dietitians is provided for medically compromised/special needs patients including individuals with an eating disorder. • Specific oral health advice for dietitians is provided for medically compromised/special needs patients including individuals with an eating disorder. Key advice includes encouraging good oral hygiene and providing advice on oral care after vomiting.	Guidelines and recommendations
Faine, M.P. (1995) USA [39]	Peer reviewed journal article	Assess the knowledge of the role of diet in dental caries aetiology in nutritionists and dental hygienists.	Cross-sectional	136 registered dietitians and 37 registered dental hygienists	• Awareness varied across different topics related to caries-preventative measures. While 95% of nutritionists recognized fluoride uptake into developing teeth makes dental enamel more resistant to dental caries, only 16% understood that fluoride may hinder bacterial activity. • Most nutritionists (53%) demonstrated awareness of the infectious nature of dental caries but only 38% recognized mothers can transmit bacteria to their children. • Nearly all nutritionists correctly	Knowledge attitudes and practices

Table 1 Included articles that identify available guidelines for dietitians, KAP of dietitians regarding oral health promotion and current models of oral health care and resources for dietitians (*Continued*)

Author (Year)/ Location	Article Type	Aims	Study Design	Details of Study	Conclusion	Focus area
					• identified high vs. low cariogenic snack foods. Nearly all (97%) of nutritionists were aware of and discussed childhood caries with clients. • Two thirds of nutritionists surveyed incorrectly linked the severity of dental decay to concentration of sugars in food. • Most nutritionists were knowledgeable on recommendations including limiting nighttime bottle feeding to reduce childhood caries risk	
Fuller, L.A. (2014) USA [40]	Peer reviewed journal article	To assess the oral health knowledge, confidence and practices of Virginia personnel in the special supplemental food program for Women, Infants and Children (WIC).	Cross-sectional 22-item investigator-designed questionnaire (content validity and reliability established). Some questions sourced from previously tested questionnaires.	159 WIC personnel including -registered dietitians (20%) -nutritionists (33%), –dietetic technicians (5%), –licensed practical nurses (~ 4%) and registered nurses (~ 1%).	• WIC respondents who were over 40 years of age and with 10+ years' experience were more knowledgeable about caries transmission and the dental decay process than younger and less experienced WIC respondents. • More than half (64%) of respondents were not confident in performing oral screening. • Respondents with higher academic qualifications were more confident (90%) in oral health counselling. • One third of respondents were performing oral screenings for decay. • Most (87%) respondents who were older and more experienced were providing oral health counselling to parents on toothbrushing and were also more likely to provide referrals to dentists.	Knowledge, attitudes and practices
Gold, J.T. (2016) USA [41]	Peer reviewed journal article	Assess the oral health knowledge, practices and attitudes of staff in the Special Supplemental Nutrition Program for Women, Infant and Children (WIC) in north central Florida.	Cross-sectional 28 item questionnaire-developed and validated from previously validated questionnaires.	39 WIC staff including, 9 nutritionists/ dietitians.	• Majority of nutritionists (> 78%) were knowledgeable about the importance of maintaining good oral health in children, risk factors and the role of caregivers. • Poor knowledge (33%) around the use of fluoridated toothpaste in children under the age of 2 and nighttime on demand breastfeeding as a risk factor. • All nutritionists were confident in	Knowledge attitudes and practices

Table 1 Included articles that identify available guidelines for dietitians, KAP of dietitians regarding oral health promotion and current models of oral health care and resources for dietitians *(Continued)*

Author (Year)/ Location	Article Type	Aims	Study Design	Details of Study	Conclusion	Focus area
					• providing oral health counselling for women and children and dental referral if required. • All nutritionists discussed the relationship between dietary choices and caries with parents. • More than two thirds (67%) of nutritionists regularly provided counselling on the importance of tooth brushing and dental visits. • None of the nutritionists were undertaking oral health risk screenings of children and less than half (44%) were referring women and children to dentists.	
Koerber, A. (2006) USA [42]	Peer reviewed journal article	Explore the attitudes and practices of health professionals in a Latino community regarding the association between diabetes and periodontitis to guide interventions for oral health promotion.	Qualitative	Participants (*N* = 14) - 50% Nurses (*n* = 7) - 36% Dentists (*n* = 5) - 14% Nutritionist (*n* = 2) Nutritionist years of experience: ~ 13-20 yrs.	• Knowledge on the relationship between diabetes and its associated symptoms and caries risk was adequate but lacked depth. • All nutritionists considered oral health and diabetes to be important. • Nutritionists were eager to provide oral health education. • None of available resources used by nutritionists discussed the need for oral health and self-care prevention measures with diabetic patients. • Nutritionists were not referring to dentists but demonstrated willingness to do so. • Nutritionists requested more training and suggested development of guidelines and new protocols on the diabetes-periodontitis association as well as patient information handouts and videotapes.	Knowledge attitudes and practices
Shick EA. (2005) USA [43]	Peer reviewed journal article	Examine the effects of knowledge and confidence on dental referral practices among WIC nutritionists in North Carolina.	Cross-sectional 118 item questionnaire-developed from previously tested questionnaires and pilot tested	324 nutritionists	• Most nutritionists were knowledgeable about basic oral hygiene and caries related diet recommendations. • Nutritionists were less aware (33%) of potential caries transmission from carers and importance of fluoride for children. • Nutritionists were very confident about providing oral health counselling and dental referrals (90–	Models of care and resources

Table 1 Included articles that identify available guidelines for dietitians, KAP of dietitians regarding oral health promotion and current models of oral health care and resources for dietitians (*Continued*)

Author (Year)/ Location	Article Type	Aims	Study Design	Details of Study	Conclusion	Focus area
					96%). They were Less confident (39.3%) about undertaking oral health risk screenings of children. • Confidence in undertaking oral health risk screenings (OR2.12), and making dental referrals (OR 3.02) was associated with more frequent referrals.	Models of care and resources
Karmally W. (2014) USA [44]	Webinar	Provide education on the association between nutrition and oral health conditions and discuss practical strategies for dietitians to integrate oral health information with nutrition counselling.	N/A	Webinar approved for continued professional education	• Webinar discusses the relationship between nutrition, disease and oral health and provides strategies on how dietitians can incorporate oral health into the nutrition assessment (including oral health screening).	Models of care and resources
Brody R.A. (2014) Israel [45]	Peer reviewed journal article	To assess the changes in knowledge and practice of dietitians, working in geriatric care in Israel, following a training program in nutrition focused physical assessment of the oral cavity.	Prospective pilot study using a pre- posttest design. Investigator designed 29 item knowledge pre-test (face and content validity established) and patient data collection forms (practices)	30 dietitians completed the pre-and post-test questionnaires. Testing conducted pre-training, immediately post-training and 12 months post-training (3 timepoints) Training was provided to dietitians which included oral related anatomy, performing extra-oral and intra-oral examination and screening for dysphagia and vitamin deficiencies	• Pretesting suggests that dietitians had limited nutrition focused physical assessment oral health knowledge. At each timepoint following training, knowledge had increased. • Three months post training, dietitians were more likely to perform oral health screenings rather than not assessing or obtaining history from the medical record. • Dietitians were 5.7 x more likely to refer to other allied health professionals 3 months post-training.	Models of care and resources
Jeganathan, S. (2010) Australia [46]	Peer reviewed journal article	Develop and validate a 3-item oral health assessment questionnaire (OHQ) for use by dietitians to screen individuals with HIV at risk of dental complications for referral to dental health services.	Cross-sectional	Tool to be validated: 3 item oral health assessment questionnaire (OHQ) and the Oral health Impact profile 14 (OHIP-14) was administered to 273 clients	• Questionnaire completed by 273 participants. • The OHQ was found to be a valid and sensitive screening tool for dietitians to initiate further investigation for oral health screening and referral to dental professionals. • The sensitivity for the OHQ was 84% and the specificity was 55%. • Compared to the 'Gold Standard' Oral health Impact profile-14 (OHIP), the OHQ demonstrated adequate validity (rho = 0.617 (95% CI 0.54, 0.69), $P < 0.0001$).	Models of care and resources
The Albion Centre, oral	Oral health	Oral health screening and referral tool for health professionals	N/A	Oral health resource includes three item oral health assessment tool, take	N/A	Models of care and resources

Table 1 Included articles that identify available guidelines for dietitians, KAP of dietitians regarding oral health promotion and current models of oral health care and resources for dietitians (*Continued*)

Author (Year)/ Location	Article Type	Aims	Study Design	Details of Study	Conclusion	Focus area
health promotion working group - NSW Health (2015) Australia [47]	resource	(including dietitians) working with individuals with HIV.		home advice for clients, referral pathways and information about common dental problems encountered by individuals with HIV		
Pac West MCH - distance Learning Network, University of Washington (2005) USA [48]	Oral health education and screening resource	Provides actions that non-dental and dental health professionals can take to identify individuals at risk of oral health complications and provides guidelines for action.	N/A	Module 5 of an online resource for actions that non-dental health professionals can consider when addressing oral health complications which includes: potential oral health screening and prevention activities, suggestions for screening tools for nutrition related oral health problems, mechanisms for referral and further resources and initiatives	N/A	Models of care and resources

Focus area I: guidelines and recommendations on the role of dietitians in oral health

Two position statements on oral health and the role of dietitians were identified: a joint position statement and guideline from the Dietitians Australia (DA, formerly Dietitians Association of Australia) and Dental Health Services Victoria (DSHV) [38], and one from the Academy of Nutrition and Dietetics (USA) [37].

Both position statements supported the belief that nutrition is an integral part of oral health across all life stages and emphasized a shift toward multidisciplinary collaboration for patient-centered care. The identified statements support and stress the need for collaboration between dietitians and dental practitioners for promoting oral health and early intervention in oral health disease [37, 38].

Scope of practice

The joint position statement by the DA and DHSV specifically provided advice and areas for intervention which the dietitian can use in addressing oral health risk factors or manifestations. Particularly, potential areas for incorporation of oral health into practice included, during a nutritional assessment, when oral health risk factors can be identified and addressed by providing guidance for management or referral to the oral health practitioner. Additionally, in community or non-acute settings, the dietitian can also participate in OHP [38].

This position statement also highlights priority life stages and risk factors for oral health [38]. In relation to the focus areas of this scoping review, ED and oral health manifestations including dental erosion, mucosal lesions, and altered salivary functions were noted, and key advice was provided to the dietitian on methods to address these issues in practice. Advice included providing education to 'at risk' individuals on oral health care after vomiting, appropriate oral hygiene practices and referral to a dental professional where appropriate [38].

Similarly, the position statements from the United States and Australia stated that oral health screening, and referral were part of the dietitian's role and responsibility in providing comprehensive patient care [37]. The statements highlighted that oral health integration into current dietetic practice can be achieved by the inclusion of oral health screening into the general nutrition assessment with referral as required. The Australian position statement further detailed that oral health screening should be undertaken particularly for at risk populations and various validated oral health screening tools were recommended depending on the setting [50]. As part of the screening process dietitians can recognize oral manifestations of systemic diseases and identify patients at-risk of poor oral health that require referal to dentists. Additionally, the American statement also encouraged the setting of patient care goals with an oral health practitioner [37].

Education

Both position statements strongly encouraged oral health education for dietitians. The Australian position statement highlighted that its purpose was to provide a framework for building the confidence and knowledge of current dietitians and for the education of future dietitians in tertiary education [38].

The Academy of Nutrition and Dietetics provided greater detail and outlined their recommendations for interprofessional education in keeping with the recommendations by the Institute of Medicine which calls for the 'improvement of access to oral health care for vulnerable populations' [37]. The latter highlighted the integration of didactic and interprofessional education within a curriculum, designed for both dietitians and oral health professionals. This included dietitians in their Bachelor programs receiving lectures and practical tutorials in oral anatomy, physiology and manifestations in disease; clinical experience targeting how to incorporate oral health screening into nutrition assessment; conducting basic nutrition physical assessments with oral and cranial nerve assessment; working with oral health professionals and creating appropriate diets for compromised oral health [37].

Focus area II: knowledge, attitudes and practices (KAP) of dietitians regarding oral health promotion

An initial search was conducted investigating KAP of dietitians regarding oral health promotion specifically for people with an eating disorder. This search returned no results and hence, a broader search was conducted to include other populations or clinical settings. A total of five articles were identified for this focus area. Due to the variation in the identification of dietitians and nutritionists in the included studies, for simplicity, both dietitians and nutritionists will be collectively referred to as 'dietitians' from here forth. One qualitative study focused generally on dietitians oral health knowledge and practice in diabetes management [42], while the remaining four cross sectional studies specifically assessed dietitian KAP in the area of women, infants and children's (WIC) populations [39–41, 43].

Knowledge

Across all the included studies in this focus area dietitians were noted to have mixed awareness of the aetiology, risks and prevention of dental caries [39–43]. Generally, knowledge of the infectious nature of caries varied widely between the cross sectional studies [39, 40, 43]. Particularly, 33 to 97% of dietitians working in the WIC populations were able to identify that mothers can transmit decay causing bacteria to their children [39–41, 43]. The authors did not report why results fluctuated significantly, however, another study did note that dietitians who were older (> 40 years old) and with more years of working experience (> 10 years) were more knowledgeable in this area (87–97%) [40].

Commonly, dietitians had adequate knowledge in their understanding of the impact of dietary choices and behaviors on caries risk [39, 41, 42]. The vast majority (82%) of dietitians involved in WIC population showed consistent awareness of the impact of high risk foods and practices such as night time bottle feeding (82%) and increased risk of dental caries [39] and either knew that periodontal disease could affect glycemic control, or were not surprised by this association [42]. Even so, 66% of dietitians incorrectly identified that the severity of dental caries was linked to the concentration of sugars in food [39].

Awareness of caries prevention strategies was in congruence with the mixed knowledge of caries risks. While one cross sectional study reported that over 95% of dietitians identified strategies for caries prevention such as the use of fluoridated toothpaste [39], others reported that only 'some' (33%) staff identified fluoridated toothpaste as a risk minimization strategy [41] and that 34–39% of dietitians were uncertain on the use of fluoride therapies in young children [43]. Furthermore, 60% of dietitians incorrectly identified that children with healthy dentition could make their first dental visit at age three, even though the American Academy of Pediatric Dentistry advises this should occur from as early as one year of age [39]. Finally, 89% of dietitians correctly identified that addressing dental caries in babies was important even though these are not permanent teeth [41].

Attitudes

Dietitians had mixed feelings regarding their ability to perform oral health screening. More than half of the dietitians in two cross sectional studies (64–67%) reported not feeling confident in their ability to perform oral screening or identifying tooth decay in children [40, 41]. However, in another cross sectional study, within the same population group, the majority (91%) of dietitians reported they were confident in identifying early childhood caries [43].

In general, dietitian attitudes towards providing OHP education to clients was positive. All dietitians reported feeling confident in their ability to provide education to pregnant women and parents about their child's oral health [41, 43]. Specifically, dietitians were confident in discussing the role of oral health related dietary habits [40], providing education to families on child dental care, oral health risks during pregnancy and postpartum dental care, dietary and feeding considerations

for reducing the risk of dental caries and the need for dental referrals [41, 43].

Additionally, dietitians were noted to be 'eager to pass this information (OHP) on to patients' and felt that their clients would find OHP information useful [42]. All dietitians were also confident in referring to dentists where appropriate [41] and were confident (76%) that consumers would take their advice and follow through their referral to dental services [43].

Practice

Most dietitians were providing OHP in their practice. Dietitians were generally found to provide counselling on issues such as toothbrushing and fluoride use (70–87%) [39, 40], the role of sugary snacks and drinks in dental decay (67–100%) [39, 40], bottle feeding before bed (100%) [41] and the impact of 'baby bottle tooth decay' (97%) [39]. Only 11% of dietitians discussed the role of caries transmission between baby and mother [41]. Although inclusion of OHP in practice was noted to be consistent amongst the included cross sectional studies, dietitians highlighted insufficient access to interpreter services for non-English speaking members, time constraints, inappropriate health insurance cover and resource constraints as common barriers for OHP in clinical practice [42, 43].

Ambivalence of performing oral screening was highlighted in their limited application of the skill in practice. The general consensus was that dietitians did not often perform oral health screening with only up to half of them including these assessments in practice [40, 41]. An even smaller percentage of dietitians (33%) attempted to assess women and caregiver dental health [41].

Interestingly, despite dietitian involvement in basic oral health screening and counselling, there were inconsistencies in the practice of making referrals to dentists. Cross sectional studies reported none to nearly all dietitians (96%) providing referrals for dental care/follow up [41–43]. Dietitians who had more years of working experience (> 10 years) were noted to be more likely to provide referrals [40].

Focus area III: current models of oral health care and resources for dietitians

Five articles were identified that met focus area III. As sources specific to populations with ED were not identified, the search was broadened to include general and other populations where dietitians are actively involved in oral health care.

General population

There is evidence to show that dietitians can play an active role in promoting oral health in the general population. An online continuing professional development training program approved by the Academy of Nutrition and Dietetics in the United States assists dietitians to understand the synergistic relationship between oral health and nutrition, the role of nutrition in the integrity of the oral cavity or progression of oral health related disease, and nutritional counselling [44]. The training specifically outlined nutritional deficiencies/risk and their associated oral manifestations, and oral health considerations through the life stages. Additionally, it also identified the existence of dietetic diagnostic terms for oral health, and encourages proficiency and competency in examining the oral cavity for nutritional deficiencies during screening [44]. An additional training module was identified from the United States on how dietitians can screen for oral health issues, refer to dental health professionals and provide education on nutrition for oral health to the general population [48]. The module also identifies 'at risk' populations that would benefit from screening, including populations with an ED, and provides guidance for non-dental health professionals with regard to information required by dental health professionals for making an appropriate and informative referral to dental services.

Aged care

The aged care population is an area where dietitians have been shown to play a role in promoting oral health. Brody et al., investigated the impact of a pilot training program for dietitians performing oral nutrition physical assessments in long term residential aged care facilities in Israel [45]. Dietitians were provided a one-and-a-half-day training program on 'nutrition focused physical assessment'. Dietitians were trained to screen symptoms such as xerostomia (dry mouth), dysgeusia (taste disorder) and pain, extra-oral examination of the face and temporomandibular joint, brief cranial nerve examination, intra-oral examination of mucosa, and signs of micronutrient deficiencies such as lesions. Three to 6 months following training, dietitians were significantly more likely to perform nutrition focused oral physical assessments ($P < 0.001$) and refer to dental health professionals than before training indicating confidence in their ability to perform this role [45].

Chronic disease

Dietitians are also a key contributor in identifying People Living with Human Immunodeficiency Virus (PLHIV) who are at risk for poor oral health. A three-item oral health screening tool for dietitians working with this population has been developed and validated in Australia [46]. Jeganathan et al., validated the tool with PLHIV and found it to have high sensitivity (84%), moderate specificity (55%), and a negative predictive value of 77%.

Dietitians are currently utilizing this tool in practice in a multidisciplinary health centre for HIV management in New South Wales, Australia [47]. The resource titled 'Open your mouth' prompts dietitians and other health professionals to ask clients about their last dental visit, identify the presence of adverse oral health symptoms such as bleeding, provide basic oral health education and a referral pathway for access to dental services [47].

Discussion

The focus of this scoping review was to identify the role of dietitians in promoting oral health among individuals with an ED by reviewing the evidence and recommendations in this area and any existing oral health models of care and resources available to dietitians.

Australian and American position statements identified that dietitians are in an ideal position to provide OHP. However, importantly, they identified that OHP is in keeping with a dietitian's scope of practice, and hence, should be, if not already, integrated in standard practice [37, 38]. The scope of practice detailed in these recommendations are limited to providing oral health education, screening and dental referrals to at-risk populations and does not involve diagnosing dental problems which would infringe on the dental profession. This scope of practice is similar to those recommended for non-dental professionals in other settings like antenatal care and aged care [51, 52]. Although these statements were not specific for ED settings, they did highlight vulnerable populations groups at-risk of poor oral health which included individuals with an ED who would benefit from OHP (See Table 1) [38]. In reviews of practice in ED settings, dietitians perform analysis and risk management of nutritional deficiencies and behaviors. However, notably OHP is often not identified as part of this role [32–34]. In fact, a recent review of clinical treatment manuals for adults with an eating disorder worldwide found less than 10 % contained information about dental health [33]. The recognition of ED as a high risk population in these statements is significant, given that ED related oral health issues including impaired dentition, dental sensitivity, and facial muscle wasting [1] would likely affect treatment outcomes, and consequently, impede ED related recovery [33].

While we acknowledge that both position statements make attempts to provide advice regarding how dietitians should implement OHP into practice, the recommendations have limited details pertaining to the ED population (see Table 1) [37, 38]. The paucity of research in this area may have contributed to the lack of clinical practice guidelines which are often developed from high quality evidence [53].

In saying this, although the profession of dietetics has experienced significant growth and development on a professional and global scale since establishment of the Academy of Nutrition and Dietetics in 1917 [54, 55] the role of the dietitian/nutritionist will continue to evolve as the understanding of the scope of practice of dietitians advances [56]. The present lack of OHP guidance for dietitians in these reviews of practice could lead to the postulation that OHP may not currently be seen as a priority or may be considered a novel area of practice. With this in mind, and the scant availability of research showcasing dietetic involvement in oral health, may provide possible insight into why current recommendations for dietetic management of ED fails to include the dietitian's role in OHP [32–34].

Although no studies that reviewed dietitians providing OHP to individuals with an ED were identified, studies that reviewed OHP across other clinical areas highlighted superficial knowledge of oral health issues, risk factors, and prevention strategies [39–42]. Likely commencing with insufficient oral health education for dietitians at a tertiary level [57] and following through with limited training for professional development [58], it may be conceived that even though these position statements with recommendations are available, they have not translated into dietetic practice. By means of addressing this gap in dietetics, both position statements call for the inclusion of 'didactic' education models that demonstrate the role of the dietitian in OHP in tertiary education [37, 38]. This is however not unique to dietitians, but a finding that was shared amongst other non-dental health professionals as a salient barrier to OHP [59–62].

Despite this challenge, some dietitians still felt they were capable of including OHP in their practice [39–43]. This notion of proactivity by dietitians in light of their varying oral health knowledge [39–43] is similar to that shown by other non-dental health professionals. Research reviewing this emerging role in diabetes educators [63], child and family health nurses [61], antenatal care providers including midwives and obstetricians/gynecologists, general practitioners [60, 64], and nursing and carer staff in residential aged care facilities [65, 66] emphasize that non-dental health professionals felt promoting oral health amongst their key population groups was essential in achieving health care goals and part of their scope of practice [60, 61, 63, 64].

The identification of some dietitians already incorporating OHP in their practice was a promising finding. It showcases the skills and capability of dietitians in providing oral health screening, education and referrals to dental services in vulnerable populations [39–42]. However, this should be considered within the context that the general scarcity of evidence could be as a result of clinician hesitance due to inadequate guidelines informing practice, varying confidence in their knowledge and

skills on the subject matter, and availability/awareness of referral pathways. The establishment of a model of care can assist in informing implementation into an ED clinical setting and hence, may be considered part of a potential solution [67]. In previous models of care we can see that when dietitians are supported they are capable of delivering OHP to WIC populations [68], children in low income communities [69], an ethnic minority group with diabetes [42] and a population with HIV [46]. Similarly, in studies where child and family health nurses and midwives had a model of care for oral health in practice [61, 64], clinicians confidently and competently were able to include oral health screening and referral in practice.

The most consistent barrier to OHP as identified in this review was the limited availability of professional development materials, both generally and specifically for OHP in ED clinical settings. This is synonymous with other studies involving non-dental health professionals who have also been reported to experience a lack of resources for both the client and health professional [59–62, 64, 66]. Support in the form of training for health professionals in OHP has resulted in improved knowledge and confidence, and clinicians were more likely to incorporate OHP in their practice [64, 70]. Further, these results indicate that involvement by non-dental health professionals allowed for timely intervention and captured 'at risk' populations that otherwise may not immediately engage in dental health services due to cost, accessibility, dental anxiety and importantly, the individual's perception of need for regular dental assessment [24, 71].

In saying this, the development and inclusion of resources for dietitians for OHP in ED clinical settings may not be enough to meet the needs of these health professionals. It is recognized that individuals with a mental health condition may not see oral health as a significant health issue due to more pressing health concerns or due to compromised mental health status [24, 72]. In addition to dietetic input, further consideration of client perceptions to receiving dietitian led oral health promotion and client centered challenges, such as client accessibility and affordability of dental services [22–24], access to appropriate resources and referral pathways for clinicians [73], and the support of dental health professionals in this shared role [37, 38, 73], will all need to be addressed in order for this to be a sustainable and successful early intervention model.

Lastly, it is important to point out that current evidence around the evaluation of oral health models of care involving dietians mainly focus on clinician outcomes in terms of their knowledge, attitude and practices in this area. Curently there is no data to show the benefit of dietitians undertaking oral health promotion on patients' outcomes nor the acceptability of such interventions by individuals.

This is an area that needs further investigation in future studies particularly as capacity building non-dental professionals to promote oral health has been shown to be effective in improving the health outcomes of patients in other settings, including maternal and infant care and aged care [74–76]. For example, the rollout out of a midwifery initiated oral health (MIOH) program in Australia has resulted in a significant improvement in the oral health status and quality of life of pregnant women and was found to be acceptable and feasible to implement into antenatal care practice.

This review is not without limitations. As only articles published in the English language were included, our findings may not be representative of all available literature on this topic. With regard to the included articles, studies were predominantly conducted in the United States, and a modest number of dietitians participated in those studies, limiting the generalizability of results across other countries or regions where the scope of practice and training of dietitians may differ. In light of this novel practice for dietitians, there was no data available on the effectiveness of dietitian initiated oral health promotion on patient outcomes. Further, this review included grey literature which is not peer-reviewed and therefore, the quality of some of the findings may be poor. Nevertheless, due to the limited number of peer reviewed articles on the topic area, the inclusion of grey literature enabled the review to be as exhaustive and comprehensive as it could be.

Conclusion

Dietitians are in a pivotal position to provide preemptive education and screening of oral health and there are examples where dietitians are successfully undertaking this role across various settings. However, this is still an underdeveloped area of dietetics in the ED clinical area. Further research is needed to explore how to support dietitians to promote oral health among the ED populations including any training and screening resources that may enhance their role as well as the effectiveness of these strategies on patient outcomes. It is equally important that future research attempts to understand and evaluate challenges that not only ED patients but any patient seen by a dietitian may encounter in terms of oral health care including their acceptability of dietitian led oral health promotion and accessibility and affordability of dental services.

Abbreviations
ED: Eating disorders; DA: Dietitians Australia; DHSV: Dental Health Services Victoria; HIV: Human Immunodeficiency Virus; KAP: Knowledge Attitudes Practices; MESH: Medical Subject Headings; OHP: Oral Health Promotion; PLHIV: People Living with Human Immunodeficiency Virus; WIC: Women infants and children

Authors' contributions
AG and TPN were involved in the conception of the review and search strategy development. MSS and TPN screened and reviewed articles for eligibility for inclusion. All authors (TPN, LR, MSS, LS and AG) made significant contribution to the final manuscript, were involved in the interpretation of data and reviewed the manuscript for intellectual content. All authors have reviewed and accepted the final manuscript. The authors read and approved the final manuscript.

Competing interests
the authors declare that they have no competing interests.

Author details
Centre for Oral Health Outcomes & Research Translation (COHORT), School of Nursing and Midwifery , Western Sydney University/South Western Sydney Local Health District/ Ingham Institute for Applied Medical Research, Liverpool BC, Locked Bag 7103, Sydney, NSW 1871, Australia. ²School of Nursing and Midwifery, Western Sydney University, Centre for Oral Health Outcomes & Research Translation (COHORT), Sydney, Australia. ³IMPACCT, Faculty of Health, University of Technology Sydney, Sydney, Australia. ⁴Sydney Dental Hospital, Oral Health Services, SLHD, Sydney, Australia. Centre for Oral Health Outcomes & Research Translation (COHORT), Western Sydney University/South Western Sydney Local Health District/University of Sydney/ Ingham Institute for Applied Medical Research, Sydney, Australia.

References
1. Aranha A, Eduardo CDP, Cordás TA. Eating disorders. Part I: psychiatric diagnosis and dental implications. J Contemp Dent Pract. 2008;9(6):73–81.
2. Keski-Rahkonen A, Raevuori A, Hoek HW. Epidemiology of eating disorders: an update. Annual Review of Eating Disorders. Boca Raton: CRC Press; 2018. p. 66–76.
3. Nielsen S. Epidemiology and mortality of eating disorders. Psychiatr Clin N Am. 2001;24(2):201–14.
4. McManus S, Meltzer H, Brugha T, Bebbington P, Jenkins R. Adult psychiatric morbidity survey, 2007, vol. 30. Leeds: Health and Social Care Information Centre downloaded on; 2014.
5. National Eating Disorders Collaboration. Eating Disorders in Australia Canberra: Australians Government, Department of Health; 2016. Available from: http://www.nedc.com.au/eating-disorders-in-australia.
6. Hudson JI, Hiripi E, Pope HG, Kessler RC. The prevalence and correlates of eating disorders in the National Comorbidity Survey Replication. Biol Psychiatry. 2007;61(3):348–58.
7. Le Grange D, Swanson SA, Crow SJ, Merikangas KR. Eating disorder not otherwise specified presentation in the US population. Int J Eat Disord. 2012;45(5):711–8.
8. Wade TD, Bergin JL, Tiggemann M, Bulik CM, Fairburn CG. Prevalence and long-term course of lifetime eating disorders in an adult Australian twin cohort. Aust N Z J Psychiatry. 2006;40(2):121–8.
9. Hay P, Girosi F, Mond J. Prevalence and sociodemographic correlates of DSM-5 eating disorders in the Australian population. J Eat Disord. 2015;3(1): 19.

10. Australian Institute of Health and Welfare. In: Welfare AIoHa, editor. Australia's Health 2018. Canberra, ACT: Australian Federal Government; 2018. p. 1–3.

11. Hay P, Mitchison D, Collado AEL, González-Chica DA, Stocks N, Touyz S. Burden and health-related quality of life of eating disorders, including avoidant/restrictive food intake disorder (ARFID), in the Australian population. J Eat Disord. 2017;5(1):21.

12. Westmoreland P, Krantz MJ, Mehler PS. Medical complications of anorexia nervosa and bulimia. Am J Med. 2016;129(1):30–7.

13. Butterfly Foundation. Paying the price: the economic and social impact of eating disorders in Australia. Canberra; 2012. Available from: https://thebutterflyfoundation.org.au/assets/Uploads/Butterfly-report-Paying-the-Price-Executive-Summary.pdf.

14. Clark DB. Patients with eating disorders: Challenges for the oral health professional. Can J Dent Hyg. 2010;44(4):163–74.

15. Kantovitz KR, Pascon FM, Rontani RMP, Gaviao MBD, Pascon FM. Obesity and dental caries--A systematic review. Oral Health Prev Dent. 2006;4(2):137–44.

16. Hooley M, Skouteris H, Boganin C, Satur J, Kilpatrick N. Body mass index and dental caries in children and adolescents: a systematic review of literature published 2004 to 2011. Syst Rev. 2012;1(1):57.

17. Kisely S, Baghaie H, Lalloo R, Johnson NW. Association between poor oral health and eating disorders: systematic review and meta-analysis. Br J Psychiatry. 2015;207(4):299–305.

18. Hermont AP, Oliveira PA, Martins CC, Paiva SM, Pordeus IA, Auad SM. Tooth erosion and eating disorders: a systematic review and meta-analysis. PLoS One. 2014;9(11):e111123.

19. Locker D, Liddell A, Dempster L, Shapiro D. Age of onset of dental anxiety. J Dent Res. 1999;78(3):790–6.

20. Cash TF, Deagle EA. The nature and extent of body-image disturbances in anorexia nervosa and bulimia nervosa: a meta-analysis. Int J Eat Disord. 1997;22(2):107–26.

21. Derenne JL, Beresin EV. Body image, media, and eating disorders. Acad Psychiatry. 2006;30(3):257–61.

22. Wallace B, MacEntee MI. Access to dental care for low-income adults: perceptions of affordability, availability and acceptability. J Community Health. 2012;37(1):32–9.

23. Wallace B, Browne A, Varcoe C, Ford-Gilboe M, Wathen N, Long P, et al. Self-reported oral health among a community sample of people experiencing social and health inequities: cross-sectional findings from a study to enhance equity in primary healthcare settings. BMJ Open. 2015;5(12):e009519.

24. Slack-Smith L, Hearn L, Scrine C, Durey A. Barriers and enablers for oral health care for people affected by mental health disorders. Aust Dent J. 2017;62(1):6–13.

25. Scully CC. Drug effects on salivary glands: dry mouth. Oral Dis. 2003;9(4):165–76.

26. Marvanova M, Gramith K. Role of antidepressants in the treatment of adults with anorexia nervosa. Ment Health Clin. 2018;8(3):127–37.

27. Dynesen AW, Gehrt CA, Klinker SE, Christensen LB. Eating disorders: experiences of and attitudes toward oral health and oral health behavior. Eur J Oral Sci. 2018;126(6):500–6.

28. Silverstein LS, Haggerty C, Sams L, Phillips C, Roberts MW. Impact of an oral health education intervention among a group of patients with eating disorders (anorexia nervosa and bulimia nervosa). J Eat Disord. 2019;7(1):29.

29. Yacoub A, Karmally W. Nutrition in Oral Health. Nutrition in Lifestyle Medicine. Switzerland: Springer; 2017. p. 193–209.

30. Lifante-Oliva C, López-Jornet P, Camacho-Alonso F, Esteve-Salinas J. Study of oral changes in patients with eating disorders. Int J Dent Hyg. 2008;6(2):119–22.

31. Bapat S, Asawa K, Bhat N, Tak M, Gupta VV, Chaturvedi P, et al. Assessment of dental nutrition knowledge among nutrition/dietetics students. J Clin Diagn Res. 2016;10(11):ZC37.

32. O'Connor G, Oliver A, Corbett J, Fuller S. Developing clinical guidelines for dietitians treating young people with anorexia nervosa-family focused approach working alongside family therapists. Ann Nutr Disord Ther. 2019;6(1):1056.

33. McMaster CM, Wade T, Franklin J, Hart S. A review of treatment manuals for adults with an eating disorder: nutrition content and consistency with current dietetic evidence. Eat Weight Disord Stud Anorexia Bulimia Obes. 2020. p. 1–14. https://doi.org/10.1007/s40519-020-00850-6.

34. McMaster CM, Wade T, Franklin J, Hart S. Development of consensus-based guidelines for outpatient dietetic treatment of eating disorders: a Delphi study. Int J Eat Disord. 2020;53(9):1480–95.

35. Dietitians Association of Australia. Dietitian or Nutritionist? Canberra, ACT: DAA; 2015. Available from: https://daa.asn.au/what-dietitans-do/dietitian-or-nutritionist/.

36. Arksey H, O'Malley L. Scoping studies: towards a methodological framework. Int J Soc Res Methodol. 2005;8(1):19–32.

37. Touger-Decker R, Mobley C. Position of the academy of nutrition and dietetics: oral health and nutrition. J Acad Nutr Diet. 2013;113(5):693–701.

38. Dietitians Association of Australia (DAA) DHSVD. Joint position statement on oral health and nutrition. Canberra: Dietetics Association of Australia, Dental Health Services Victoria; 2015. p. 32.

39. Faine MP, Oberg D. Survey of dental nutrition knowledge of wig nutritionists and public health dental hygienists. J Am Diet Assoc. 1995;95(2):190–4.

40. Fuller LA, Stull SC, Darby ML, Tolle SL. Oral health promotion: knowledge, confidence, and practices in preventing early-severe childhood caries of Virginia WIC program personnel. Am Dent Hyg Assoc. 2014;88(2):130–40.

41. Gold JT, Tomar S. Oral health knowledge and practices of WIC staff at Florida WIC program. J Community Health. 2016;41(3):612–8.

42. Koerber A, Peters KE, Kaste LM, Lopez E, Noorullah K, Torres I, et al. The views of dentists, nurses and nutritionists on the association between diabetes and periodontal disease: a qualitative study in a Latino community. J Public Health Dent. 2006;66(3):212–5.

43. Shick EA, Lee JY, Rozier RG. Determinants of dental referral practices among WIC nutritionists in North Carolina. J Public Health Dent. 2005;65(4):196–202.

44. Karmally W. Nutrition and Oral health: what dietitians should know. Nutri-Bites Webinar Series. Chicago: ConAgra Foods Science Institute; 2014.

45. Brody RA, Touger-Decker R, Radler DR, Parrott JS, Rachman SE, Trostler N. A novel approach to Oral health assessment training for dietitians in Long-term care settings in Israel: a pilot study of changes in knowledge and practice. Top Clin Nutr. 2014;29(1):57–68.

46. Jeganathan S, Purnomo J, Houtzager L, Batterham M, Begley K. Development and validation of a three-item questionnaire for dietitians to screen for poor oral health in people living with human immunodeficiency virus and facilitate dental referral. Nutr Diet. 2010;67(3):177–81.

47. The Albion Centre. Nutrition, Oral Health and HIV. Australia: The Albion Centre; 2018. Available from: http://thealbioncentre.org.au/clinical-services/nutrition/.

48. Pac West MCH distance learning network. Module 5 Screening and referral for nutrition related oral health problems. Washington: University of Washington; 2005. Available from: http://depts.washington.edu/pwdlearn/oralhealth/pdfs/mod5print.pdf.

49. Oral Health Promotion Working Group. In: Centre A, editor. Open your mouth: NSW Health; 2013.

50. Chalmers J, King P, Spencer A, Wright F, Carter K. The oral health assessment tool—validity and reliability. Aust Dent J. 2005;50(3):191–9.

51. Fricker A, Lewis A. Better oral health in residential care: final report. Adelaide: Central Northern Adelaide Health Service, South Australian Dental Service; 2009.

52. Workgroup OHCDPE. Oral health care during pregnancy: a national consensus statement. Washington, DC: National Maternal and Child Oral Health Resource Center; 2012.

53. Australian Nursing & Midwifery Federation (ANMF). Definitions of policies, position statements, guidelines, issues papers and fact sheets: Australian Nursing & Midwifery Federation (ANMF); 2014. Available from: anmf.org.au/documents/policies/definitions.

54. Academy of Nutrition and Dietetics. Eatright-About us 2018. Available from: https://www.eatrightpro.org/about-us.

55. Shen X, Tang W, Yu Z, Cai W. The history and development of registered dietitian accreditation systems in China and other comparable countries. Nutr Res. 2019;70:11–7.

56. International Confederation of Dietetic Associations (ICDA). Dietitian-Nutritionists around the world: Their education and their work 2016.

57. Scardina G, Messina P. Good oral health and diet. Biomed Res Int. 2012;2012:1–10.

58. Johnson L, Boyd L, Rainchuso L, Rothman A, Mayer B. Eating disorder professionals' perceptions of oral health knowledge. Int J Dent Hyg. 2017; 15(3):164–71.

59. Poudel P, Griffiths R, Wong VW, Arora A, Flack JR, Khoo CL, et al. Perceptions and practices of general practitioners on providing oral health care to people with diabetes-a qualitative study. BMC Fam Pract. 2020;21(1):1–11.

60. George A, Dahlen HG, Reath J, Ajwani S, Bhole S, Korda A, et al. What do antenatal care providers understand and do about oral health care during pregnancy: a cross-sectional survey in New South Wales, Australia. BMC Pregnancy Childbirth. 2016;16(1):382.

61. Veale M, Ajwani S, Johnson M, Nash L, Patterson T, George A. The early childhood oral health program: a qualitative study of the perceptions of child and family health nurses in South Western Sydney, Australia. BMC Oral Health. 2016;16(1):56.

62. Barnett T, Hoang H, Stuart J, Crocombe L, Bell E. Utilisation of oral health services provided by non-dental health practitioners in developed countries: a review of the literature. Community Dent Health. 2014;31(4):224–33.

63. Poudel P, Griffiths R, Wong VW, Arora A, Flack JR, Khoo CL, et al. Perceptions and practices of diabetes educators in providing oral health care: a qualitative study. Diabetes Educ. 2018;44(5):454–64.

64. Dahlen HG, Johnson M, Hoolsema J, Norrie TP, Ajwani S, Blinkhorn A, et al. Process evaluation of the midwifery initiated oral health-dental service program: perceptions of midwives in greater Western Sydney, Australia. Women Birth. 2019;32(2):e159–e65.

65. Hoad-Reddick G. A study to determine oral health needs of institutionalised elderly patients by non dental health care workers. Community Dent Oral Epidemiol. 1991;19(4):233–6.

66. Chalmers JM, Pearson A. A systematic review of oral health assessment by nurses and carers for residents with dementia in residential care facilities. Special Care Dent. 2005;25(5):227–33.

67. Agency for Clinical Innovation (ACI). A practical guide on how to develop a Model of Care at the Agency for Clinical Innovation. Chatswood; 2013.

68. Taylor E, Marino D, Thacker S, DiMarco M, Huff M, Biordi D. Expanding oral health preventative services for young children: a successful interprofessional model. J Allied Health. 2014;43(1):5E–9E.

69. Biordi DL, Heitzer M, Mundy E, DiMarco M, Thacker S, Taylor E, et al. Improving access and provision of preventive oral health care for very young, poor, and low-income children through a new interdisciplinary partnership. Am J Public Health. 2015;105(S2):e23–e9.

70. Heilbrunn-Lang AY, De Silva AM, Lang G, George A, Ridge A, Johnson M, et al. Midwives' perspectives of their ability to promote the oral health of pregnant women in Victoria, Australia. BMC Pregnancy Childbirth. 2015; 15(1):110.

71. Freeman R. The psychology of dental patient care: barriers to accessing dental care: patient factor. Br Dent J. 1999;187(3):141.

72. BSDH Bsfdaoh. Oral health care for people with mental health problems: guidelines and recommendations. United Kingdom: British Society for Disability and Oral Health; 2000.

73. Marshall R, Spencer A. Accessing oral health care in Australia; 2006.

74. Nyongesa NN. Implementing an evidence-based oral health assessment tool (OHAT) in a nursing home. North Dakota: North Dakota State University; 2013.

75. Maher L, Phelan C, Lawrence G, Dawson A, Torvaldsen S, Wright C. The early childhood Oral health program: promoting prevention and timely intervention of early childhood caries in NSW through shared care. Health Promot J Aust. 2012;23(3):171–6.

76. George A, Sousa MS, Kong AC, Blinkhorn A, Norrie TP, Foster J, et al. Effectiveness of preventive dental programs offered to mothers by non-dental professionals to control early childhood dental caries: a review. BMC Oral Health. 2019;19(1):172.

17

Reduction in depressive symptoms predicts improvement in eating disorder symptoms in interpersonal psychotherapy: results from a naturalistic study

Malin Bäck[1,2]* ⓘ, Fredrik Falkenström[1], Sanna Aila Gustafsson[3], Gerhard Andersson[1,4] and Rolf Holmqvist[1]

Abstract

Background: Interpersonal psychotherapy (IPT) can be effective for both Bulimia Nervosa (BN) and co-occurring depression. While changes in symptoms of Eating disorder (ED) and depression have been found to correlate, it is unclear how they interact during treatment and in which order the symptoms decrease.

Methods: Thirty-one patients with BN and depressive symptoms received IPT using the manual IPT-BNm in a naturalistic design. The outcome was measured with the Eating Disorder Examination Questionnaire (EDE-Q) and the Montgomery Åsberg Depression Rating Scale (MADRS-S). Symptom improvement at each session was measured with Repeated Evaluation of Eating Disorder Symptoms (REDS) and the Patient Health Questionnaire-9 (PHQ-9).

Results: Significant improvements with large effect sizes were found on both ED symptoms and depression. The rates of change were linear for both BN and depression. A strong correlation between reduction of depressive symptoms and ED symptoms was found. Depressive symptom reduction at one session predicted improvement of ED symptoms at the next session.

Conclusions: IPT-BNm had an effect on both BN and co-occurring depressive symptoms. The analyses indicated that reduction in depressive symptoms preceded reduction in bulimic symptoms.

Keywords: IPT, Interpersonal psychotherapy, Bulimia nervosa, IPT-BN, IPT-BNm

Plain English summary

Interpersonal Psychotherapy (IPT) is an effective treatment for major depression and eating disorders. In this study, 31 patients suffering from Bulimia nervosa (BN) and co-occurring depression received 16 weeks of IPT. In the therapy, bulimic symptoms were linked to ongoing interpersonal events. The therapy is based on the assumption that if patients' interpersonal stress is reduced, if they receive social support, process their feelings, and improve interpersonal skills; their eating disorder symptoms will decrease. The results in our study showed that the treatment was effective for symptoms of BN and depression. The average rate of change was linear. Even though early response was associated with favourable treatment outcome, the effect took place continuously during the whole treatment, indicating that there were different paths to recovery. Symptom improvement in BN and depression was strongly correlated. Reductions of depressive symptoms at one session

* Correspondence: relatera@me.com; malin.back@rjl.se
[1]Department of Behavioural Sciences and Learning, Linköping University, Linköping, Sweden
[2]Futurum: Academy for Health and Care, Jönköping, Region Jönköping County, Sweden
Full list of author information is available at the end of the article

were correlated with a reduction in eating disorder symptoms at the next session. As comorbid depression is common in eating disorders (ED) and may jeopardize the ED treatment, this is an urgent topic and further research is needed to validate the findings of this study.

Background

Patients with Bulimia Nervosa (BN) often have recurrent relapses and a life-long vulnerability for eating disorder (ED) behaviour. Even with recommended treatments, only about half of the patients recover [1, 2]. One factor that may complicate treatment of BN and has a negative effect on the outcome is the high co-morbidity with depression [3]. The association between depression and ED symptoms can be intricate, with depression initiating eating problems for some patients and eating problems initiating or worsening a depression for others. Often, the relationship is best described as a vicious circle between these symptoms. A meta-analysis on the longitudinal relationship between ED-pathology and depression showed a bi-directional relationship, indicating that depression and ED affect each other, and that they might be influenced by shared risk factors [4]. In the light of these findings the next important step is to understand how the two conditions influence each other during ED-treatment. Cognitive Behavioural Therapy (CBT) is the primary recommended psychological treatment for patients with BN and binge eating disorder (BED) [5]. In the most studied form of CBT treatment for bulimia [6], it is recommended that co-occurring depression should be treated before focusing on ED [6, 7], given that mood intolerance as well as interpersonal difficulties, low self-esteem and perfectionism may be maintaining processes that inhibit ED treatment [6]. Interpersonal psychotherapy (IPT) has been suggested as a valuable treatment option for patients with BN or BED, as IPT focuses particularly on such problems as mood and interpersonal stress [6, 8, 9].

In a previous study using an IPT manual for depression, the authors examined the effect of IPT on ED with co-morbid major depression and found significant improvements with large effect sizes on both ED and depression measures [10]. Symptom reductions for the two diagnoses were strongly correlated, which indicate that the mechanisms of change in IPT for depressive symptoms may also work on ED symptoms or that change in one syndrome promotes change in the other. There is limited research on whether improvement in depression during psychological treatment precedes improvement in ED symptoms, or if it is the other way around with improvement in ED symptom preceding improvement in depression.

IPT was created as a treatment for depression and has also shown positive results for other mental disorders, such as social anxiety disorder, post-traumatic stress disorder (PTSD) and ED [11–13]. In ED research, IPT was first used as a control treatment for CBT in a randomised controlled trial on individuals with BN [14]. In this trial, Fairburn et al. (1991) used an IPT-manual that was not specifically adapted for BN. Beyond initial psychoeducation; eating problems were not addressed during the treatment. However, as the IPT treatment showed positive results, a manual called IPT-BN was created [15]. Using this manual, positive results have been attained in both individual and group settings for patients with full or sub-threshold BN and BED [7]. In comparison with CBT, IPT seems to have a delayed effect on ED-symptoms. Long-term follow-up studies have shown that patients who have been treated with IPT continue to improve after treatment [8, 9, 16]. IPT focuses on current interpersonal stressors associated with ED symptoms [7, 17]. The interventions in IPT promote interpersonal problem solving, emotional processing and practicing communication of need of social support [7, 18], which can help patients improve their interpersonal life and may have a positive effect on their self-image [7]. This is supposed to lead to improvements in ED-symptoms secondary to relational improvements. The fact that IPT only indirectly focuses on behavioural change may lead to slower changes in eating behaviours [19].

A central component in IPT is the explicit exploratory linking between current symptoms and relational issues [20, 21]. However, the original IPT-BN manual did not include this central aspect of IPT [7, 9]. There was also no monitoring of ED symptoms after the initial sessions, as is usually the case in IPT (see below and under Method section). Techniques such as problem solving were not used. This has been proposed as another explanation for the delayed treatment response in IPT-BN compared to CBT [22]. In order to improve IPT for BN, a manual was created where the ED problems were in focus by including original components of IPT such as psychoeducation, weekly evaluation of current symptoms (in this case eating problems), directive techniques, problem solving, modelling and role play [23]. In this modified version of IPT-BN (IPT-BNm; Wight et al., 2011 [23], ED symptoms are viewed as interpersonal markers that are monitored and discussed during each session. For instance; if the therapist and patient note that the patient has deviated from the intended schedule of food and exercise, or if the patient reports changes in frequency of binge eating or vomiting, the therapist encourages exploration of potentially emotionally stressful interpersonal events that may have preceded change in ED symptoms. In a deepened cyclic process, explicit conceptualisations of associations between ED symptoms and interpersonal events are being made. The aim is to facilitate awareness, hope and resolutions in the chosen interpersonal focus area [18].

Two studies have shown initial support for this treatment [24, 25]. An open trial by Arcelus including 59 patients with BN found significant reductions in ED symptoms at the end of treatment [25]. The three-month follow-up found that the symptom reduction had continued. The patients also suffered from co-morbid moderate depression, which improved significantly during treatment [25].

In many psychotherapies, rapid symptom reduction predicts final treatment response [26]. The preliminary results of IPT-BNm showed a more rapid response [25] compared to earlier studies of IPT-BN by Agras [8]. By the middle of therapy (session 8), the patients had made significant improvements in terms of ED and depressive symptoms [25]. Furthermore Arcelus et al. compared a brief form of IPT-BNm with 10 sessions (IPT-BN10) with IPT-BNm (16 sessions) and a waiting-list control group in a small-randomised trial including 30 patients. Significant differences were found for patients treated with IPT-BN10 and the waiting-list control. No significant differences were found on any of the EDE-Q scales when comparing IPT-BN10 and IPT-BNm. The authors suggested that IPT-BN10 may work faster than previous research on IPT-BN has shown and that IPT also can be delivered in a briefer format [24].

The primary aim of this study was to evaluate the effectiveness of IPT-BNm by Whight et. al [23]. on ED symptoms and depressive symptoms in a Swedish treatment context. In addition, we also analysed a) whether early improvement in ED symptoms and/or depressive symptoms predicted better outcome, and b) whether change in ED symptoms preceded change in depressive symptoms or vice versa.

Methods

Thirty-one bulimic patients were included in this naturalistic study, which was performed in conjunction with an implementation project by the Swedish Eating Disorder Register (SwEat) in IPT-BNm. The data collection was conducted at seven outpatient psychiatric services specialising in ED treatment in Sweden. The patients received ED focused IPT with an explicit focus on the links between interpersonal issues and ED symptoms, according to the manual IPT-BNm (23, 24, 25,). Therapy sessions were videotaped, and the supervisor rated at least three sessions in every therapy for competence and adherence. According to the adherence rating procedure (supervisor ratings), the therapists conducted IPT-BNm in an adherent and competent way [20]. The Ethics Review Board in Örebro/Uppsala approved the study 2012-12-05, registration number; 2012/471. Written informed consent was obtained from all participants.

Participants
Patients
Inclusion criteria were age 16–50 years and meeting the DSM-IV criteria for Bulimia nervosa [27]. The frequency and duration criteria were not used. Exclusion criteria were a body mass index (BMI) lower than 17.5, other on-going psychological treatment and/or inpatient care, a need for intense medical treatment or drug abuse. Thirty-one bulimic patients with co- occurring depressive symptoms were included in the study. The patients were recruited at outpatient services where the therapists worked. All 31 patients completed the treatment. They were all women, in the age between 19 and 50 years. Patients were initially assessed at the ED services according to the routine by SwEat (SEDI and EDE) [28], which was complemented with a clinical interview made by the therapist in a pre-treatment assessment session. This assessment session was part of the treatment protocol of the study, called *session zero* and it included, among other items, questions based on the DSM-IV [27], the self-assessment instruments EDE-Q and REDS. Even if co-morbid depression was not an inclusion criterion, the patients were also assessed for co-occurring depressive symptoms based on the MADRS-S and PHQ-9. The patients were diagnosed with Bulimia nervosa [27]. They also presented a mild or moderate depressive psychopathology. For most of the patients, this was their first BN treatment. However, according to the medical records, five of the patients had had a former assessment more than 6 months earlier, so they may have received treatment-related information/psychoeducation earlier.

Therapists
Seventeen therapists participated in the study. Nine therapists had one patient and eight therapists had two to four patients. The data collection was conducted during the years 2013–2016, and was made in conjunction with an IPT-project by SwEat which had the aim to teach therapists IPT-BNm [22, 23]. The therapists received weekly internet-based group supervision by accredited IPT-supervisors. All 17 therapists were experienced ED therapists before starting the IPT training but had not conducted IPT therapies focusing on ED symptoms using IPT-BNm. All had completed at least one previous IPT-therapy with a depression focus for a patient with co-occurring ED [20, 21]. One third of the therapists had previous training in CBT, one third had training in psychodynamic therapy and one third had an integrative training. Ten therapists were clinical psychologists, three were social workers, three were occupational therapists, two were nurses, and one auxiliary psychiatric nurse. Therapists were between 31 and 61 years old and had between 2- and 16-years' experience of psychotherapeutic work. Among those therapists who collected data in more than one IPT-therapy, they all had the opportunity to receive regular supervision and had support from their managers and workplaces to work with IPT and make preparations for data collection and supervision.

Description of the treatment IPT-BNm

Interpersonal psychotherapy for Bulimia nervosa modified version, IPT-BNm, consists of 12–16 weekly sessions of 45 min duration. The initial four sessions cover a detailed assessment and review of the patient's ED symptomatology, linking to the interpersonal context and how that maintains the ED. The initial phase also provides psychoeducation regarding patients' ED and associated symptomatology. A timeline of symptoms and life events is also completed along with an interpersonal inventory. In collaboration between patient and therapist, an interpersonal focus area is chosen that will form the basis of the work of the treatment phase. IPT recognizes four focus areas: interpersonal dispute, interpersonal role transition, complicated grief and interpersonal deficit/sensitivity. The treatment phase consists of discussing the relationship between the interpersonal focus area and current ED symptoms. ED symptoms are tracked during each session. Specific techniques used during these sessions include: communication analysis, role-play, clarification, exploration and encouragement of affect, use of the therapeutic relationship and behavioural change techniques; such as decision analysis and problem solving. In the final two sessions explicit discussion of the ending of therapy takes place as well as contingency planning for the future and a reflection on the interpersonal skills learned during therapy [23].

Outcome measures

The Eating Disorder Examination Questionnaire (EDE-Q) is a widely used self-report measure of ED psychopathology [29, 30], derived from the EDE- interview [31], and has satisfactory validity and reliability [32, 33]. In addition to a total score, the EDE-Q generates four subscales; Restraint, Eating Concern, Shape Concern and Weight concern. Clinical norms for a female Swedish bulimic population have suggested cut off as following scores; Restraint: M = 2.9 (SD = 1.1), Eating Concern: M = 2.9 (SD = 0.9), Shape concern: M = 4.4 (SD = 1.3), Weight Concern: M = 3.4 (SD = 1.6), and finally EDE-Q total: M = 3.4 (SD = 1.0) [34]. EDE-Q was administered at the first, eighth and last session.

The *Montgomery Åsberg Depression Rating Scale* (MADRS-S) is the self-rated version of MADRS, especially developed to be sensitive to changes in depression severity [35]. The MADRS-S consists of nine items corresponding to the nine DSM-IV major depression criteria. By MADRS-S standards, 13–19 points indicate mild depression, 20–34 moderate depression, and more than 34 points severe depression [36]. The instrument, which has good reliability and validity [35], was administered at the first, the eighth and the last session.

The *Repeated Evaluation of Eating Disorder Symptoms* (REDS) is a self-rating questionnaire, which measures

the most common ED-symptoms [37]. The 14 REDS items comprise thoughts and ideas about food, impulses, weight and body image. The patient gives responses on a 5-point scale ranging from 'never' to 'very often' and indicates how often he/she has experienced each symptom during the past week. The REDS has demonstrated good reliability and validity in a Swedish study [37]. The cut-off between clinical and non-clinical populations is 22 points. In this study, REDS was used weekly to measure symptom changes. The REDS was completed before each session.

The *Patient Health Questionnaire-9 (*PHQ-9) consists of questions corresponding to the nine DSM-IV major depression criteria [38]. The PHQ-9, a validated and reliable instrument, has proved suitable for screening as well as repeated measurements. The cut-off limits for symptom severity are: 0–4 none/minimal depression, 5–9 mild depression, 10–14 moderate depression, 15–19 intermediate depression and 20–27 severe depression [39–41]. A cut-off score of 10 points has been suggested for differentiating clinical from non-clinical individuals [42, 43]. This study used the PHQ-9 to measure weekly symptom changes and was completed before each session.

Data analysis

Paired samples *t*-tests were used to compare the start and end values. Effect sizes were calculated as within-group Cohen's *d*. If patients completed their treatment before the sixteenth session, last observation carried forward (LOCF) was used for the final PHQ-9 and REDS scores. Reliable change was assessed using the Reliable Change Index (RCI) [44]. The RCI indicates whether the symptom change exceeds measurement error. Jacobson and Truax's third definition was used to determine the RCI with Cronbach's alpha used as estimation of the reliability [45]. Seven points on the REDS and five points on the PHQ-9 were found to be RCI limits by this method. The cut-off for clinical significance (CS) was 10 on the PHQ-9 and 22 on the REDS. Patients who improved more than the RCI limits and also scored below the CS cut-off after treatment were considered to have attained a reliable, clinically significant change and were considered *remitted* [44], while patients with reliable change who did not reach the CS level were classified as *improved*. Patients whose symptoms increased more than the RCI limit were labelled *deteriorated*, and the remaining patients were labelled *unchanged*. The significance of early response was tested by regression analyses and by testing correlations between early and final responders. Patients who had reached a reliable symptom change at session four (REDS with seven or more point and on PHQ-9 with five or more points) were considered as early responders. Session four was targeted based on that the interpersonal focus area in IPT should be formulated in this session and is the final session in the initial phase [21]. Final responders were also defined of reliable symptom change (RCI). Pearson correlations were used to examine associations between outcome scores for eating disorder (REDS) and depression (PHQ-9). Within-patient analyses were done using Dynamic Structural Equation Modeling (DSEM). DSEM is based on time-series analysis but can be used with panel data due to the possibility of adding random effects to model between-patient components [46]. As such, DSEM is a kind of Multilevel Model (MLM), but with two important differences to traditional multilevel models: 1) random effects can be modeled for both predictors and outcome variables, and 2) lagged effects are modeled using latent variables [47]. These two additions are essential for avoiding the so-called dynamic panel bias, which arises when regressing a variable on its own lagged component, while using manual methods for separating within- and between patient components [48]. The part of the DSEM model of most interest is the within-patient part, which is a cross-lagged panel model in which lagged time-series relationships among variables are estimated. The within-patient cross-lagged paths, which are the ones of most interest in this study, represent the average effect of one variable at any given session on the other variable by the following session. This path is adjusted for autoregression, i.e. the effect of the outcome variable at the prior occasion. This is important since it means that the cross-lagged effects can be interpreted as effects on (residualized) change in the other variable. Specifically, in the present study the relationships between depression and ED symptoms are analyzed. At a between-patient level, different patients may have different average levels of depression and/or ED symptoms across the whole study. It may also be that different patients have different linear trajectories across the

whole study, in that some improve more/faster, while others remain more or less on the same level or even deteriorate. At a within-patient level, we analyze whether deviations from each person's average level (or average linear trajectory over time) in depression/ED at a given session can predict change in depression/ED by the next session. This is a test of which symptom 'drives' change in the other symptom. DSEM models are estimated using Markov Chain Monte Carlo estimation, which is a simulation-based estimation method for Bayesian analysis. Two chains were run, and Potential Scale Reduction value (PSR) was calculated to check for convergence between the chains. PSR values were required to be below 1.05 and remain so for at least 2000 iterations. Estimation was done using Mplus version 8.1.7, with default infinite variance priors to ensure that analyses are not unduly influenced by prior information [49]. In panel data, there are two dimension of sample size, the number of participants (N) and the number of repeated measurements (T). For within-person coefficients, statistical power and coefficient bias are determined roughly by the product of these dimensions. A recent simulation study [50] on a similar SEM model as the one used in the present study showed that with $N = 50$ and T = 5, i.e. 250 observations in total, statistical power was well above 80% for finding a medium-sized effect, and average coefficient bias was negligible. In the present study we had $N = 31$ and T = 16, i.e. 496 observations, which should be sufficient even for smaller effect sizes.

Results

Eating disorders and depressive symptoms outcome
As shown in Table 1, both ED symptoms and depressive symptoms decreased significantly, with large effect sizes, during the treatment. The patients improved significantly

Table 1 Pre- and post-ratings of ED and depressive symptoms for the 31 patients

Measure	Pre- Treatment		Post-Treatment		t	p	Cohen's d
	M	SD	M	SD			
Eating disorder problems:							
EDE-Q							
Global	3.95	0.76	2.38	1.36	5.32	<.001	1.48
Restraint	3.55	1.48	1.88	1.36	4.70	<.001	1.17
Eat concern	3.7	1.4	1.7	1.26	4.64	<.001	1.5
Shape concern	4.65	1.4	3.28	1.89	4.00	<.001	0.83
Weight concern	3.86	1.24	2.64	1.62	3.30	.003	0.85
REDS	32.58	9.69	15.52	8.24	8.59	< .001	1.90
Depression:							
MADRS-S	18.24	8.91	11.30	5.97	4.15	< .001	0.93
PHQ-9	13.81	5.34	5.48	4.53	7.36	< .001	1.68

Note: EDE-Q Eating Disorder Examination Questionnaire, *REDS* Repeated Evaluation of Eating Disorder Symptoms, *MADRS-S* Montgomery Åsberg Depression Rating Scale and PHQ-9 = Patient Health Questionnaire-9

Reduction in depressive symptoms predicts improvement in eating disorder symptoms in interpersonal...

185

on all EDE-Q subscales from a clinical to a non-clinical level, with large effect sizes.

Ratings on the EDE-Q, REDS, MADRS-S and PHQ-9 are presented in Table 1.

Symptom changes during treatment

In Fig. 1, symptom improvement on REDS and PHQ-9 are shown.

The symptom reduction of ED (REDS) during treatment was linear, with the standardized beta coefficient − .45 (t [28] = − 11.16, $p < .001$). Symptom improvement was marginally larger in the first part of the therapy than in the second, with a reduction of 10 points to session 8 and a further reduction with 8 points to session 16 but a quadratic regression model was not significant. The average participant reached the cut off score of 22 for REDS at session nine. The symptom reduction of depression (PHQ-9) was also linear with the standardized beta coefficient − .41 (t (30) = − 9.41, $p < .001$). The quadratic coefficient was not significant.

Reliable symptom change

The results in Table 2 show the numbers of remitted, improved, unchanged and deteriorated patients.

Twenty-two of the 31 patients were remitted [17] or improved [5] in their ED-symptoms. Two more passed the cut-off for CS [22] but were not considered remitted due to low entry values. Six remained unchanged and one had reliably deteriorated in ED symptoms. However, this patient went from clinically depressed to remitted in depression.

Fifteen patients were remitted [12] or improved [3] in both ED and depression. All but two patients were below the clinical level of depression at termination of treatment. Twenty-three were remitted and another five were below the clinical level but were not considered remitted because of low entry values. Among the two

Table 2 Numbers of deteriorated, unchanged, improved and remitted patients ($n = 31$)

	Deteriorated	Unchanged	Improved	Remitted
REDS	1	6	5	17
PHQ-9	1	7	0	23

Note: *REDS* Repeated Evaluation of Eating Disorder Symptoms, and *PHQ-9* Patient Health Questionnaire-9

patients who were still clinically depressed, both had achieved a reliable change in ED symptoms.

The relationship between early response and final outcome

In order to study the significance of early response an assessment of patients' symptom change at session 4 was made. Those who had reached a reliable change in ED-symptoms at session 4 on REDS (change ≥7 points) were considered as early responders. The association between early responders and final responders was close to significance (χ^2 (1) = 3.70, $p = .054$). There were seven early response patients; all of those were also final responders. There were 13 early responders on PHQ-9 (change ≥5 points); 12 of them were also final responders. The association between early response and final responding was significant (χ^2 (1) = 3.84, $p = .05$). Early response on REDS was not associated with final responding on PHQ-9 ($p = .43$); early response on PHQ-9 was not associated with final responding on REDS ($p = .56$).

Associations between symptom change in ED and depression

Change in gain scores on ED-symptoms (REDS) and depressive symptoms (PHQ-9) were strongly correlated ($r = .60$, $p = .001$). In order to further analyze the associations between ratings on REDS and PHQ-9 between sessions, the associations were analysed using DSEM. Model 1 was a basic cross-lagged panel model, with

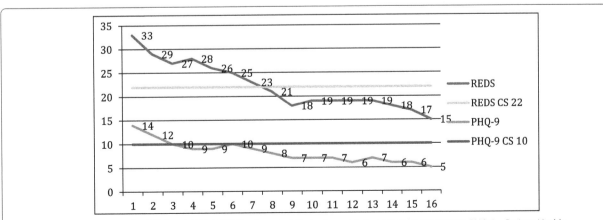

Fig. 1 Symptom trajectories for REDS and PHQ-9. REDS = Repeated Evaluation of Eating Disorder Symptoms, PHQ-9 = Patient Health Questionnaire-9, and CS = cut off score for clinical significance

REDS and PHQ-9 at session $t-1$ predicting REDS and PHQ-9 at session t. In Model 2, we adjusted for linear change over time in both variables. REDS and PHQ-9 were standardized before analysis, to make coefficients for these comparable. Results are presented in Table 3. The coefficients of most interest in Table 3 are the cross-lagged within-patient effects, i.e. $REDS_{t-1} \rightarrow PHQ\text{-}9_t$ and $PHQ\text{-}9_{t-1} \rightarrow REDS_t$. As can be seen from Table 3, in Model 1 both of these paths were statistically significant. Although the $REDS_{t-1} \rightarrow PHQ_t$ path seemed numerically larger, the difference between these two coefficients was not itself statistically significant (difference = 0.11, se = 0.08, p = 0.18, 95% CI -0.05, 0.26). In Model 2, which adjusts coefficients for the person-specific linear slope of session number, the $PHQ_{t-1} \rightarrow REDS_t$ path remained about the same as in Model 1 (0.13, se = 0.06, p = .04 95% CI 0.00, 0.25), while the $REDS_{t-1} \rightarrow PHQ_t$ path disappeared completely (– 0.01, se = 0.08, p = .92, 95% CI -0.16, 0.16). Still, the difference between these two coefficients remained statistically non-significant (– 0.14, se = 0.12, p = .26, 95% CI -0.35, 0.10).

Discussion

The aim of this study was to analyse the effects of IPT on symptom reduction in patients with bulimia nervosa with co-occurring depression. The results indicate that the treatment was effective. Based on EDE-Q results, patients on average improved from a clinical level in ED symptoms to a non-clinical level. This finding is in line with previous research showing that IPT is an effective treatment for BN. Effect sizes were similar to those in previous IPT-studies regarding BN [8, 9, 25]. Both ED symptoms and depressive symptoms decreased substantially and significantly, with

most patients reaching clinically significant change. Twenty-four (77%) of the 31 patients were remitted or improved in bulimic symptoms at the end of treatment. Fifteen of the patients (48%) were remitted or improved on both diagnoses.

There was a trend for patients with early response to improve to a larger extent than the other patients. These results are parallel to results of CBT for BN, where early responding also usually predicts final outcome [7, 14, 17]. However, the clinical implications of this finding must be used with caution since the improvement trajectories differ between patients in this study and a number of patients improved although they were not early responders. It has been suggested that IPT could be delivered in a briefer format, since many of the patients in the studies by Arcelus [24, 25] improved more during the first eight sessions. However, ED often implies life-long vulnerability with recurrent relapses [1] and thus it could be argued that IPT-BNm of 16 sessions is not an unnecessary extensive intervention, especially if the treatment targets several co-occurring conditions. In our study, symptom reduction was linear during the whole treatment, and there was no indication that improvement took place at different rates early and late in treatment. Research suggests that patients improve in different rates but on the average linearly [51] and that the long-term effects of IPT are stable [15, 16, 19]. Downsizing treatment duration may therefore not be cost-effective in the long run. Maybe the question we should be asking ourselves is how well the results can be maintained, rather than the speed of recovery.

There is a substantial comorbidity between ED pathology and depression [4]. The relations between these

Table 3 Fixed effects from Dynamic Structural Equation Models testing the session-wise lagged relationships between symptoms of eating disorder and depression

Fixed effects, within level	Model 1				Model 2			
	Estimate	sd	p	95% CI	Estimate	sd	p	95% CI
$PHQ_{t-1} \rightarrow PHQ_t$	0.58	0.05	<.001	0.48, 0.69	0.44	0.08	<.001	0.29, 0.59
$REDS_{t-1} \rightarrow PHQ_t$	0.24	0.05	<.001	0.14, 0.34	−0.01	0.08	.92	−0.16, 0.16
$REDS_{t-1} \rightarrow REDS_t$	0.73	0.05	<.001	0.63, 0.83	0.20	0.08	.02	0.04, 0.36
$PHQ_{t-1} \rightarrow REDS_t$	0.13	0.05	.008	0.04, 0.23	0.13	0.06	.04	0.00, 0.25
$PHQ_t \leftrightarrow REDS_t$	0.15	0.017	<.001	0.12, 0.19	0.12	0.01	<.001	0.10, 0.16
Fixed effects, between level								
$PHQ_{intercept} \leftrightarrow REDS_{intercept}$	0.089	0.211	0.52	−0.10, 0.69	0.68	0.41	.01	0.15, 1.71
$PHQ_{slope} \leftrightarrow REDS_{slope}$					0.00	0.00	.04	0.00, 0.01
$PHQ_{intercept} \leftrightarrow REDS_{slope}$					−0.02	0.02	.26	−0.07, 0.02
$PHQ_{slope} \leftrightarrow REDS_{intercept}$					−0.02	0.02	.08	−0.07, 0.00
$PHQ_{intercept} \leftrightarrow PHQ_{slope}$					−0.03	0.02	.002	−0.09, − 0.01
$REDS_{intercept} \leftrightarrow REDS_{slope}$					−0.06	0.03	<.001	−0.13, − 0.02

Note. PHQ_{t-1} and $REDS_{t-1}$ are the PHQ-9 and REDS scores, respectively, at session t-1, while PHQ_t and $REDS_t$ are the PHQ-9 and REDS scores at scores at session t. Unidirectional arrows ($\rightarrow$) represent regression paths (potentially causal), while bidirectional arrows ($\leftrightarrow$) represent covariances

syndromes are intricate, as depression may initiate eating problems and eating problems may initiate a depression. Often, the development is a vicious circle between these symptoms. In CBT treatment of comorbid ED and depression, therapists are often encouraged to first help the patient with the depression, as depressive thoughts and feelings may hamper the therapeutic work with the eating behaviour [6]. In order to enhance effective treatment of combined conditions, it is important to better understand whether decrease in depression predicts improvement of eating problems, or it is the other way, i.e. ED improvement precedes improvement in depressive symptoms. The cross-lagged analyses of symptom reduction showed that when adjustment for individual linear change trajectories was made, reduction in depressive symptoms predicted reduction in ED symptoms at the next session whereas reduction in ED symptoms did not predict reduction in depressive symptoms. The difference between these coefficients was not significant, probably due to low statistical power. It can be argued that depression should be targeted before ED symptoms in comorbid conditions [6]. General models of psychotherapy emphasize the need to restore hope and motivation in the patient before more specific symptoms are focused [52, 53]. In this study, decrease in depressive symptom at one session was correlated with decrease in ED symptoms at the next session. IPT-BNm focuses especially on ED symptoms. The fact that the treatment was also effective for depression, and that reduction in depressive symptoms seemed to correlate with subsequent reduction in ED symptoms, is interesting. One perspective is that IPT, by focusing on interpersonal issues, has a more general impact on emotional suffering than treatments that target specific symptoms. The treatment can have a remoralizing effect, influencing depressive symptoms such as hopelessness, alienation and distrust. If interpersonal issues become more understandable and manageable, a general reduction of the sense of being stuck and hopeless might be achieved. A reasonable suggestion is that the treatment first leads to a decrease of depressive symptoms and subsequently reduces ED-symptoms. Furthermore, since the IPT approach focuses on processing interpersonal stressors and negative affects which is hypothesized to lead to improvements in ED symptoms [7], it seems natural that this process of change may appear in different pace depending on the patients' interpersonal context. Thus, more research concerning what, how and when change takes place in IPT for eating disorders needs to be done. This is the first study to our knowledge to analyse correlations between weekly ratings of symptoms in co-occurring conditions, both with regard to ED treatment in general and in IPT research. Although this study is small, these results suggest that change in depressive symptoms is strongly correlated with change in ED symptoms the next session. Since depressive co-morbidity with BN is common and may complicate or obstacle ED treatment [4, 6], this is a clinical important finding showing that IPT-BNm may be an especially suitable treatment option for patients suffering from BN and co-occurring depression.

Strengths and limitations

The main strength of this study was the weekly ratings of symptoms, which made it possible to analyse the interaction in symptom reduction. The study was naturalistic with a limited number of patients. This may obstruct the generalizability of the results. Another limitation was the lack of follow-up data. Since the patients presented with mild to moderate depressive symptomatology, we do not know whether the findings can be generalized to more severe forms of mood disorders. For future studies, it would be important to measure change in identified interpersonal problems.

Conclusions

The modified version of IPT-BN used in this study is an effective treatment for BN, especially with co-occurring depression. Symptom improvement in ED and depressive symptoms was strongly correlated, with reduction of depressive symptoms at one session driving symptom reduction in ED at the next session. Even though early response was associated with favourable treatment outcome, effect took place continuously during the whole treatment, indicating that there were different paths to recovery.

Abbreviations
APA: American psychiatric association; BED: Binge eating disorder; BN: Bulimia Nervosa; BMI: body mass index; CBT: Cognitive Behavioural therapy; CS: Clinical significance; ED: Eating disorder; EDE: Eating Disorder examination; EDE-Q: Eating Disorder examination Querstionnarie; DSEM: Dynamic Structural Equation Modelling; DSM-IV: Diagnostic and statistical manual of mental disorders - 4th edition; IPT: Interpersonal Psychotherapy; IPT-BN: Interpersonal Psychotherapy for Bulimia nervosa; IPT-BNm: Interpersonal Psychotherapy for Bulimia nervosa, modified version; IPT-BN10: Interpersonal Psychotherapy for Bulimia nervosa, ten sessions; LOCF: Last observation carried forward; MADRS-S: Montgomery Åsberg Depression Rating Scale; MLM: Multi level model; PHQ-9: Patient Health Questionnaire-9; PSC: Potential Scale Reduction value; PTSD: Post traumatic stress disorder; RCI: Reliable change index; REDS: Repeated Evaluation of Eating Disorder Symptoms; SEDI: Structured Eating Disorder Interview; SWEAT: Swedish Eating Disorders clinical quality register

Acknowledgements
This study was part of a larger IPT project in Sweden and is supported by SwEat – Swedish Eating Disorder Register. We want to thank all the therapists, patients, teachers and supervisors who contributed to the data of this study.

Authors' contributions
All authors contributed to the planning and design of the study. MB took primary responsibility for the manuscript, including reviewing relevant literature and drafting the paper for publication. MB and SAG collected the data. MB, FF and RH performed statistical analyses. All authors assisted with

literature review and editing of the manuscript. All authors read and approved the final manuscript.

Competing interests
The authors declare that they have no competing interests.

Author details
[1]Department of Behavioural Sciences and Learning, Linköping University, Linköping, Sweden. [2]Futurum: Academy for Health and Care, Jönköping, Region Jönköping County, Sweden. [3]Faculty of Medicine and Health, University Health Care Research Center, Örebro University, Örebro, Sweden. [4]Department of Clinical Neuroscience, Karolinska Institute, Stockholm, Sweden.

References
1. Wade TD. Recent research on bulimia nervosa. Psychiatr Clin North Am. 2019;42(1):21–32.
2. Berkman ND, Lohr KN, Bulik CM. Outcomes of eating disorders: a systematic review of the literature. Int J Eat Disord. 2007;40(4):293–309.
3. Brown TA, Keel PK. Current and emerging directions in the treatment of eating disorders. Subst Abuse. 2012;6:33–61.
4. Puccio F, Fuller-Tyszkiewicz M, Ong D, Krug I. A systematic review and meta-analysis on the longitudinal relationship between eating pathology and depression. Int J Eat Disord. 2016;49(5):439–54.
5. (UK) NGA. Eating disorders: recognition and treatment. London: National Institute for Health and Care Excellence (UK); 2017. Contract No.: NICE Guideline, No. 69. https://www.ncbi.nlm.nih.gov/books/NBK436876/.
6. Fairburn CG, Cooper Z, Shafran R. Cognitive behaviour therapy for eating disorders: a "transdiagnostic" theory and treatment. Behav Res Ther. 2003; 41(5):509–28.
7. Murphy R, Straebler S, Basden S, Cooper Z, Fairburn CG. Interpersonal psychotherapy for eating disorders. Clin Psychol Psychother. 2012;19(2):150–8.
8. Agras WS, Walsh T, Fairburn CG, Wilson GT, Kraemer HC. A multicenter comparison of cognitive-behavioral therapy and interpersonal psychotherapy for bulimia nervosa. Arch Gen Psychiatry. 2000;57(5):459–66.
9. Fairburn CG, Bailey-Straebler S, Basden S, Doll HA, Jones R, Murphy R, et al. A transdiagnostic comparison of enhanced cognitive behaviour therapy (CBT-E) and interpersonal psychotherapy in the treatment of eating disorders. Behav Res Ther. 2015;70:64–71.
10. Bäck M, Gustafsson-Aila S, Holmqvist R. Interpersonal psychotherapy for eating disorders with co-morbid depression: a pilot study. Eur J Psychother Couns. 2017;19(4):378–95.
11. Cuijpers P, Geraedts AS, van Oppen P, Andersson G, Markowitz JC, van Straten A. Interpersonal psychotherapy for depression: a meta-analysis. Am J Psychiatry. 2011;168(6):581–92.
12. Cuijpers P, Donker T, Weissman MM, Ravitz P, Cristea IA. Interpersonal psychotherapy for mental health problems: a comprehensive meta-analysis. Am J Psychiatry. 2016;173(7):680–7.
13. Markowitz JC, Petkova E, Neria Y, Van Meter PE, Zhao Y, Hembree E, et al. Is exposure necessary? A randomized clinical trial of interpersonal psychotherapy for PTSD. Am J Psychiatry. 2015;172(5):430–40.
14. Fairburn CG, Jones R, Peveler RC, Carr SJ, Solomon RA, O'Connor ME, et al. Three psychological treatments for bulimia nervosa. A comparative trial. Arch Gen Psychiatry. 1991;48(5):463–9.
15. Fairburn CG, Jones R, Peveler RC, Hope RA, O'Connor M. Psychotherapy and bulimia nervosa. Longer-term effects of interpersonal psychotherapy, behavior therapy, and cognitive behavior therapy. Arch Gen Psychiatry. 1993;50(6):419–28.
16. Linardon J. Rates of abstinence following psychological or behavioral treatments for binge-eating disorder: meta-analysis. Int J Eat Disord. 2018; 51(8):785–97.
17. Murphy R, Cooper Z, Hollon SD, Fairburn CG. How do psychological treatments work? Investigating mediators of change. Behav Res Ther. 2009; 47(1):1 5.
18. Lipsitz JD, Markowitz JC. Mechanisms of change in interpersonal therapy (IPT). Clin Psychol Rev. 2013;33(8):1134–47.
19. Miniati M, Callari A, Maglio A, Calugi S. Interpersonal psychotherapy for eating disorders: current perspectives. Psychol Res Behav Manag. 2018;11:353–69.
20. Law R. Curriculum for practitioner training in interpersonal psychotherapy (trainee). IAPT/NHS/UK. 2011. Available from: http://www.iapt.nhs.uk/silo/files/curriculum-for-practitioner-training-in-interpersonal-psychotherapy-trainer.pdf.
21. Weissman M, Markowitz JC, Klerman G. The guide to interpersonal psychotherapy. New York: Oxford University Press; 2017.
22. Arcelus A, Whight D, Haslam SM. Interpersonal problems in people with bulimia nervosa and the role of interpersonal psychotherapy. In: Hay PJ, editor. New insights into the prevention and treatment of bulimia nervosa; 2011. https://www.intechopen.com/books/new-insights-into-the-prevention-and-treatment-of-bulimia-nervosa.
23. Whight D, Meadows L, McGrain L, Langham C, Baggott J, Arcelus J. IPT-BN (m) interpersonal psychotherapy for bulimia spectrum disorders: a treatment guide. Leicestershire: Troubador; 2011.
24. Arcelus J, Whight D, Brewin N, McGrain L. A brief form of interpersonal psychotherapy for adult patients with bulimic disorders: a pilot study. Eur Eat Disord Rev. 2012;20(4):326–30.
25. Arcelus J, Whight D, Langham C, Baggott J, McGrain L, Meadows L, et al. A case series evaluation of a modified version of interpersonal psychotherapy (IPT) for the treatment of bulimic eating disorders: a pilot study. Eur Eat Disord Rev. 2009;17(4):260–8.
26. Linardon J, Brennan L, de la Piedad Garcia X. Rapid response to eating disorder treatment: a systematic review and meta-analysis. Int J Eat Disord. 2016;49(10):905–19.
27. APA. Diagnostic and statistical manual of mental disorders. 4th ed. Washington, DC: American Psychiatric Association; 1994.
28. Birgegard A, Bjorck C, Clinton D. Quality assurance of specialised treatment of eating disorders using large-scale internet-based collection systems: methods, results and lessons learned from designing the stepwise database. Eur Eat Disord Rev. 2010;18(4):251–9.
29. Fairburn CG, Beglin SJ. Assessment of eating disorders: interview or self-report questionnaire? Int J Eat Disord. 1994;16(4):363–70.
30. Fairburn CG, Beglin SJ. Eating disorder examination questionnaire (6.0). In: Fairburn CG, editor. Cognitive behavior therapy and eating disorders. New York: Guilford Press; 2008.
31. Cooper Z, Fairburn CG. The eating disorder examination: a semi-structured interview for the assessment of the specific psychopathology of eating disorders. Int J Eat Disord. 1987;6(1).
32. Mond JM, Hay PJ, Rodgers B, Owen C. Eating disorder examination questionnaire (EDE-Q): norms for young adult women. Behav Res Ther. 2006;44(1):53–62.
33. Reas DL, Grilo CM, Masheb RM. Reliability of the eating disorder examination-questionnaire in patients with binge eating disorder. Behav Res Ther. 2006;44(1):43–51.
34. Welch E, Birgegard A, Parling T, Ghaderi A. Eating disorder examination questionnaire and clinical impairment assessment questionnaire: general population and clinical norms for young adult women in Sweden. Behav Res Ther. 2011;49(2):85–91.
35. Svanborg P, Asberg M. A new self-rating scale for depression and anxiety states based on the comprehensive psychopathological rating scale. Acta Psychiatr Scand. 1994;89(1):21–8.
36. Hawley CJ, Gale TM, Sivakumaran T. Hertfordshire neuroscience research g. defining remission by cut off score on the MADRS: selecting the optimal value. J Affect Disord. 2002;72(2):177–84.
37. Falsdalen Riegler U, Sundin S. Standardization and validation of the self-report questionnaire KUS-P: How normal is your eating disturbance? Normering och validering av självskattnings-formuläret kus-p. Hur ätstörd är normalt att vara? [Master]. 2009. http://www.diva-portal.org/smash/record.jsf?pid=diva2:220788: Örebro University.
38. Spitzer RL, Kroenke K, Williams JB. Validation and utility of a self-report version of PRIME-MD: the PHQ primary care study. Primary care evaluation of mental disorders. Patient health questionnaire. JAMA. 1999;282(18):1737–44.

39. Kendel F, Wirtz M, Dunkel A, Lehmkuhl E, Hetzer R, Regitz-Zagrosek V. Screening for depression: Rasch analysis of the dimensional structure of the PHQ-9 and the HADS-D. J Affect Disord. 2010;122(3):241–6.

40. Kroenke K, Spitzer RL, Williams JB. The PHQ-9: validity of a brief depression severity measure. J Gen Intern Med. 2001;16(9):606–13.

41. Lowe B, Kroenke K, Herzog W, Grafe K. Measuring depression outcome with a brief self-report instrument: sensitivity to change of the patient health questionnaire (PHQ-9). J Affect Disord. 2004;81(1):61–6.

42. Gyani A, Shafran R, Layard R, Clark DM. Enhancing recovery rates: lessons from year one of IAPT. Behav Res Ther. 2013;51(9):597–606.

43. Manea L, Gilbody S, McMillan D. Optimal cut-off score for diagnosing depression with the patient health questionnaire (PHQ-9): a meta-analysis. CMAJ. 2012;184(3):E191–6.

44. Jacobson NS, Truax P. Clinical significance: a statistical approach to defining meaningful change in psychotherapy research. J Consult Clin Psychol. 1991; 59(1):12–9.

45. Frank E, Prien RF, Jarrett RB, Keller MB, Kupfer DJ, Lavori PW, et al. Conceptualization and rationale for consensus definitions of terms in major depressive disorder. Remission, recovery, relapse, and recurrence. Arch Gen Psychiatry. 1991;48(9):851–5.

46. Asparouhov T, Hamaker EL, Muthén B. Dynamic structural equation models. Struct Equ Model Multidiscip J. 2018;25(3):359–88.

47. Snijders TAB, Bosker RJ. Multilevel analysis: an introduction to basic and advanced multilevel modeling: Sage Publishers; 2012.

48. Nickell S. Biases in dynamic models with fixed effects. Econometrica. 1981; 49(6):1417–26.

49. Muthén LK, Muthén BO. Mplus user's guide. Los Angeles: Muthén & Muthén; 1998-2017.

50. Falkenström F, Solmonov N, Rubel J. Do therapist effects really impact estimates of within-patient mechanisms of change? A Monte Carlo simulation study. Psychother Res. 2000. https://doi.org/10.1080/10503307. 2020.1769875.

51. Falkenström F, Josefsson A, Beggren T, Holmqvist R. How much therapy is enough? Comparing dose-effect and good-enough models in two different settings. Psychotherapy. 2016;53:130–9.

52. Bohart AC. The client is the most important common factor: Clients' self-healing capacities and psychotherapy. J Psychother Integr. 2000;10:127–49.

53. Fonagy P, Allison E. The role of mentalizing and epistemic trust in the therapeutic relationship. Psychotherapy (Chic). 2014;51:372–80.

18

Family-related non-abuse adverse life experiences occurring for adults diagnosed with eating disorders

Katie Grogan[1]*[iD], Diarmuid MacGarry[1], Jessica Bramham[1], Mary Scriven[2], Caroline Maher[2] and Amanda Fitzgerald[1]

Abstract

Background: Although previous reviews suggest a strong association between abuse and eating disorders, less is known about non-abuse adverse life experiences, such as parental mental illness or family discord, which occur frequently for this population. The aim of the current study was to identify family-related non-abuse adverse life experiences occurring for adults with eating disorders, and to establish whether they occur for people with anorexia nervosa, bulimia nervosa or binge-eating disorder more than the general population and other psychiatric populations.

Method: A systematic review of studies focusing on family-related non-abuse adverse life experiences and eating disorders was conducted in accordance with PRISMA guidelines. The search string was applied to four electronic databases including Psycinfo, PubMed/Medline, CINAHL Plus and EMBASE.

Results: Of the 26 studies selected for inclusion, six types of family-related non-abuse adverse life experiences were identified: adverse parenting style; family disharmony; loss of a family member, relative or close person; familial mental health issues; family comments about eating, or shape, weight and appearance; and family disruptions. Findings provided tentative evidence for eating disorder specific (i.e. parental demands and criticism) and non-specific (i.e. familial loss and family disruptions) non-abuse adversities, with findings also suggesting that those with bulimia nervosa and binge-eating disorder were more impacted by loss, family separations and negative parent-child interactions compared to those with anorexia nervosa.

Conclusions: This review provides a clear synthesis of previous findings relating to family-related non-abuse adverse life experiences and eating disorders in adults. Implications for trauma-informed care in clinical practice were discussed (e.g. considering the impact of past life events, understanding the function of ED behaviours, reducing the risk of potential re-traumatisation).

Keywords: Anorexia nervosa, Bulimia nervosa, Binge eating disorders, Eating disorders, Non-abuse adverse life experiences, Family adversity, Adults

* Correspondence: katie.grogan@ucdconnect.ie
[1]School of Psychology, University College Dublin, Dublin, Ireland
Full list of author information is available at the end of the article

Plain English summary

There is evidence to suggest the significance of family factors beyond abuse in the lives of people with eating disorders. Yet, there have been few attempts in previous literature to demonstrate the importance of these family factors in eating disorder prognosis and recovery. This is the first systematic review completed on the topic of adversity that explores adverse life experiences beyond abuse in the context of eating disorders. Six types of family-related non-abuse adverse life experiences were identified: adverse parenting style; family disharmony; loss of a family member, relative or close person; familial mental health issues; family comments about eating, or shape, weight and appearance; and family disruptions. This study demonstrated that adversities occurring in the context of home and family environments are associated with having bulimia nervosa and binge-eating disorder to a greater extent than anorexia nervosa. These findings suggest that the course of anorexia nervosa may be less influenced by psychosocial factors such as family background issues. The paper discussed how the shared feature of bingeing among bulimia nervosa and binge eating disorder may occur as a reaction to family-related stress, or may have emerged as a coping mechanism for dealing with complex family backgrounds. This review provides evidence for the suitability and usefulness of trauma-informed approaches and recovery-oriented perspectives in clinical practice during the treatment of eating disorders. Avenues for future research have been clearly indicated in order to present more conclusive findings regarding specific family adversities.

Review

Adversity, also known as 'adverse life experiences' (ALEs) within a mental health setting, includes any experiences or life events that have the potential to result in undesirable outcomes by disrupting normal functioning [61], and can be diverse in source, intensity and manifestation [47]. These experiences can be socially induced (e.g. child maltreatment, family discord), or they may occur naturally over time (e.g. parental loss, family illness). ALEs can occur at any point in a person's life, but those occurring in the formative years (i.e. from age 0–18 years) are referred to as adverse childhood experiences (ACEs). Recent research has brought about increased awareness of the consistent relationship between exposure to ACEs or ALEs and long-term, negative mental health outcomes (e.g. [24, 33, 41, 58]).

Although the definition of ALEs is broad and encapsulates many diverse forms of adversity, research investigating ALEs in relation to eating disorders (EDs) has focused predominantly on childhood abuse, to the extent that various systematic reviews and meta-analyses have been conducted (e.g. [12, 43, 51]). These reviews collectively support the association between various forms of childhood abuse (i.e. sexual abuse, physical abuse, physical neglect, emotional abuse and emotional neglect) and bulimia nervosa (BN), binge eating disorder (BED), and to a lesser extent anorexia nervosa (AN). The inclusion of psychiatric control groups (i.e. participants with psychiatric disorders other than EDs) in these reviews allowed for the identification of disorder-specific (i.e. applying to people with EDs only) and non-specific (i.e. applying to people with psychiatric illnesses in general) results so that findings can be applied in clinical practice to better match treatment choices to specific clinical presentations [56]. Caslini et al. [12] also conducted ED subgroup comparisons (i.e. AN versus BN versus BED) to determine whether these three ED groups have underlying commonalities or differences, which in turn helps to establish the suitability of a 'transdiagnostic approach' to ED treatment [21, 23].

Although the association and impact of the relationship between childhood abuse and EDs appear to be firmly established, less research has examined the relationship between other non-abuse forms of ALEs and EDs. Non-abuse ALEs include any of the previously noted ALEs (e.g. parental loss, family discord etc.) but exclude abuse (i.e. sexual abuse, physical abuse, emotional abuse and neglect). These non-abuse ALEs, which are commonly family-based in nature, have sometimes been referred to as 'cumulative adversity' or 'micro-traumas' due to their negative impact over time, despite appearing less severe than abuse. The detrimental effects of these forms of trauma are further enhanced when the perpetrator is unaware of the impact of their actions, and moreover, if the victim feels ashamed when they cannot attribute their psychological distress to a major trauma or horrific event, leading to higher levels of emotional suffering and self-blame [13].

There are distinct reasons why we need to be better informed about non-abuse ALEs in relation to mental health outcomes. Firstly, non-abuse ALEs may occur more frequently than more extreme forms of adversity, such as abuse. For instance, Kessler et al. [33] completed surveys in nine countries (Belgium, France, Germany, Israel, Italy, Japan, The Netherlands, Spain and USA) to assess levels of childhood adversity. Results demonstrated that rates were higher for parental death during childhood (12.5%) compared to physical abuse (8.0%), sexual abuse (1.6%) or neglect (4.4%) among their sample of 51,945 adults, and that other non-abuse ALEs such as parental divorce (6.6%), family violence (6.5%) and parental mental health illness (6.2%) occurred in a significant proportion of cases. Secondly, there is evidence to suggest that just as abuse is associated with multiple psychiatric outcomes, so too are non-abuse ALEs. For instance, odd ratios (ORs) showed significant associations between DSM-IV disorders and abuse (i.e. physical abuse OR = 1.8; sexual abuse OR = 1.8; neglect OR = 1.5) as well as non-abuse ALES (e.g. parental mental illness OR = 2.0; parental substance misuse OR = 1.6; family violence OR = 1.6) [33]. Importantly, Kessler et al. [33] demonstrated that adversities associated with maladaptive family functioning, specifically (e.g. parental mental illness, parental substance misuse, family violence) had a greater impact on mental health disorders, compared with 'other childhood adversities' (e.g. serious physical illness).

There are clear clinical implications for adversity findings in the context of EDs. Mental health researchers and clinicians worldwide are now moving towards recovery centred approaches in working with people with various mental health diagnoses, which involves viewing recovery as a process, and not an end goal to be reached [29]. In line with the introduction of recovery-oriented principles in the care of people with mental health diagnoses in recent years, clinicians are encouraged to utilise a trauma-informed perspective in the management and treatment of various disorders [73]. Trauma-informed perspectives involve a consideration of the relevance of trauma and adversity in not only the development and maintenance (i.e. risk) of various mental health diagnoses, but also in terms of prognosis. In other words, instead of focusing on how adversity might impact on ED onset alone, knowledge about the role of adversity will also aid clinicians in their selection of appropriate interventions and treatments by generating a clearer clinical picture of the contextual factors contributing to client's difficulties. Such trauma-informed work can help clinicians to facilitate a person to regain control and personal responsibility in working through their difficulties, resulting in resilience and improved recovery outcomes [73]. In this sense, such adversity research is not invested in exploring the causal relationship between certain adversities and later ED onset (i.e. risk), but instead to benefit patient prognosis by allowing clinicians to work from a more trauma-informed and recovery-oriented perspective.

The aim of the current study was to identify the various non-abuse ALEs occurring for adults with EDs by conducting a systematic review of the literature, with a particular focus on family-related non-abuse ALEs. This is the first systematic review examining adversity in the context of EDs that is not focused on abuse. The objective of this study was to provide information for clinicians regarding the potential family-related non-abuse ALEs which may impact individuals throughout their ED recovery. The four specific research questions were 1) What were the various family-related non-abuse ALEs reported to have occurred for adults with EDs? 2) What differences in these ALEs were reported by those with EDs compared to non-clinical samples (i.e. members of the general population without an ED diagnosis)? 3) What differences in these ALEs were reported by those with EDs compared to other psychiatric control groups? And 4) What differences in these ALEs were reported between the various ED subgroups (i.e. AN vs. BN vs. BED)?

Method
Study design
The current study was completed in accordance with Preferred Reporting Items for Systematic Reviews and Meta-Analysis (PRISMA [42];) guidelines. A protocol for this systematic literature review was registered with Prospero (protocol ID: CRD42019121905). Both qualitative and quantitative studies were included, and PICOTS parameters were used to assist in defining further inclusion and exclusion criteria in relation to study population, intervention/exposure, comparison, outcome, timing and setting (see Table 1).

Search strategy
Four electronic databases were chosen for the literature search; Psycinfo, PubMed/Medline, CINAHL Plus and EMBASE. Searches were refined using filters which limited search results to English language only, peer-reviewed articles and articles published from the year 1980-present. Similar to previous adversity systematic reviews (e.g. [50, 64]), we chose to limit the search to research published from 1980 in order to ascertain relatively up-to-date findings. Furthermore, the DSM-III [1] was published in 1980, with earlier versions of the DSM having categorised EDs considerably differently compared to later versions. Each electronic database required slight adjustments to the search string depending on the database index terms, keywords and/or mesh terms (see Additional file 1 for sample search string). However, boolean searching, and methods for both broadening and narrowing the searches were utilized across all databases based on the two concepts being searched; EDs and ALEs. The search strategies for each of the four database searches were reviewed and checked by two librarians with expertise in systematic reviews.

Study selection
Database searches and importing of selected studies for screening took place on 1st May 2019. Figure 1 depicts the search and selection process which occurred for the current study. A total of 2684 studies were identified by applying the search string to the four databases, and an additional 26 studies were identified by scanning reference lists of included studies. This resulted in 2710 articles being imported for screening to Covidence [32], an online systematic review management software. This figure was reduced to 2021 once duplicates ($n = 689$) were

Table 1 PICOTS parameters outlining inclusion/exclusion criteria for the database searches

Parameter	Inclusion	Exclusion
Population	Adults who report adverse life experiences in childhood or adulthood Adults with eating disorders including anorexia, bulimia, eating disorder not otherwise specified/ unspecified feeding or eating disorder, binge eating disorder Adults with obesity who also have a diagnosis of an eating disorder	Children (age < 18) Populations who do not have a diagnosed eating disorder Populations with obesity but no ED Populations not exposed to adverse/traumatic life experiences Animal studies
Intervention/ Exposure	Family-related adverse/traumatic childhood experiences Family related adverse/traumatic adulthood experiences	Childhood abuse (including sexual abuse, physical abuse, emotional abuse or neglect) Adulthood abuse (including sexual abuse, physical abuse, emotional abuse or neglect) Health problems Social adversity (e.g. bullying at school)
Comparator	Healthy control participants Psychiatric control participants No comparison	
Outcome	No restriction on outcome Participants may or may not have recovered from their eating disorder	
Timing	No restriction on duration of negative life event Negative life event can be experienced in either childhood or adulthood	
Setting	No restriction on setting of intervention, but article must be published in English Articles must be peer reviewed	Articles published in language other than English Non peer-reviewed articles

removed. Titles and abstracts were screened by two independent authors (K.G and D.M.G), with an 88% agreement rate between authors. Disagreements between authors were resolved through discussion, and where consensus was not reached, a third author was consulted (A.F). A total of 1877 abstracts did not meet inclusion criteria, resulting in 144 studies remaining for full-text screening. Full-texts were obtained from various sources (i.e. multiple university libraries, Google Scholar and Library Genesis). For a minority of studies, full-text article download was unavailable, and so the authors were contacted in order to request access. If no response was received within 4 weeks, the article was deemed unavailable. Full-text screening was conducted by the same authors, with an agreement rate of 79% (*Kappa coefficient* = .58; moderate range), again with any conflicts being resolved via consensus or consultation with a third author. One hundred and twelve studies were excluded after this stage, with reasons provided in the flow diagram (see Fig. 1). An updated search was completed across databases once again on 17th March 2020, which led to one further study being identified which met inclusion criteria.

Quality assessment

All remaining studies at this point (n = 33) were assessed using the Mixed Methods Appraisal Tools (MMAT) screening criteria [28] in order to critically appraise methodological quality. MMAT has been found to be an easy-to-use tool with moderate to perfect inter-rater reliability [49]. The two screening criteria were 'Are there

clear research questions?' and 'Do the collected data allow to address the research questions?' The authors suggest that further appraisal might not be feasible or appropriate if answering 'No' or 'Can't tell' to one or both of these screening questions. Seven studies failed to meet these screening criteria resulting in exclusion from the review. The methodological quality of the final set of studies for inclusion (n = 26) was assessed using MMAT criteria [28]. For the purpose of assessing studies included in the current literature review, the qualitative, quantitative non-randomised and quantitative descriptive tools were utilised and findings were reported (see Table 2).

Data extraction and synthesis

Data from selected studies were extracted by one author (K.G.) using a data extraction template form. A second author (D.M.G) completed double-extraction of 20% of papers for reliability purposes, demonstrating 87% agreement. Data extracted from each study included author, year, country, methodology/design, data source, percentage female, sample information, methodological quality score, measure of adversity and findings (Table 2). This table also took account of whether or not the studies included findings on abuse, which will not be discussed further in this review as this was not the focus of the research questions.

Owing to the heterogeneity of study designs, the inclusion of both qualitative and quantitative methods and the inclusion of diverse ED (AN, BN and BED)

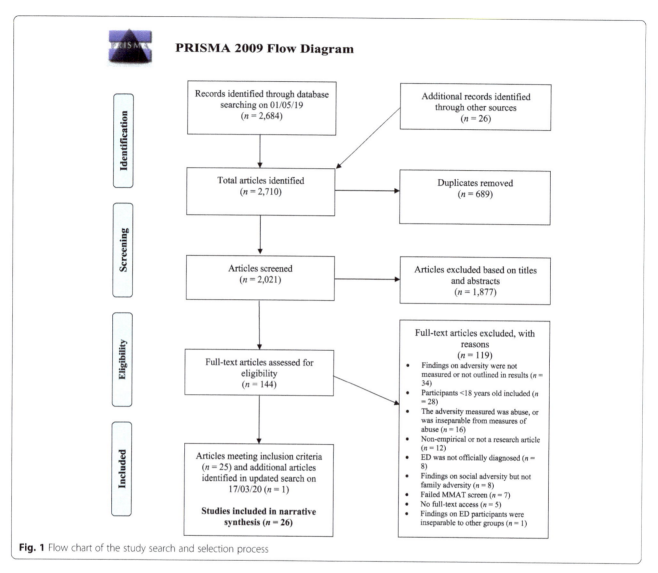

Fig. 1 Flow chart of the study search and selection process

and control (psychiatric control and non-clinical controls[1]) populations in the final studies selected, meta-analysis was not appropriate for the data included in this review. Furthermore, there was a broad set of adversities included in this review, and various tools used to measure the adversity within the original studies. Narrative synthesis was therefore deemed the most appropriate form of analysis for these diverse data types so that nuances across studies can be captured adequately [62]. Narrative synthesis was conducted in line with Popay et al.'s [55] *'Guidance on the conduct of narrative synthesis in systematic reviews'*. Specific tools and techniques outlined by the authors were utilised in the synthesis including

'grouping and clusters' and *'tabulation'*. Research question 1 was addressed by identifying the various forms of non-abuse ALEs occurring for adults with EDs as reported in previous studies, and by grouping and clustering each variable into meaningful non-abuse ALE subheadings. Research questions 2, 3 and 4 were addressed using tabulation methods, whereby specific non-abuse ALE findings associated with ED versus controls, ED versus psychiatric controls, and ED subgroup comparisons were separated, described and synthesised. This allowed for a more succinct narrative synthesis of findings. Findings from the five non-comparative studies included rates of the adversity under investigation, with no between group comparisons made. Therefore, these studies were not referred to in the narrative synthesis, as they did not serve to answer research questions 2, 3 and 4, but findings on rates for these studies can be located in Additional file 2.

---

[1]From here on out, the term 'controls' will refer to non-clinical participants whereas 'psychiatric controls' will refer to participants who do not have ED diagnoses, but do have other psychiatric diagnoses. In some instances, 'control participants' include non-clinical siblings of people with EDs, but this will be clearly outlined when discussed.

Table 2 Description of included studies, quality ratings of study methodologies and information on study findings

Study information	Participant information			Quality	Details and findings reported	Findings (Adversity domain)						Abuse (y/n)
Author (year) Country	Data source / Total sample / (age in years)	% female	Comparisons	MMAT	Measure of adversity	A1	A2	A3	A4	A5	A6	
A. Qualitative design												
1. Arthur-Cameselle et al. (2017) [2] USA	College sample N = 29 (M = 20.1; range = 18–24)	100%	Athletes with ED (A: n = 12; M = 20.5) **vs.** Non-athletes with EDs (NA: n = 17; M = 19.8). [EDs: AN (n = 17), BN (n = 3), BED (n = 1), AN+BN (n = 8)]	1.1 ◉ 1.2 ● 1.3 ● 1.4 ● 1.5 ●	Semi-structured interview				✓	✓		Y
2. Reid et al. (2019) [60] UK	ED charity in Northern England N = 16 (Range = 19–58)	94%	No comparisons [EDs: not specified]	1.1 ● 1.2 ● 1.3 ◉ 1.4 ● 1.5 ●	Adjusted version of Dan McAdams Life Story Interview			✓	✓			Y
B. Descriptive/ non-comparative design												
3. Duarte & Pinto-Gouveia (2017) [20] Portugal	Treatment seekers from a university hospital N = 114 (M = 36.62; SD = 37.62; range = 20–63)	100%	No comparison [EDs: BED = 100%]	4.1 ● 4.2 ● 4.3 ● 4.4 ◉ 4.5 ●	Shame Experiences Interview					✓		Y
4. Noordenbos et al. (2002) [46] The Netherlands	Dutch Foundation of AN and BN N = 41 (M = 34.3; SD = 7.6; range = 25–53)	100%	No comparison [EDs: AN = 44%, AN+BN = 41%, BN = 15%]	4.1 ● 4.2 ● 4.3 ○ 4.4 ● 4.5 ○	Self-report questionnaire		✓					Y
5. Sweetingham & Waller (2008) [68] UK	Specialist ED service N = 92 (M = 28.5; SD = 8.17; range = 18–58)	100%	No comparison [EDs: ANR = 13%, AN-BP = 8%, BN-P = 27%, BN-NP = 8%, EDNOS = 44%]	4.1 ● 4.2 ● 4.3 ● 4.4 ◉ 4.5 ●	Experience of Shame Scale					✓		Y
C. Observational/ comparative design												
6. Boumann & Yates (1994) [5] USA	University hospital, ED clinic and advertisement in general population N = 50 (Range 18–43)	100%	BN (n = 25) **vs.** Control (n = 25)	3.1 ● 3.2 ● 3.3 ● 3.4 ○ 3.5 ●	Family History Research Diagnostic Criteria interview		✓		✓			N
7. Calam et al. (1990) [10] UK	Clinical practice, self-help groups, university and places of employment N = 380	100%	ED (n = 98) **vs.** Control (n = 242) [EDs: AN = 31%, BN/Hx AN = 35%,	3.1 ● 3.2 ● 3.3 ● 3.4 ● 3.5 ●	Parental Bonding Instrument	✓						N

Table 2 Description of included studies, quality ratings of study methodologies and information on study findings (*Continued*)

Study information	Participant information		% female	Comparisons	Quality	Details and findings reported	Findings						Abuse (y/n)
Author (year) Country	Data source Total sample (age in years)				MMAT	Measure of adversity	Adversity domain						
							A1	A2	A3	A4	A5	A6	
8. Connan et al. (2007) [15] UK	Specialist inpatient unit, register, university advertisement N = 47 (Range = 18–45)		100%	AN (n = 18, M = 26.4, SD = 6.4) **vs.** R-AN (n = 13, M = 27.4, SD = 4.5) **vs.** Controls (n = 16, M = 27.5, SD = 4.6) [BNX = 34%]	3.1 ● 3.2 ● 3.3 ● 3.4 ● 3.5 ●	Measure of Parental Style	✓						Y
9. Cuijpers et al. (1999) [16] The Netherlands	Netherlands Mental Health Survey and Incidence Study N = 7046		49%	ACOA (n = 586) **vs.** non-ACOA (n = 6460)	3.1 ● 3.2 ○ 3.3 ● 3.4 ◉ 3.5 ●	Interview				✓			Y
10. Dalle Grave et al. (1996) [17, 18] Italy	Inpatient treatment unit N = 103		100%	ANR (n = 30, M = 21.9, SD = 6.0) **vs.** ANB (n = 12, M = 25.7, SD = 4.0) **vs.** BN (n = 17, M = 22.1, SD = 2.9) **vs.** BED (n = 30, M = 36.4, SD = 13.2) **vs.** Obese (n = 14 M = 40.5, SD = 13.5)	3.1 ● 3.2 ○ 3.3 ● 3.4 ○ 3.5 ●	Semi-structured Interview			✓				Y
11. Dalle Grave et al. (1996) [17, 18] Italy	ED treatment unit N = 238		100%	ANR (n = 30, M = 21.9, SD = 6.0) **vs.** ANB (n = 22, M = 24.9, SD = 4.2) **vs.** BN (n = 24, M = 22.3, SD = 2.7) **vs.** BED (n = 30, M = 36.4, SD = 13.2) **vs.** Sch. (n = 20, M = 33.9, SD = 7.1) **vs.** Controls (n = 112, M = 18.1 years, SD = 0.8 years)	3.1 ● 3.2 ○ 3.3 ● 3.4 ○ 3.5 ●	Semi-structured interview		✓					Y

Table 2 Description of included studies, quality ratings of study methodologies and information on study findings (Continued)

Study information — Author (year) Country	Participant information — Data source / Total sample (age in years)	% female	Comparisons	Quality MMAT	Details and findings reported — Measure of adversity	Findings — Adversity domain A1	A2	A3	A4	A5	A6	Abuse (y/n)
12. Degortes et al. (2014) [19] Italy	Outpatient ED unit N = 214	un.	BED (n = 107; M = 31.1; SD = 11.1) **vs.** BN (n = 107; M = 25.4; SD = 5.6)	3.1 ● 3.2 ● 3.3 ● 3.4 ● 3.5 ●	Semi-structured interview	✓	✓	✓			✓	Y
13. Gonçalves et al. (2016) [25] Portugal	Specialised ED treatment setting, other treatment settings and schools/universities N = 180	100%	BN (n = 60, M = 21.52, SD = 4.86) **vs.** Controls (n = 60, M = 21.50, SD = 4.81) **vs.** PC (n = 60, M = 21.45 SD = 4.86)	3.1 ● 3.2 ● 3.3 ○ 3.4 ● 3.5 ●	Oxford Risk Factor Interview	✓	✓		✓	✓	✓	Y
14. Lehoux & Howe (2007) [36] Canada	Outpatient ED unit N = 80 (Range = 18–38)	100%	BN (n = 40, M = 25.13, SD = 5.26) **vs.** Sisters (n = 40, M = 26.32, SD = 5.25)	3.1 ● 3.2 ● 3.3 ● 3.4 ● 3.5 ●	Sibling Inventory of Differential Experience	✓						Y
15. Machado et al. (2014) [38] Portugal	Specialised ED treatment setting, other treatment settings and schools/universities N = 240	100%	AN (n = 86, M = 20.02, SD = 4.49) **vs.** Controls (n = 86, M = 20.08, SD = 4.24) * **vs.** AN (n = 68, M = 19.74, SD = 4.76) **vs.** PC (n = 68, M = 19.79, SD = 4.74)	3.1 ● 3.2 ● 3.3 ● 3.4 ● 3.5 ●	Oxford Risk Factor Interview		✓		✓	✓		Y
16. Mangweth et al. (1997) [39] Austria	University advertisement N = 85	0%	Austrian ED (n = 30, M = 25.7, SD = 4.8) **vs.** Austrian control (n = 30, M = 23.8, SD = 3.1) **vs.** American ED (n = 25, M = 21.2, SD = 3.3)	3.1 ● 3.2 ● 3.3 ● 3.4 ◉ 3.5 ●	Semi-structured interview	✓	✓					Y
17. Manwaring et al. (2006) [40] USA	Advertisement in the community N = 155 (M = 31.17; SD = 5.73; range = 18–40)	100%	Binge-first BED (n = 125, M = 30.70, SD = 5.83)	3.1 ● 3.2 ● 3.3 ●	Oxford Risk Factor Interview			✓				Y

Table 2 Description of included studies, quality ratings of study methodologies and information on study findings (*Continued*)

Study information	Participant information			Quality	Details and findings reported	Findings						Abuse
						Adversity domain						
Author (year) Country	Data source Total sample (age in years)	% female	Comparisons	MMAT	Measure of adversity	A1	A2	A3	A4	A5	A6	(y/n)
			vs. Diet-first BED (n = 30, M = 32.07, SD = 5.46)	3.4 ● 3.5 ●								
18. Monteleone et al. (2019) [44] Italy	ED centre N = 177	100%	ANR (n = 41, M = 25.45, SD = 8.02) vs. BP (n = 59, M = 27.14; SD = 9.78) vs. Control (n = 77, M = 25.58, SD = 2.31)	3.1 ● 3.2 ● 3.3 ● 3.4 ● 3.5 ●	Parental Bonding Instrument	✓						Y
19. Pike et al. (2006) [54] USA	Database and advertisement N = 431 (Range = 18–40)	100%	BED (n = 162, M = 30.8, SD = 5.8) vs. Control (n = 162, M = 30.0, SD = 5.6) *** vs. BED (n = 107, M = 30.6, SD = 5.9) vs. PC (n = 107, M = 29.5, SD = 6.7)	3.1 ● 3.2 ● 3.3 ● 3.4 ● 3.5 ●	Oxford Risk Factor Interview	✓	✓	✓			✓	Y
20. Pike et al. (2008) [53] USA	Database and advertisement N = 150 (Range = 18–40)	100%	AN (n = 50, M = 26.70, SD = 6.23) vs. Control (n = 50, M = 26.56, SD = 5.51) vs. PC (n = 50, M = 27.02, SD = 6.05)	3.1 ● 3.2 ● 3.3 ● 3.4 ● 3.5 ●	Oxford Risk Factor Interview, Parental Bonding Instrument	✓	✓	✓	✓		✓	Y
21. Schmidt et al. (1993) [63] UK	ED treatment unit N = 203	99%	ANR (n = 64, M = 24.0, SD = 6.2) vs. ANB (n = 23, M = 24.7, SD = 6.9) vs. BN/Hx AN (n = 37, M = 23.6, SD = 5.3) vs. BN (n = 79, M = 24.4, SD = 5.4)	3.1 ● 3.2 ● 3.3 ● 3.4 ● 3.5 ●	Semi-structured interview	✓	✓	✓	✓		✓	Y
22. Striegel-Moore et al. (2005) [65] USA	Consumer database and advertisement N = 321 (Range = 18–40)	100%	BED (n = 107) vs. PC (n = 107) vs. Control (n = 107)	3.1 ● 3.2 ● 3.3 ● 3.4 ○ 3.5 ●	Oxford Risk Factor Interview	✓	✓		✓		✓	N

Table 2 Description of included studies, quality ratings of study methodologies and information on study findings (*Continued*)

Study information	Participant information			Quality	Details and findings reported	Findings						Abuse
Author (year) Country	Data source Total sample (age in years)	% female	Comparisons	MMAT	Measure of adversity	Adversity domain						(y/n)
						A1	A2	A3	A4	A5	A6	
23. Swanson et al. (2010) [67] UK	Inpatient treatment facility and university campus N = 119 (Range = 18–48)	100%	AN (n = 43, M = 24.67, SD = 6.81) vs. Controls (n = 76, M = 20.53, SD = 5.1)	3.1 ● 3.2 ● 3.3 ● 3.4 ○ 3.5 ●	Parental Bonding Instrument	✓						N
24. Tagay et al. (2014) [69] Germany	Inpatient clinic and private practice N = 103 (M = 29.11; SD = 10.53; range = 18–68)	100%	AN (n = 52; M = 28.32; SD = 11.67) vs. BN (n = 51; M = 29.88; SD = 9.34)	3.1 ● 3.2 ● 3.3 ● 3.4 ● 3.5 ●	Essen Trauma Inventory			✓				Y
25. Wade et al. (2007) [72] Australia	Twin Registry N = 1056 (M = 35; SD = 2.11; range 28–40)	100%	AN = 23 vs. BN = 20 vs. MD = 186 vs. Control = 393	3.1 ● 3.2 ○ 3.3 ● 3.4 ● 3.5 ●	Family Life Events interview, Oxford Risk Factor Interview, Parental Bonding Instrument, Revised Moos Family Environment Scale	✓	✓		✓			N
26. Webster & Palmer (2000) [74] UK	ED services, psychiatric unit of general hospital, general medical practices N = 160 (Range = 18–49)	100%	AN (n = 28, M = 29) vs. BN (n = 32; M = 30) vs. AN+BN (n = 20; M = 30) vs. MD (n = 40; M = 34) vs. Control (n = 40, M = 34)	3.1 ● 3.2 ● 3.3 ● 3.4 ● 3.5 ●	Childhood Experience of Care and Abuse Interview	✓	✓					Y

A1 = Adverse parenting style; A2 = Family disharmony; A3 = Loss of a family member, relative or someone close; A4 = Familial mental health issues; A5 = Family comments about weight, eating or appearance; A6 = Family disruptions
MMAT = Mixed Methods Appraisal Tool; N = number of participants in total sample; M = mean age; SD = standard deviation; range = age range; un. = unknown; n = number of participants in sub-samples; ● = yes; ○ = no; ◉ = can't tell
ED Eating disorder, AN anorexia nervosa, BN bulimia nervosa, BED binge eating disorder, AN+BN mixed anorexia and bulimia, ANR AN restrictive subtype, AN-BP AN binging/ purging subtype, BN-P BN purging subtype, BN-NP BN non-purging subtype, EDNOS Eating Disorder Not Otherwise Specified, BN/Hx AN BN with a history of AN, BNX BN with no history of AN, R-AN Recovered AN, ACOA adult children of alcoholics, Non-ACOA non adult children of alcoholics, ANB AN binge eating/purging type, sch. schizophrenia, PC psychiatric controls, BP bingeing-purging, MD major depression

Results
Study characteristics
Twenty-six studies reported on family-related non-abuse ALEs in the ED literature (see Table 2), two of which were qualitative and the remaining were quantitative. The quantitative studies consisted of three descriptive/ non-comparative studies and the remaining were observational/ comparative designs. The majority of studies were conducted in the UK (n = 7), followed by USA (n = 6), Italy (n = 4), Portugal (n = 3) and The Netherlands (n = 2), with only one study being conducted in each of Canada, Australia, Germany and Austria. The vast majority of these studies included female only samples (n = 21), however there was one study which included males only, one study whereby the gender of participants was not noted and three others which included 49, 94 and 99% female samples. The majority of the studies included mixed ED samples (n = 15), four studies included BED only samples, four studies included AN only samples, and three included BN only samples.

Methodological quality of included studies
Twelve of the included studies met full criteria as assessed using MMAT, 10 studies met four of five criteria, and the remaining four studies obtained three of five criteria. No studies obtained fewer than three of five criteria. The limitations of the studies which obtained three of five criteria (n = 4) were identified during the synthesis of findings below so that results can be interpreted with caution by the reader.

Findings on research question 1: family-related non-abuse ALEs occurring for adults with ED as reported in previous literature
Across the 26 studies, family-related non-abuse ALEs could be grouped under six broad subheadings: adverse parenting style; family disharmony; loss of a family member, relative or someone close; familial mental health issues; family comments about eating or weight, shape and appearance; and disruptions in family structure. Twenty-one of these 26 studies reported findings on abuse.

Findings on research question 2: differences between people with EDs and non-clinical controls in relation to family-related non-abuse ALEs
Parenting style
Generally, ED groups demonstrated less favourable parent-child interactions during childhood compared to control groups, with evidence suggesting lack of care/ lack of affection/ increased parental indifference for people with AN [15, 44, 67], BN [10, 25, 44, 74] and mixed ED diagnoses [39, 74]. In contrast, Webster and Palmer [74] showed no differences between AN and

control groups, and similarly Wade et al. [72] demonstrated no differences between AN, BN and control groups in terms of parental care. Two studies investigated these same parent variables by comparing adults with EDs to their siblings without EDs. Lehoux & Howe [36] showed that there were no differences in levels of parental affection between those with BN and sibling controls. Wade et al. [72] showed no differences between people with AN or BN and their unaffected twin comparisons for maternal care, but showed that people with BN experienced greater levels of paternal care than their unaffected twin comparisons.

Some studies demonstrated that those diagnosed with AN [15, 44, 72] and BN [36, 44] showed greater levels of parental over-control/overprotection when compared to non-clinical controls. However there was also evidence of the contrary, that there were no differences in levels of parental control for those with AN [10, 67, 74], BN [10, 25, 72, 74] or a mixed AN and BN group (i.e. AN/ BN [74];) when compared to control participants.

In terms of other parenting factors, those with AN reported greater levels of paternal and maternal parenting problems [53] and higher parental demands [53]; people with BN (but not AN) reported greater levels of parental criticism [25, 72]; and people with general ED diagnoses reported lower quality relationships with fathers [39] when compared to controls. Wade et al. [72] reported no differences in relation to parental expectations between people with AN or BN and controls [72] whereas Gonçalves et al. [25] reported higher rates among those with BN compared to controls.

Family disharmony
Studies showed that rates of unresolved/ unaddressed family disagreements were higher among those with AN [38] and BN [25]; rates of witnessing inter-parental violence as well as perceived parental marital dissatisfaction were higher for those with general EDs [39]; and rates of family discord were higher for those with AN [53], BN and AN/BN (but not AN) [74], when compared to control participants. Boumann and Yates [5] showed that the odds of having divorced parents was 4.9 times higher for those with BN compared to controls. Machado et al. [38] failed to find differences between ED and control participants in terms of parental arguments, participant arguments with parents, arguments within the home and sibling rivalry. Moreover, Wade et al.'s [72] study which employed three different designs within their research (i.e. Design 1 = Diagnostic group comparisons; Design 2a = Monozygotic twin pairwise comparisons; Design 2b = Monozygotic twin case control) demonstrated conflicting findings with Design 2b suggesting that people with AN experience greater levels of parental conflict

compared to controls and the other designs reporting no differences.

Loss

Pike et al. [54] demonstrated that people with BED reported more loss compared to controls whereas Pike et al. [53] reported that rates of loss did not differ between those with AN compared to controls.

Familial mental health issues

It was demonstrated that individuals with BN experienced higher rates of parental psychiatric disorder, major depression, personality disorders [5] and familial depression [25] compared to controls, but that rates of alcoholism [5, 25] or drug abuse [25] did not differ between the two groups. Machado et al. [38] also demonstrated no differences between their AN and control groups in relation to either family alcoholism or parental alcoholism. With a different design compared to other studies, Cuijper et al. [16] provided evidence that being an adult son of a parent with alcohol dependence was associated with ED psychopathology compared to adult sons of a parent without alcohol dependence, but that there were no differences between daughters of parents with or without alcohol dependence. However, these results should be interpreted with caution as authors measured parental alcohol dependence via self-report rather than using a standardised measure, and there was limited information on the demographics of study populations making it difficult to generalise findings. It was demonstrated that rates of familial EDs were higher for those with AN [38] and BN [25] compared to control families, however Pike et al. [53] showed that rates of familial AN and BN did not differ between their AN and control samples.

Family comments about eating, or weight, shape and appearance (i.e. physical appearance)

Machado et al. [38] demonstrated that there were no differences between their AN and control groups in terms of family comments about physical appearance. However, other studies demonstrated that individuals with AN [72] as well as those with BN [25, 72] experienced more parental comments about physical appearance when compared to a control group. Regarding comments about amounts eaten, increased rates of these sorts of comments were shown for those with AN [38, 72] as well as BN [72] when compared to control groups, but Gonçalves et al. [25] found no differences in family comments about eating between their participants with BN and controls.

Disruptions in family structure

Individuals with BED [54], but not those with AN [53], experienced more members leaving or joining the family structure (e.g. sibling being born, parents leaving home etc.) when compared to controls. There were no differences between individuals with BN and controls in relation to changes in parental figures [25].

Summary of ED vs. control findings

Greater levels of loss and family disruptions were experienced by those with BED compared to controls. There was evidence to suggest greater levels of family comments about physical appearance and eating for those with AN and BN compared to controls, but caution is warranted as not all studies supported this finding consistently. Although there are numerous studies suggesting a parental lack of care and over-control for people with EDs compared to controls, there is also a minority of studies suggesting no differences, implying a need for research to confirm these findings. Other parenting factors such as parental demands and criticisms appear to impact those with EDs compared to controls, but these findings must be replicated in order for them to be confirmed. Findings on family disharmony (i.e. family discord and disagreements) and familial mental health (i.e. familial ED and alcoholism) are inconclusive due to conflicting findings among included studies.

Findings on research question 3: differences between people with EDs and psychiatric controls in relation to family-related non-abuse ALEs

Parenting style

Wade et al.'s [72] study demonstrated no differences between participants with AN or BN and major depression (MD) regarding parental care or control. Similarly, Gonçalves et al. [25] showed no differences between their participants with BN and psychiatric controls in terms of parental non-involvement. Webster and Palmer [74] demonstrated that there were no differences between four groups (AN, BN, AN/BN and depression) in terms of parental control, but that people with depression had higher levels of parental indifference and reported a lack of parental care compared to those with AN (but not BN or mixed AN/BN). In terms of other parental variables, it was demonstrated that people with AN and BN had higher levels of parental criticism than those with MD; that those with BN (but not AN) had higher levels of parental expectations when compared to psychiatric controls [25, 72], and that those with AN [53] and BED [65] reported higher levels of parental demands compared to psychiatric controls.

Family disharmony

Family discord was shown to be greater for those with AN [53] and BED [65] as compared to other psychiatric disorders. Similarly, higher rates of unresolved/ unaddressed family disagreements was reported for those with BN compared to psychiatric controls [25] and a trend towards a significant difference was demonstrated for those with AN compared to psychiatric controls [38]. In contrast, other studies reported no differences between those with ED versus psychiatric controls in terms of family discord (BN = AN/BN = AN = depression [74];), arguments with parents [38], sibling rivalry [38] and parental conflict [72].

Loss
No differences in loss were established between people with BED [54] or AN [53] compared to psychiatric controls. Across two other studies, rates of loss of a family member were reported at 17% for people with BED compared to 0–9% for people with obesity and schizophrenia, as well as AN-restrictive, AN-binge/purge and BN [17, 18]. However, the authors commented that values were too low to conduct statistical analysis and so these findings were not tested for statistical significance. It also must be noted that the methodological quality of these studies was weakened due to the measures used and a lack of consideration of confounding variables, as assessed using MMAT criteria.

Familial mental health issues
It was demonstrated that individuals with AN [38] and BN [25] had higher rates of familial ED compared to psychiatric controls, however Pike et al. [53] reported that rates of familial AN and BN did not differ between their AN and psychiatric control samples. Pike et al.'s [53] study showed that parental mood and substance disorder were experienced by those with AN and psychiatric controls combined more than controls, but that there were no differences between the AN and psychiatric control groups.

Family comments about eating, or weight, shape and appearance (i.e. physical appearance)
Machado et al. [38] demonstrated no differences between their AN and psychiatric control groups in terms of family comments about physical appearance or eating. However, it was demonstrated that individuals with BN experienced more comments about physical appearance [25, 72] and that people with both BN and AN experienced more comments about eating [72] when compared to psychiatric comparison groups.

Disruptions in family structure
Individuals with BED [54], but not those with AN [53], experienced more members leaving or joining the family structure compared to psychiatric controls. Striegel-Moore et al. [65] demonstrated that a mixed group of individuals with BED and psychiatric controls together reported higher ratings of parental separation when

compared with controls, but no differences were shown between BED and psychiatric control groups. There were no differences between individuals with BN and psychiatric controls in relation to changes in parental figures [25].

Summary of ED versus psychiatric control findings
There is evidence to suggest higher levels of adverse parenting styles such as parental demands and criticism among people with EDs compared to psychiatric controls. Findings also suggest that people with BED experienced more members leaving or joining family structure compared to psychiatric controls. Further replication of these findings is required before drawing any strong conclusions. Findings on family disharmony are inconclusive, with some studies suggesting that this adversity is reported by those with EDs more than those with psychiatric controls, particularly for family dissonance (i.e. discord and disagreements), but there were also findings to suggest no differences between the groups. There was some evidence that family comments about physical appearance and comments about eating are reported more for those with BN compared to psychiatric controls, but there were conflicting findings regarding whether this adversity was experienced by those with AN more than psychiatric controls. Loss and family mental health issues were not experienced by those with EDs more than psychiatric control groups. There was some evidence to suggest that family mental health issues might be associated with psychiatric disorders in general, but not ED specific. Parental care and parental control findings mostly suggest no differences between ED and psychiatric control groups, with some evidence that parental indifference might be more significant to those with depression than AN.

Findings on research question 4: differences among ED subgroups in relation to family-related non-abuse ALEs
Parenting style
Studies on parenting style consistently demonstrated that people with BN experience poorer child-parent interactions compared to those with AN. Webster and Palmer [74] showed that people with BN reported increased levels of parental indifference and a greater lack of care compared to their AN counterparts, but the groups did not differ in terms of control (over- or under-control). Similarly, Schmidt [63] assessed differences between the childhood experiences of four groups of ED participants including restricting AN, bulimic AN, BN with a history of anorexia and normal-weight BN, and demonstrated that normal-weight BN patients had experienced higher levels of parental indifference and over-control (but not under-control) than the other three groups. Monteleone et al. [44] demonstrated no

differences between their AN restricting and bingeing-purging (BP) subgroups in relation to parental care or control, however it must be noted that the BP group consisted of people with both AN and BN diagnoses. Moreover, Connan [15] demonstrated no differences in parental indifference between active versus recovered AN groups, but because rates were higher in both these groups compared to controls, it can be concluded that these negative parental styles may occur for people with AN regardless of whether they recover or not.

Family disharmony
Findings showed that there were no differences in rates of family conflicts between a BED and BN group [19] and there were no differences in rates of family discord between those with AN and BN [74]. However, Schmidt et al. [63] showed that a normal-weight BN group reported a trend towards higher levels of intrafamilial discord compared to the restricting AN, bulimic AN or BN with a history of anorexia groups [63].

Loss
In terms of ED subgroup comparisons, loss was assessed as a precipitating factor in two of the studies, with Degortes et al. [19] having demonstrated that participants with BED reported more bereavements in the 6 months preceding ED onset compared to BN comparisons, and Manwaring et al. [40] having shown that a binge-first (i.e. bingeing symptoms began before dieting) group of BED participants were more likely to report having lost someone close to them in the year preceding ED onset when compared to a diet-first group (i.e. dieting symptoms began before bingeing). These studies considered the temporal sequencing of loss and ED onset, with findings suggesting that loss preceded bingeing behaviours, and therefore presents itself as a likely risk factor for the later onset of an ED, specifically BED. When comparing samples of those with AN and BN, Tagay et al. [69] demonstrated no statistical differences in relation to number of deaths experienced, however they reported that death of a close person or family member was considered the most traumatic form of life event by both groups, over-and-beyond other forms of adverse experiences including abuse/assault, imprisonment, natural disasters or having been involved in accidents such as a fire.

Parental mental health issues
Schmidt et al. [63] demonstrated that there were no differences between ED subgroups (i.e. restricting AN, bulimic AN, BN with a history of anorexia and BN) in relation to the frequency of maternal or paternal mental health difficulties.

Family comments about eating, or weight, shape and appearance (i.e. physical appearance)
None of the original studies included in this review conducted analyses on ED subgroup differences for this adversity subtype and so no findings can be reported here.

Disruptions in family structure
ED subgroup comparisons showed that individuals with BED experienced more separation from family members in the 6 months preceding ED onset than those with BN [19]. Schmidt et al. [63] analysed comparisons in four ED subgroups (i.e. restricting AN, bulimic AN, BN with a history of anorexia and BN) and showed that the three BN groups had 3 or more total changes in family arrangements (e.g. boarding school, adoption, parental separation, parental death and other) compared to the AN-restricting group, with parental separation being the most commonly reported reason for these changes.

Summary of ED subgroup findings
There was evidence to suggest that loss of someone close is linked to the later onset of bingeing behaviour/BED and therefore might pose an ED risk, due to the consideration of temporal sequencing in the studies which assessed their relationship. Similarly, findings on separation of family members and parental separation also demonstrated that this adversity is reported more often for those with BED than BN, and more often for those with BN than AN, suggesting that perhaps the bingeing behaviours involved in BN and BED might result from people's attempt to cope with these specific family adversities. Findings suggested that those with BN experience more negative parent-child interactions compared to those with AN in the form of parental indifference, in particular. Family disharmony or parental mental health issues did not appear to be associated with any particular ED subgroup. No ED subgroup analyses were conducted on family comments about eating or physical appearance and so no conclusions can be draw about this variable in terms of ED subgroup specificity.

Discussion
Summary of research aims and findings
The aim of the current systematic review was to identify the various forms of family-related non-abuse ALEs reported to have occurred for adults diagnosed with EDs. The four specific research questions were 1) What were the various family-related non-abuse ALEs reported to have occurred for adults with EDs? 2) What differences in these ALEs were reported by those with EDs compared to non-clinical samples? 3) What differences in these ALEs were reported by those with EDs compared to other psychiatric control groups? And 4) What differences in these ALEs were reported between the various

ED subgroups (i.e. AN vs. BN vs. BED)? Six types of family-related non-abuse ALEs were reported in the ED literature, which included adverse parenting style; family disharmony; loss of a family member, relative or close person; familial mental health issues; family comments about eating or physical appearance; and disruptions in family structure. This is the first systematic review in the ED literature to identify adversities other than abuse which may impact people with EDs. Findings on these adversities will be summarised and discussed as per the remaining research questions.

Differences between ED versus control groups

There was evidence to suggest that experiences of loss [54], family disruptions [54] and family comments about amounts eaten [38, 72] occurred more often for people with EDs compared to control participants. However, it must be noted that there was more consistent support for these findings for those with BED and BN compared to AN, and that replication studies are necessary in order to confirm these findings. However, these findings were not surprising considering the association that has been established between ALEs and various mental health issues (e.g. [24, 33, 41, 58]), suggesting a potential role of family-related non-abuse ALEs in the trajectory of EDs. Findings were more inconclusive for other variables such as family disharmony, familial mental health and parenting style. Studies investigating these variables were limited and conflicting findings were demonstrated among included studies, suggesting a need for further research on these adversities.

Differences between ED versus psychiatric control groups

There was evidence that adverse parenting styles in the forms of parental demands and criticism [53, 65, 72] occur for those with EDs more than psychiatric controls; that people with BN [25, 72] but not those with AN [38, 72] experienced more parental comments about weight when compared to psychiatric controls; and that those with BED [54] but not AN [53] experienced more family disruptions in the form of family members leaving or joining the family structure compared to psychiatric controls. Replication studies are required to provide confirmation of these findings, though they provide tentative evidence of ED-specific family adversities. Again, these findings might suggest a relationship between family problems with BN and BED over-and-beyond AN.

Findings on loss were consistent, demonstrating no differences in rates of loss between those with AN or BED and psychiatric control participants [53, 54], suggesting that loss may be a non-specific adversity experienced by people with psychiatric difficulties in general compared to the general population. In terms of parental mental health issues, it appeared that results were varied

depending on the type of mental health issues assessed. There was evidence to suggest that whereas familial mood, substance disorders and alcoholism might be general risk factors for various psychiatric illnesses [38, 53], parental EDs is associated with offspring ED but not other offspring psychiatric disorders [25, 38]. This finding is easily understood considering the "unequivocal evidence" of heritability of EDs, as suggested by Klump, Bulik, Kaye, Treasure & Tyson ([34], p.97), but it must be noted that Pike et al.'s [53] study failed to support this finding. However, Pike et al. [53] note that child-reporting of familial psychiatric illness might not fully capture true rates of the disorders that might exist within families. Findings on family disharmony (i.e. family discord and unresolved disagreements) were conflicting, resulting in an inability to draw conclusions on these variables.

Differences between ED subtypes

There was evidence to suggest that loss of someone close and separation of family members are linked to the later onset of bingeing behaviour and BED when compared to dieting behaviours or BN [19, 40]; that separations within families were reported more often for those with BED than BN [19], and more for those with BN than AN [63]; and that those with BN experienced more negative parent-child interactions compared to those with AN, particularly parental indifference [63, 74]. This again suggests that these family adversities are significant in the lives of those with BED and BN to a greater extent than people with AN. Finally, findings on family disharmony and parental mental health difficulties suggested that these variables were not specific to any ED subtype. Although the distinction of ED subtype differences is useful for clinical purposes, research confirming no differences between ED subtypes across multiple variables supports the transdiagnostic approach to working with EDs due to apparent indistinct features across ED subtypes [21, 23].

Considerations for the interpretation of results

Regarding the findings implying elevated rates of critical comments about physical appearance and eating for people with EDs, it must be considered that personal factors might also influence perception and subsequent reporting. For instance, research has suggested that people with EDs overvalue their body weight and shape [11, 22] and that people with EDs are prone to attentional biases to disorder salient stimuli (e.g. body size, food) that are perceived as potential threats [3]. This could impact recall bias whereby an ambiguous cue such as someone commenting on appearance might be interpreted in a more negative light due to its perceived threat for people with EDs. Alternatively, another consideration is that those with EDs may be accessing treatment that is oriented around increasing food intake and these comments are therefore likely to be elevated in such a setting. However, regardless of the purpose of the comments, previous research has demonstrated that such comments have been linked to adverse effects such as poorer self-esteem, lower perceived social support and larger perceived body size [70]. Similarly, caution must be advised in interpreting the finding that adverse parental styles were experienced by those with BN more than those with AN. Previous research has suggested that BN is associated with increased interpersonal sensitivity, including criticism and rejection sensitivities [26], so it must also be considered that increased reporting of these parenting styles might have been influenced by child perspectives and behaviours resulting from this increased sensitivity or poor attachment. This results in a difficulty in drawing conclusions on such results as the definition of ALEs suggests that these experiences be external and verifiable, and not internal or psychological [52, 57, 64].

A common finding evident across the research questions addressed was that these differences in family-related non-abuse ALEs were more prevalent for people with BN and BED than AN. It is therefore likely that the inclusion of AN groups in addition to other ED groups in studies assessing these questions in this current review may have impacted on or led to insignificant findings with regard to the two research questions relating to ED versus control and psychiatric control differences. Despite this, we can make the following inferences from these findings: that AN is less influenced by familial factors and that the trajectory of AN may be less connected to family environment of childhood upbringing when compared to BN or BED. This may provide an explanation for why family therapies demonstrate better efficacy for people with AN compared to other EDs due to more positive and intact family relations [31, 37]. Furthermore, the function of self-starvation, one of the hallmark symptoms of AN, has been associated with evading hurtful feelings, relational problems and high expectations in previous research [8, 48]. Starvation also leads to impairments of cognitive functioning, including memory and attention, for people with AN who are currently ill as well as weight-restored [45]. Therefore it must be considered that the lack of significant findings for the AN group in relation to non-abuse ALEs might reflect a buffering of such experiences as a consequence of functional avoidance of hurtful feelings or cognitive impairment impacting the accuracy of reporting. Despite this, this finding is in line with previous research which suggested that genetic influences are more significant for AN compared to BN [71]. Various authors have formed similar conclusions that individuals with BN and BED

might experience more family-related ALEs compared to those with AN (e.g. [63, 74]), and similarly, findings on abuse suggested a clear association between abuse with both BN and BED, but to a lesser extent with AN [12]. The common symptom of bingeing for BN and BED might explain this association as it has been previously described as a manifestation of greater reactivity to stress [27] and is positively related to poorer interpersonal problem solving skills [66], suggesting that bingeing may come about as a reaction to family-related problems or as a coping mechanism for dealing with such situations. However, careful consideration is warranted in deciding whether to focus on such family problems during treatment, as a focus on these can be counterproductive to recovery, especially when treatment involves engaging the family.

Implication of findings
There are a number of clinical implications stemming from the findings of this study, application of which would result in clinicians working from a trauma-informed perspective in line with recovery-oriented practice [7, 29, 73]. First, considering the relevance of adversity in the lives of people with EDs, clinicians may wish to use a life events checklist in order to assess for the presence of these adversities in the lives of their clients. For instance, if a person has experienced loss of a parent at a young age, experiential trauma-focussed work in combination with, prior to or subsequent to ED treatment may be effective. The order of treatment focus should be decided together with the client, in line with best practice recovery-oriented guidelines [14]. Second, according to the self-medication hypothesis, eating behaviours may serve a function for managing or avoiding trauma-related memories or cues [6]. Therefore, any attempts at removing or lessening such behaviours should take account of the function they serve so that people with EDs are not left without an alternative means to cope. Third, in relation to increased reporting of comments about weight or appearance, clinicians must take extra care of the language and choice of wording so as to minimise the risk of inadvertent re-traumatisation. Other treatment actions that should be carefully considered to avoid re-traumatisation include routine weighing and medical rescue interventions deemed aggressive and coercive, such as force feeding [7]. In summary, this trauma-informed approach to ED care should result in (i) a better understanding of the context of client's difficulties, (ii) a better selection of appropriate treatment types and onward referral if necessary, and (ii) a reduction of the risk of accidental re-traumatisation by service-providers [9].

Finally, findings from this review demonstrated that certain distinctions may exist between the three disorders (particularly for BN and BED versus AN), suggesting the need for research to investigate these disorders separately to allow for the identification of disorder-specific findings. This is not necessarily to say that this research cautions against the use of a transdiagnostic approach to ED treatment which has been proposed by many experts [22], but that at least from a research perspective, empirical findings relating to subtype similarities and differences can assist with identifying features of the three disorders which may be addressed from transdiagnostic perspectives versus those which are specific to an ED subtype. For instance, previous research has demonstrated that not all processes identified in the transdiagnostic CBT-E model operate in the same manner across ED subtypes, but that the model provides guidance for clinicians on a range of factors which may be important in the maintenance of any ED subtype [35]. Lampard et al. [35] conclude that an understanding of both transdiagnostic mechanisms and mechanisms specific to ED subtypes can inform clinical practice.

Quality of included studies

Included studies demonstrated good to excellent methodological quality as rated by MMAT, however studies were not without their limitations. All adversities were measured via retrospective self-report (i.e. standardised questionnaires, interviews etc.). Negative recall bias might skew results whereby individuals who are suffering with mental health issues may have a high tendency for threat detection [2] as well as a subjectively negative report of past experiences [4, 59]. Other issues regarding the methodologically weaker studies were mentioned previously, which include a lack of information on study demographics, small sample sizes, and a lack of consideration for confounding variables.

Strengths, limitations and future recommendations

This review was conducted in line with best practice guidelines including PRISMA [42] and Cochrane [62]. The study aimed to minimise bias through the use of multiple reviewers during the screening, extraction and analysis phases, with evidence of moderate to high interrater reliability throughout. This review had a broad focus which was beneficial in terms of providing a representative view of the current literature base on a topic of adversity that has not been systematically reviewed in the ED context to date.

However, the studies included were highly heterogeneous due to the inclusion of diverse research designs, measures of adversity and ED populations. Future research could aim to use meta-analytical approaches by narrowing the scope of the research question to focus on distinct forms of family-related non-abuse ALEs (e.g.

loss of family member). This might allow for the inclusion of further relevant studies which were not captured in the current search due to the broad research focus. Meta-analytical approaches would also help to determine whether the familial adversity is related to BN and BED more strongly than AN using statistical means. In terms of taxonomy, this review established correlates of EDs important for treatment considerations rather than risk, due to the lack of information on timing. As suggested by Jacobi et al. [30], reviews which aim to identify risk factors would benefit from establishing the interaction between biological and psychosocial factors, ideally through the utilisation of longitudinal design in place of retrospective cross-sectional designs. Furthermore, the use of ecological momentary assessment methods or other qualitative approaches would help reduce recall bias in the reporting of adversity, or similarly the use of informant reporting of events (e.g. sibling report). Literature published from 1980 onwards was reviewed in the current article, meaning that some relevant research published before this date may have been missed. The search was also restricted to articles in the English language only, which represents a potential selection bias as some authors may have published relevant findings which were not available for inclusion in this review. However, as the majority of studies appeared to be undertaken in the US and UK, we estimate that this risk of bias would be low. Furthermore, as DSM criteria for EDs have changed throughout the years, there may be issues relating to the classification of ED subtypes inherent in this research. As can be seen from the findings reported, older studies use terminology to describe EDs that do not exist today, and may result in an overlap of symptom presentations across ED subtypes. As the classification of mental disorders is ever-changing, there is strong encouragement through the research framework, Research Domain Criteria (RDoC), that future research should focus on symptoms rather than the categorisation of symptoms in investigating mental health disorders to overcome this issue. Finally, future research should investigate adversities occurring in those under age 18, which was beyond the scope of the current review.

Summary and conclusions

Overall, these findings help us understand the role of ALEs, above and beyond abuse, in the overall trajectory of EDs. This review confirmed, as hypothesised, that adults with EDs are subject to higher rates of various forms of family-related non-abuse ALEs compared to non-clinical samples, with findings on loss and disruptions of family structure providing most compelling evidence. The review identified potential ED-specific ALEs, such as parental demands and parental criticism, which may occur more frequently when compared to other psychiatric groups. ED subgroup findings suggest that those with BN and BED in particular, may experience a greater level of family-related non-abuse ALEs, such as loss, family separation and negative parent-child interactions compared to those with AN. Collectively, findings suggested that AN may be less influenced by psychosocial factors connected to family environment during childhood compared to BN and BED [63, 74]. These findings are important to consider for clinicians working from trauma-informed and recovery-oriented approaches in ED treatment, as they will help to form a clearer picture of client's difficulties and targets for intervention, which will benefit recovery outcomes.

Abbreviations
ACE: Adverse childhood experiences; ALE: Adverse life experiences; AN: Anorexia Nervosa; BED: Binge-eating disorder; BN: Bulimia Nervosa; BP: Bingeing-purging; DSM: Diagnostic and Statistical Manual of Mental Disorders; ED: Eating disorder; MD: Major depression; MMAT: Mixed Methods Appraisal Tools; OR: Odd ratio; PICOTS: Population, Intervention, Comparators, Outcome/exposure, Timing, Setting; PRISMA: Preferred Reporting Items for Systematic Review and Meta-Analyses; RDoC: Research Domain Criteria

Authors' contributions
The authors listed were the sole contributors of this manuscript, and all agreed for the manuscript to be submitted for publication. The authors read and approved the final manuscript.

Competing interests
The authors declare no competing interests.

Author details
[1]School of Psychology, University College Dublin, Dublin, Ireland. [2]Elm Mount Unit, St. Vincent's University Hospital, Dublin, Ireland.

References
1. American Psychiatric Association. Diagnostic and statistical manual of mental disorders. 3rd ed. Washington DC: APA press; 1980.
2. Arthur-Cameselle J, Sossin K, Quatromoni P. A qualitative analysis of factors related to eating disorder onset in female collegiate athletes and non-athletes. Eat Disorde. 2017;25(3):199–215. https://doi.org/10.1080/10640266.2016.1258940.
3. Aspen V, Darcy AM, Lock J. A review of attention biases in women with eating disorders. Cogn Emot. 2013;27(5):820–38. https://doi.org/10.1080/02699931.2012.749777.
4. Baumeister RF, Bratslavsky E, Finkenauer C, Vohs KD. Bad is stronger than good. Rev Gen Psychol. 2001;5(4):323.
5. Boumann CE, Yates WR. Risk factors for bulimia nervosa: a controlled study of parental psychiatric illness and divorce. Addict Behav. 1994; 19(6):667–75.
6. Brewerton TD. Posttraumatic stress disorder and disordered eating: food addiction as self-medication. J Women's Health. 2011;20(8):1133–4.
7. Brewerton TD. An overview of trauma-informed care and practice for eating disorders. J Aggress Maltreat Trauma. 2019;28(4):445–62.
8. Brockmeyer T, Holtforth MG, Bents H, Kämmerer A, Herzog W, Friederich H-C. Starvation and emotion regulation in anorexia nervosa. Compr Psychiatry. 2012;53(5):496–501.
9. Butler LD, Critelli FM, Rinfrette ES. Trauma-informed care and mental health. Dir Psychiatry. 2011;31(3):197–212.
10. Calam R, Waller G, Slade P, Newton T. Eating disorders and perceived relationships with parents. Int J Eat Disord. 1990;9(5):479–85.
11. Carr A, McNulty M. The handbook of adult clinical psychology: an evidence based practice approach. London: Routledge; 2016.
12. Caslini M, Bartoli F, Crocamo C, Dakanalis A, Clerici M, Carrà G. Disentangling the association between child abuse and eating disorders: a systematic review and meta-analysis. Psychosom Med. 2016;78(1):79–90 https://doi.org/10.1097/PSY.0000000000000233.
13. Cavelzani A. "What doesn't kill you makes you stronger" micro-trauma and dyadic expansion of consciousness. PiscoMed Publishing online, 1-7. 2018.
14. Commonwealth of Australia. A national framework for recovery-oriented mental health services: policy and theory. Canberra: Australian Health Ministers Advisory Council; 2013.
15. Connan F, Troop N, Landau S, Campbell IC, Treasure J. Poor social comparison and the tendency to submissive behavior in anorexia nervosa. Int J Eat Disord. 2007;40(8):733–9.
16. Cuijpers P, Langendoen Y, Bijl RV. Psychiatric disorders in adult children of problem drinkers: prevalence, first onset and comparison with other risk factors. Addiction. 1999;94(10):1489–98.
17. Dalle Grave R, Oliosi M, Todisco P, Bartocci C. Trauma and dissociative experiences in eating disorders. Dissociation. 1996;IX(4):274–81.
18. Dalle Grave R, Rigamonti R, Todisco P, Oliosi E. Dissociation and traumatic experiences in eating disorders. Eur Eat Disord Rev. 1996b;4(4):232–40.
19. Degortes D, Santonastaso P, Zanetti T, Tenconi E, Veronese A, Favaro A. Stressful life events and binge eating disorder. Eur Eat Disord Rev. 2014; 22(5):378–82. https://doi.org/10.1002/erv.2308.
20. Duarte C, Pinto-Gouveia J. The impact of early shame memories in Binge Eating Disorder: The mediator effect of current body image shame and cognitive fusion. Psychiat Res. 2017;258:511–517.
21. Fairburn CG. Eating disorders: the transdiagnostic view and the cognitive behavioral theory. In: Cognitive behavior therapy and eating disorders. New York: Guilford Press; 2008. p. 7–22, chapter xii, 324 pages.
22. Fairburn CG, Cooper Z, Shafran R. Cognitive behaviour therapy for eating disorders: a "transdiagnostic" theory and treatment. Behav Res Ther. 2003; 41(5):509–28.
23. Fairburn CG, Cooper Z, Shafran R, Wilson GT. Eating disorders: a transdiagnostic protocol; 2008.
24. Fergusson DM, Horwood LJ, Lynskey MT. Childhood sexual abuse and psychiatric disorder in young adulthood: II. Psychiatric outcomes of childhood sexual abuse. J Am Acad Child Adolesc Psychiatry. 1996;35(10):1365–74.
25. Gonçalves S, Machado BC, Martins C, Hoek HW, Machado PP. Retrospective correlates for bulimia nervosa: a matched case–control study. Eur Eat Disord Rev. 2016;24(3):197–205.
26. Hamann DM, Wonderlich-Tierney AL, Vander Wal JS. Interpersonal sensitivity predicts bulimic symptomatology cross-sectionally and longitudinally. Eat Behav. 2009;10(2):125–7.
27. Hilbert A, Vögele C, Tuschen-Caffier B, Hartmann AS. Psychophysiological responses to idiosyncratic stress in bulimia nervosa and binge eating disorder. Physiol Behav. 2011;104(5):770–7.
28. Hong QN, Pluye P, Fàbregues S, Bartlett G, Boardman F, Cargo M, et al. Mixed methods appraisal tool (MMAT), version 2018. Montreal: IC Canadian Intellectual Property Office, Industry Canada; 2018.
29. Jacob K. Recovery model of mental illness: a complementary approach to psychiatric care. Indian J Psychol Med. 2015;37(2):117.
30. Jacobi C, Hayward C, de Zwaan M, Kraemer HC, Agras WS. Coming to terms with risk factors for eating disorders: application of risk terminology and suggestions for a general taxonomy. Psychol Bull. 2004;130(1):19.
31. Jewell T, Blessitt E, Stewart C, Simic M, Eisler I. Family therapy for child and adolescent eating disorders: a critical review. Fam Process. 2016;55(3):577–94.
32. Kellermeyer L, Harnke B, Knight S. Covidence and Rayyan. J Med Libr Assoc. 2018;106(4):580.

33. Kessler RC, McLaughlin KA, Green JG, Gruber MJ, Sampson NA, Zaslavsky AM, et al. Childhood adversities and adult psychopathology in the WHO world mental health surveys. Br J Psychiatry. 2010;197(5):378–85 https://doi.org/10.1192/bjp.bp.110.080499.

34. Klump KL, Bulik CM, Kaye WH, Treasure J, Tyson E. Academy for eating disorders position paper: eating disorders are serious mental illnesses. Int J Eat Disord. 2009;42(2):97–103.

35. Lampard AM, Tasca GA, Balfour L, Bissada H. An evaluation of the transdiagnostic cognitive-behavioural model of eating disorders. Eur Eat Disord Rev. 2013;21(2):99–107.

36. Lehoux PM, Howe N. Perceived non-shared environment, personality traits, family factors and developmental experiences in bulimia nervosa. Br J Clin Psychol. 2007;46(1):47–66.

37. Lock J, Le Grange D. Family-based treatment: where are we and where should we be going to improve recovery in child and adolescent eating disorders. Int J Eat Disord. 2019;52(4):481–7.

38. Machado BC, Gonçalves SF, Martins C, Hoek HW, Machado PP. Risk factors and antecedent life events in the development of anorexia nervosa: a Portuguese case-control study. Eur Eat Disord Rev. 2014;22(4):243–51. https://doi.org/10.1002/erv.2286.

39. Mangweth B, Pope HG, Hudson JI, Olivardia R, Kinzl J, Biebl W. Eating disorders in Austrian men: an intracultural and crosscultural comparison study. Psychother Psychosom. 1997;66(4):214–21.

40. Manwaring JL, Hilbert A, Wilfley DE, Pike KM, Fairburn CG, Dohm FA, Striegel-Moore RH. Risk factors and patterns of onset in binge eating disorder. Int J Eat Disord. 2006;39(2):101–7.

41. McLafferty M, O'Neill S, Murphy S, Armour C, Bunting B. Population attributable fractions of psychopathology and suicidal behaviour associated with childhood adversities in Northern Ireland. Child Abuse Negl. 2018;77:35–45 https://doi.org/10.1016/j.chiabu.2017.12.015.

42. Moher D, Liberati A, Tetzlaff J, Altman DG, Group, P. Preferred reporting items for systematic reviews and meta-analyses: the PRISMA statement. PLoS Med. 2009;6(7):e1000097.

43. Molendijk ML, Hoek HW, Brewerton TD, Elzinga BM. Childhood maltreatment and eating disorder pathology: a systematic review and dose-response meta-analysis. Psychol Med. 2017;47(8):1402–16 https://doi.org/10.1017/S0033291716003561.

44. Monteleone AM, Ruzzi V, Patriciello G, Pellegrino F, Cascino G, Castellini G, Maj M. Parental bonding, childhood maltreatment and eating disorder psychopathology: an investigation of their interactions. Eating and Weight Disorders-Studies on Anorexia, Bulimia and Obesity. 2019;25:577–89.

45. Nikendei C, Funiok C, Pfüller U, Zastrow A, Aschenbrenner S, Weisbrod M, et al. Memory performance in acute and weight-restored anorexia nervosa patients. Psychol Med. 2011;41(4):829–38.

46. Noordenbos G, Oldenhave A, Muschter J, Terpstra N. Characteristics and treatment of patients with chronic eating disorders. Eat Disord. 2002;10(1):15–29.

47. Noltemeyer AL, Bush KR. Adversity and resilience: a synthesis of international research. Sch Psychol Int. 2013;34(5):474–87.

48. Nordbø RH, Espeset EM, Gulliksen KS, Skårderud F, Holte A. The meaning of self-starvation: qualitative study of patients' perception of anorexia nervosa. Int J Eat Disord. 2006;39(7):556–64.

49. Pace R, Pluye P, Bartlett G, Macaulay AC, Salsberg J, Jagosh J, Seller R. Testing the reliability and efficiency of the pilot mixed methods appraisal tool (MMAT) for systematic mixed studies review. Int J Nurs Stud. 2012;49(1):47–53.

50. Palmier-Claus J, Berry K, Bucci S, Mansell W, Varese F. Relationship between childhood adversity and bipolar affective disorder: systematic review and meta-analysis. Br J Psychiatry. 2016;209(6):454–9.

51. Palmisano GL, Innamorati M, Vanderlinden J. Life adverse experiences in relation with obesity and binge eating disorder: a systematic review. J Behav Addict. 2016;5(1):11–31 https://doi.org/10.1556/2006.5.2016.018.

52. Paykel ES. Life events, social support and depression. Acta Psychiatr Scand. 1994;89:50–8.

53. Pike KM, Hilbert A, Wilfley DE, Fairburn CG, Dohm F, Walsh BT, Striegel-Moore R. Toward an understanding of risk factors for anorexia nervosa: a case-control study. Psychol Med. 2008;38(10):1443–53.

54. Pike KM, Wilfley D, Hilbert A, Fairburn CG, Dohm FA, Striegel-Moore RH. Antecedent life events of binge-eating disorder. Psychiatry Res. 2006;142(1):19–29. https://doi.org/10.1016/j.psychres.2005.10.006.

55. Popay J, Roberts H, Sowden A, Petticrew M, Arai L, Rodgers M, et al. Guidance on the conduct of narrative synthesis in systematic reviews. A product from the ESRC methods programme Version, vol. 1; 2006. p. b92.

56. Racine SE, VanHuysse JL, Keel PK, Burt SA, Neale MC, Boker S, Klump KL. Eating disorder-specific risk factors moderate the relationship between negative urgency and binge eating: a behavioral genetic investigation. J Abnorm Psychol. 2017;126(5):481.

57. Rafanelli C, Roncuzzi R, Milaneschi Y, Tomba E, Colistro MC, Pancaldi LG, Di Pasquale G. Stressful life events, depression and demoralization as risk factors for acute coronary heart disease. Psychother Psychosom. 2005;74(3):179–84 https://doi.org/10.1159/000084003.

58. Raposo SM, Mackenzie CS, Henriksen CA, Afifi TO. Time does not heal all wounds: older adults who experienced childhood adversities have higher odds of mood, anxiety, and personality disorders. Am J Geriatr Psychiatry. 2014;22(11):1241–50 https://doi.org/10.1016/j.jagp.2013.04.009.

59. Ready RE, Weinberger MI, Jones KM. How happy have you felt lately? Two diary studies of emotion recall in older and younger adults. Cognit Emot. 2007;21(4):728–57.

60. Reid M, Wilson-Walsh R, Cartwright L, Hammersley R. Stuffing down feelings: Bereavement, anxiety and emotional detachment in the life stories of people with eating disorders. Health Soc Care Commun. 2020;28(3):979–987.

61. Riley JR, Masten AS. Resilience in context. In: Resilience in children, families, and communities. Boston: Springer; 2005. p. 13–25.

62. Ryan, R. (2013). Cochrane consumers and communication review group: data synthesis and analysis. Cochrane Consumers and Communication Review Group, available at: http://cccrg.cochrane.org (Accessed 8 Mar 2016). [Google Scholar].

63. Schmidt U, Tiller J, Treasure J. Setting the scene for eating disorders: childhood care, classification and course of illness. Psychol Med. 1993;23(3):663–72 https://doi.org/10.1017/S0033291700025447.

64. Serafini G, Muzio C, Piccinini G, Flouri E, Ferrigno G, Pompili M, et al. Life adversities and suicidal behavior in young individuals: a systematic review. Eur Child Adolesc Psychiatry. 2015;24(12):1423–46.

65. Striegel-Moore RH, Fairburn CG, Wilfley DE, Pike KM, Dohm F-A, Kraemer HC. Toward an understanding of risk factors for binge-eating disorder in black and white women: a community-based case-control study. Psychol Med. 2005;35(6):907–17.

66. Svaldi J, Dorn C, Trentowska M. Effectiveness for interpersonal problem-solving is reduced in women with binge eating disorder. Eur Eat Disord Rev. 2011;19(4):331–41.

67. Swanson H, Power K, Collin P, Deas S, Paterson G, Grierson D, et al. The relationship between parental bonding, social problem solving and eating pathology in an anorexic inpatient sample. Eur Eat Disord Rev. 2010;18(1):22–32.

68. Sweetingham R, Waller G. Childhood experiences of being bullied and teased in the eating disorders. Eur Eat Disord Rev. 2008;16(5):401–407.

69. Tagay S, Schlottbohm E, Reyes-Rodriguez ML, Repic N, Senf W. Eating disorders, trauma, PTSD, and psychosocial resources. Eat Disord. 2014;22(1):33–49. https://doi.org/10.1080/10640266.2014.857517.

70. Taylor CB, Bryson S, Doyle AAC, Luce KH, Cunning D, Abascal LB, et al. The adverse effect of negative comments about weight and shape from family and siblings on women at high risk for eating disorders. Pediatrics. 2006;118(2):731–8.

71. Treasure J, Schmidt U, Van Furth E. Handbook of eating disorders. West Sussex: Wiley Online Library; 2003.

72. Wade TD, Gillespie N, Martin NG. A comparison of early family life events amongst monozygotic twin women with lifetime anorexia nervosa, bulimia nervosa, or major depression. Int J Eat Disord. 2007;40(8):679–86.

73. Wand T. Recovery is about a focus on resilience and wellness, not a fixation with risk and illness. Aust N Z J Psychiatry. 2015;49(12):1083–4. https://doi.org/10.1177/0004867415614107.

74. Webster JJ, Palmer RL. The childhood and family background of women with clinical eating disorders: a comparison with women with major depression, or women without psychiatric disorder. Psychol Med. 2000;30(1):53–60 https://doi.org/10.1017/S0033291799001440.

19

"I'm truly free from my eating disorder": Emerging adults' experiences of FREED, an early intervention service model and care pathway for eating disorders

Rachel Potterton[1]* (iD), Amelia Austin[1], Michaela Flynn[1], Karina Allen[1,2], Vanessa Lawrence[1], Victoria Mountford[1,2,3], Danielle Glennon[2], Nina Grant[2], Amy Brown[2,4], Mary Franklin-Smith[5], Monique Schelhase[5], William Rhys Jones[5], Gabrielle Brady[6], Nicole Nunes[6], Frances Connan[6], Kate Mahony[7], Lucy Serpell[7,8] and Ulrike Schmidt[1,2]

Abstract

Background: Eating disorders (EDs) typically start during adolescence or emerging adulthood, periods of intense biopsychosocial development. FREED (First Episode Rapid Early Intervention for EDs) is a service model and care pathway providing rapid access to developmentally-informed care for emerging adults with EDs. FREED is associated with reduced duration of untreated eating disorder and improved clinical outcomes, but patients' experiences of treatment have yet to be assessed.

Objective: This study aimed to assess emerging adults' experiences of receiving treatment through FREED.

Method: This study triangulated qualitative data on participants' experiences of FREED treatment from questionnaires and semi-structured interviews. Participants were 106 emerging adults (aged 16–25; illness duration < 3 yrs) (questionnaire only = 92; interview only = 6; both = 8). Data were analysed thematically.

Results: Most participants reported psychological and behavioural changes over the course of treatment (e.g. reduction in symptoms; increased acceptance and understanding of difficulties). Participants identified five beneficial characteristics of FREED treatment: i) rapid access to treatment; ii) knowledgeable and concerned clinicians; iii) focusing on life beyond the eating disorder; iv) building a support network; v) becoming your own therapist.

Conclusion: This study provides further supports for the implementation of early intervention and developmentally-informed care for EDs. Future service model development should include efforts to increase early help-seeking.

Keywords: Eating disorders, Anorexia nervosa, Bulimia nervosa, Binge eating disorder, Early intervention

* Correspondence: rachel.h.potterton@kcl.ac.uk
[1]Institute of Psychiatry, Psychology and Neuroscience, King's College London, London, UK
Full list of author information is available at the end of the article

Plain English Summary

FREED is a service model and care pathway providing rapid access to developmentally-informed care for emerging adults with EDs in the United Kingdom (UK). Whilst previous studies have demonstrated FREED's effectiveness in reducing ED symptoms, it is also vitally important to also explore patients' experiences of receiving treatment through this service. To this end, we interviewed and / or collected questionnaire data from 106 emerging adults who had received treatment through FREED. The vast majority of participants reported that treatment had been helpful, and that they had experienced reductions in their symptoms and / or increased acceptance and understanding of their ED. They identified several aspects of treatment that were particularly helpful. Emerging adults reported that treatment had been provided rapidly and the clinicians were knowledgeable and concerned about their ED. Additionally, participants liked that treatment had focused on life beyond their ED and had helped them build a support network and become their own therapist. This study provides further evidence that service models such as FREED should be implemented widely.

Introduction

Incidence and prevalence of eating disorders (EDs) peak during late adolescence and emerging adulthood, periods of intense psychosocial development [1–6]. Mean age of onset for anorexia nervosa (AN), bulimia nervosa (BN) and other specified feeding and eating disorders (OSFED) is between 15 and 19 years, whilst binge eating disorder (BED) typically occurs slightly later, between 23 and 24 years [1, 2, 4, 7]. Approximately 14% of female and 4% of male university students (18–22 years of age) screen positive for clinically significant EDs, compared to 12-month prevalence estimates amongst the general population of 2.2% for women and 0.7% for men [6, 8].

Timely and effective ED treatment can prevent derailment of development, yet emerging adults' treatment needs are typically less well met than those of both adolescents and adults [9]. Emerging adults tend to present to specialist ED services with longer duration of untreated ED than adolescents and report less positive treatment outcomes and more negative treatment experiences [10–13]. There are likely several contributing factors to such shortfalls in existing services. In the UK and many other countries, patients receiving ED treatment are required to transition from child and adolescent ED services (CAEDS) to adult ED services (AEDS) at or around 18 years of age [14]. Many young people fall in the gap i.e. are discharged from CAEDs and choose not to seek a referral to AEDS from their GP [15, 16]. Additionally, in the UK statutory wait-time targets do not apply to adult services, and individuals aged 18 years or over wait longer than those aged under 18 years for treatment (NHS Royal College of [17–19]). Even when treatment is received, AEDS can present difficulties for emerging adults [10, 20, 21]. Incompatibility between the distinctive developmental needs of emerging adults and the culture of adult services may contribute to reluctance to access, dissatisfaction, disengagement, and poor clinical outcomes [22]. This incompatibility is particularly relevant to ED services, as there is a clear shift in treatment philosophy— primarily relating to how personal responsibility is understood and managed—in services for under 18s compared to ED services for 18 years and over [23].

First Episode Rapid Early Intervention for Eating Disorders (FREED) was developed as a service model and care package for 16 to 25-year-olds presenting for their first specialist treatment ("first-episode") with an ED of less than 3 years duration ("recent-onset") [24]. FREED aims to reduce the length of time between treatment-seeking and receipt of specialist evidence-based treatment, with most patients starting treatment within 4 weeks of referral to the service. FREED also adapts said treatment to the specific developmental needs of emerging adults, for instance by taking a flexible approach to appointment scheduling, increasing involvement of family/friends, and focusing on managing transitions (e.g. to university) [25]. The key characteristics of FREED compared to treatment as usual are outlined in more detail in Table 1.

FREED's effectiveness and scalability has been evaluated in a pilot study and in a larger scale study (FREED-Up), both using a similar pre-post quasi-experimental design comparing patients receiving FREED with similar patients seen in the same service(s) previously [26–29]. The single-centre pilot study found that FREED patients had a shorter duration of untreated ED and significantly better treatment uptake than controls [27]. Additionally, FREED anorexia nervosa patients (AN) showed significantly greater clinical improvement and reduced need for intensive additional treatment (inpatient, day-patient) up to 2 years later [26, 28]. The multi-centre FREED-Up study replicated these findings [29, 30].

Alongside quantitatively-based evaluation, it is vitally important to consider patients' experiences of treatment process and outcomes [31, 32]. Studies of treatment experience can provide insights into the "active ingredients" to achieve change and inform future improvement in service delivery and treatment, as well as assessing fidelity of implementation [31]. Qualitative methodologies are particularly well-suited to understanding phenomena from the individual's perspective, and are therefore well-placed to explore emerging adults' experiences of FREED [9]. This is the first study to use qualitative methodologies to explore patients' views of FREED, and indeed any ED early intervention service adapted to emerging adults' developmental needs.

Table 1 Comparison of FREED service model with treatment as usual (TAU) as delivered before the introduction of FREED (adapted from Fukutomi et al., [26])

Characteristic	Service Model	
	FREED	**TAU**
Target group	Prioritisation of patients aged 16–25 years old with duration of ED of less than 3 years	No prioritisation according to illness stage Priority determined by diagnosis and severity
Referral and engagement	Person-centred, user-friendly, flexible approach reaching out to young people and families	Barriers to access seen as useful gatekeeping / test of patient motivation
	Actively remove barriers to access	Initial appointment communicated via letter
	Engagement call within 48 h of referral from FREED clinician	Patient's responsibility to contact service prior to assessment
	Multiple methods of contact (e.g. text; emails)	Strict discharge policy if not engaging
	Flexible approach to initial and subsequent appointments (e.g. accommodating cancellations)	
Waiting times	Target of 2 weeks from referral to assessment and 4 weeks from referral to treatment	Statutory waiting time targets
Assessment	Assessment of biopsychosocial needs, including focus on young person's strengths and priorities	Assessment of biopsychosocial needs Assessment is separate from treatment
	Explore social media use as potential illness maintaining factor	Patient prepared to wait between assessment and treatment, focus on staying safe during this time
	Psychoeducation using personal feedback and information about malleable changes to brain, body and behaviour to encourage early action on change	Limited psychoeducation at assessment Variable involvement of family and friends
	Instil a sense of hope for recovery and at the same time of urgency of action to make changes now (e.g. through goal setting)	
	Assessment is seen as part of treatment	
	Active involvement of family and friends	
Treatment	Evidence-based psychological therapy tailored to stage of illness and emerging adulthood	One-size-fits-all; standard packages of evidence-based treatment determined by diagnosis and severity
	Early dietitian involvement with focus on nutritional change	Medical and dietetic input when necessary
	Emphasis on transitions (e.g. moving to university) with flexible, supportive transition arrangements to provide a safety net. If necessary, continuation of treatment via distance methods (e.g. email, skype) with joint management arrangements with university-based services	Variable focus on nutritional change. Variable family involvement. Variable use of technology. Discharge to other services at transition of care
	Encourage joint sessions (e.g. with a family member)	

Study aim

To assess emerging adults' experiences of receiving treatment for their ED through FREED, a service model and care pathway providing rapid access to developmentally-informed care for emerging adults with first-episode, recent-onset EDs.

Method

Design

This research was embedded within the FREED-Up study, which was granted approval by the relevant ethics committees. It used a qualitative design, informed by a critical realist philosophical framework [33, 34]. Critical realism occupies a middle-ground between positivist and constructivist paradigms and is therefore interested both in empirical descriptions of phenomena (e.g. patients' descriptions of their treatment experiences), and in considering how the broader social context may impinges on and construct those descriptions. Critical realism is

particularly well-suited to studies related to clinical interventions, as increased understanding of both experiences and their construction can suggest targets for intervention development. Data from semi-structured interviews were triangulated with questionnaire-based data to develop a comprehensive understanding of patient experiences [35].

Participants

Participants for this research were drawn from the FREED-Up study, which focused on the continued evaluation of the effectiveness and scalability of the FREED service model (see [25, 29] for further details). The FREED-Up study included 278 emerging adults (18–25 years old) with first-episode, recent-onset (< 3 years) (as ascertained by a structured onset interview) DSM-5 EDs (AN, BN, BED or OSFED) who presented for treatment at four specialist ED services in England between 2016 and 2018. The present study specifically focused on exploring emerging adults' experiences of receiving treatment through FREED.

Procedure
Questionnaires
All FREED-UP study participants who received the FREED intervention (N = 278) completed detailed online questionnaires at 3, 6, and 12 months post-entry to the study. As part of these questionnaires, participants were asked optionally at 6 and 12 months "If you would like to share something about your experience with the FREED early intervention service please feel free to write this below. If not please move onto the next section." 100 participants (36%) responded at both or either time-points.

Semi-structured interviews
Selected FREED-Up study participants were informed of the opportunity to participate in an optional interview by phone or email by one researcher (RP). Potential participants were told that the study was about their experiences of getting help and receiving treatment for their ED. No time-limit was placed on consideration of participation. A purposive sampling strategy was used; this involves identification and selection of participants who are likely to be especially knowledgeable or provide diverse perspectives on the phenomenon of interest [36]. In practice, the researcher accessed existing FREED-Up demographic and clinical data and approached participants with characteristics of putative relevance to the research question (e.g. age; diagnosis; gender, ethnicity; living situation, geographic location). Participants were made aware that participation was voluntary, and their decision to participate (or not) would not affect their care or treatment in any way. The researcher also emphasised that both positive and negative experiences were of interest. No monetary incentive was offered for participation. Estimated sample size was informed by the approximate number of participants required in previous comparable studies of emerging adults' ED care experiences (i.e. between 15 and 20 participants) [10, 37]. However, recruitment continued until saturation; that is, until the themes devised in concurrent data analysis had been fully explored and new data were easily accommodated within them. In total, 45 emerging adults were approached to participate to reach the final sample size of 14 (31%).

Semi-structured interviews were conducted on a one-to-one basis by RP (a PhD researcher with a psychology background) either over the phone (71%) or in person. RP was not involved in treatment of study participants and had no prior relationship to participants. Care was taken to establish rapport and promote open discussion over the phone (e.g. ensuring the participant was in a private location). Interviews were structured around a topic guide, which was developed by RP. The topic guide was informed by evidence-based conceptualisations of FREED and emerging adulthood, and focused on exploring patients' experiences of their treatment and its impact (see Appendix for interview topic guide). The topic guide was used flexibly and revised iteratively. The average length of the interview was 33 min. All interview audio was recorded and transcribed verbatim. All identifying information was removed at point of transcription.

Data analysis
Quantitative data was analysed using SPSS software, version 26. Qualitative data from both questionnaires and semi-structured interviews were analysed collectively. Data analysis was undertaken concurrently with data collection using NVivo version 10. Data analysis used the six steps of thematic analysis [38](see Table 2). Consistent with the critical realist framework, the study used a primarily deductive yet flexible coding process. Coding was therefore informed by existing theory and literature on FREED and emerging adults' experiences of ED treatment [33]. For example, it was expected that participants would report positive experiences of the short waiting-times characteristic of FREED and this was reflected in the initial coding frame. However, coding was not constrained by such expectations, and codes were deleted, reconceptualised, and added as required. Steps three, four and five of the thematic analysis process focused on exploring latent themes i.e. underlying ideas, assumptions and conceptualisations which shape or inform emerging adults' descriptions of their treatment experiences [33, 38]. For instance, care was taken to consider the ways in which broader societal discourses about EDs impinged on and constructed participants' descriptions. The dataset was repeatedly reviewed and discussed by the authors to ensure the emerging themes fit with the original data. Researchers also reflected upon their own personal and professional perspectives to increase awareness of/minimise how these beliefs shaped data analysis.

Results
Participant characteristics
The final study sample consisted of 106 participants (questionnaire = 92; interview = 6; both questionnaire and interview = 8) (see Table 3 for summary of participant characteristics, compared to those who did not provide qualitative data). All participants were emerging adults (16–26 years old) with first-episode, recent-onset (< 3 years) DSM-5 EDs (AN, BN, BED or OSFED), and had received treatment through FREED at four specialist ED services in England between 2016 and 2018.

Table 2 Steps of thematic analysis

Step	Process
1. Familiarization with data	Transcribe; read and re-read data-set; note down initial ideas
2. Generation of initial codes	Code data-set
3. Search for themes	Collate codes into potential themes
4. Review themes	Check themes against coded extracts and the entire data set; generate a thematic map
5. Define and name themes	Refine the specifics of each theme; generate clear names and definitions
6. Write up	Select and analyse quotations; write a report of the analysis

Thematic analysis

One theme regarding psychological and behavioural changes which the participants had noticed and attributed to the treatment process was identified. Additionally, five themes relating to features of the treatment process were identified. A thematic map is presented in Fig. 1. The data were examined for differences according to participant characteristics (e.g. diagnosis; stage of treatment, data collection time-point [6 months vs. 12 months]), but these did not appear to be associated with differences in the themes identified. Data collection method (interview vs. questionnaire) did appear to be associated with themes identified, such that questionnaire responses tended to relate to treatment impact (i.e. theme 1), whereas the theme related to treatment process was largely derived from the interview data.

Psychological and behavioural change

The majority of participants (~75% of those providing questionnaire data) reported noticeable psychological and behavioural changes over the course of treatment. All such changes were positively-framed; no participants reported negative treatment-related change. About one-third of participants described dramatic changes (e.g. describing themselves as "recovered", or treatment as "life-changing").

"Comparing myself now to myself at the beginning of [treatment] is like night and day." (James, questionnaire)

Other participants were positive about treatment, but more hesitant about the progress they had made. They expressed beliefs that treatment had been an important step in an ongoing journey towards recovery.

"I may not be completely healed... but I don't feel like the ED is controlling me anymore." (Gaia, questionnaire)

"I have so far to go still but I have also come so far." (Jenny, questionnaire)

A small minority (~3%) of participants believed treatment was not associated with change but did not tend to elaborate on their beliefs.

"Although I am grateful to have received treatment quickly, I don't feel that it has been helpful so far." (Amelia, questionnaire)

Some of those reporting changes elaborated on the specific nature of these. About 10% of those providing questionnaire data explicitly commented upon reduction of symptoms (e.g. preoccupation with weight and shape, bingeing, purging, restriction) or related improvements in their physical health over the course of treatment.

"I look back at the last 28 days and how little my eating disorder behaviours have shown up. I have not purged once, and binge-eating thoughts take up a lot less of my time." (Luke, questionnaire)

More commonly (about one-quarter of those providing questionnaire data), participants commented on how treatment had changed their perspective on their ED. Many participants described accepting that they had an ED, and increased understanding of their difficulties.

"I'm finally coming to terms with having an eating disorder." (Zira, questionnaire).

"I have learned lots about my condition." (Lydia, questionnaire)

Many participants described how therapy helped them understand their ED as a coping mechanism for stress and difficult emotions. This enabled them to adopt more adaptive strategies when struggling.

"I have gained skills that I can sometimes apply to cope with difficult situations." (Briana, questionnaire)

Some participants (~15%) described how treatment helped them understand that their ED was not who they were. Participants described how treatment helped them build an identity separate from their ED.

"[treatment] helped me to see that, although my eating disorder had infiltrated into all aspects of my life, it wasn't who I was." (Amy, questionnaire)

Table 3 Participant (and non-participant) demographics at first specialist contact

	FREED-UP participants with experience data (interview and/or questionnaire) (N = 106)	FREED-Up participants with experience data (interview) (N = 14)	FREED-Up participants with no experience data (N = 172)
Age (M ± SD)	20.75 ± 2.56*	20.86 ± 1.99	19.84 ± 2.20*
DUED (M ± SD)	18.62 ± 10.69	21.50 ± 10.55	17.36 ± 10.18
BMI (M ± SD)	20.06 ± 4.63	18.87 ± 3.23	20.11 ± 4.33
EDE-Q score (M ± SD)	4.16 ± 1.10	4.53 ± 0.72*	4.03 ± 1.28*
Gender (% female)	92.5%	93%	93.6%
ED Diagnosis			
AN	38.7%	35.7%	44.2%
BN	31.1%	35.7%	22.7%
BED	0.9%	7.1%	1.2%
OSFED	29.2%	21.4%	32.0%
Ethnicity			
White	71.7%	71.4%	61.0%
Asian	6.6%	0%	11.6%
Black	1.9%	0%	5.2%
Mixed	4.7%	14.3%	8.7%
Other / Unspecified	9.4%	14.3%	10.3%
Occupation			
Student	58.3%	50.0%	67.9%
Employed	35.9%	50.0%	20.8%
Unemployed	5.8%	0.0%	11.3%
Living Situation			
With family	42.5%	35.7%	58.7%
With friends / in halls	35.8%	50.0%	27.9%
With partner	5.7%	0.0%	4.1%
Alone	4.7%	0.0%	5.2%
Other / Unspecified	11.3%	14.3%	4.1%
Treatment			
Completion rate	84.9%	92.9%	57.6%
No. of sessions (M ± SD)	23.27 ± 12.87*	24.71 ± 10.36*	15.77 ± 11.63*

Asterisk indicates that these figures were significantly different at $p < 0.05$
Abbreviations: *AN* anorexia nervosa, *BED* binge eating disorders, *BMI* body mass index, *BN* bulimia nervosa, *DUED* duration of untreated eating disorder, *EDE-Q* Eating Disorder Examination Questionnaire, *M* mean, *OSFED* other specified feeding and eating disorder, *SD* standard deviation

Relatedly, several participants described feeling freer, and more able to be themselves.

> *"It's such a relief to wake up in the morning not thinking about it, or throughout the day and at night. I have to be careful not to get too obsessive, but I do feel much freer."* (Zainab, questionnaire)

Several participants (~ 10%) described how since treatment they had been able to pursue goals and interests that were not weight or shape-related (e.g. university studies, travelling).

> *"[treatment] has changed my life and has got me back to university."* (Emma, questionnaire)

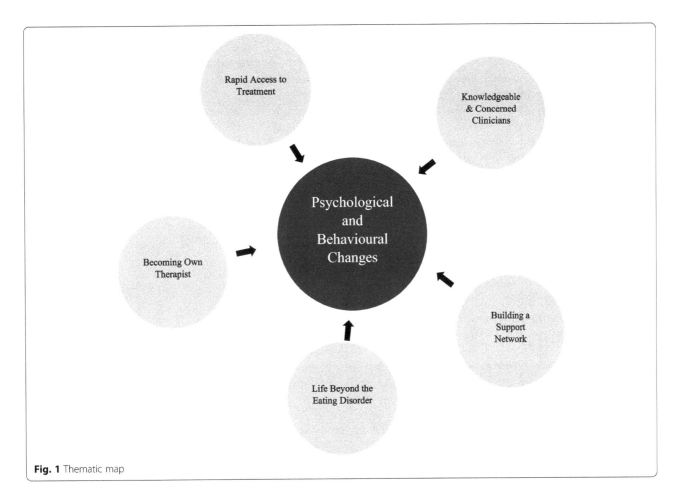

Fig. 1 Thematic map

"Thanks to FREED I managed to do my A-levels and thus maintain my prospects. Without this service it is likely my life would have been very different". (Lucy, questionnaire)

Of those who ascribed subtle changes to treatment, or did not believe treatment had helped them, some participants (~ 2% of those providing questionnaire data) felt they had been discharged from treatment before change had been achieved, and they felt hopeless and abandoned.

"I feel a sense of hopelessness. I was discharged a few months ago - because they felt there was nothing more they could do to help me, with my weight remaining the same, and my depression worsening." (Roisin, questionnaire)

More commonly, participants (~ 10%) identified that they came to treatment without any hope of recovery, and that FREED had instilled a sense of hope. Rather than feeling abandoned, they felt empowered and well-equipped to move forward in their recovery without a therapist.

"The FREED team have given me hope that I can make a full recovery." (Victoria, questionnaire)

"I still have a lot of work to do but I can see that I'm going somewhere now." (Chloe, questionnaire)

Treatment process

Five key themes relating to participants' experiences of treatment process were identified in the data: i) rapid access to treatment; ii) knowledgeable and concerned clinicians; iii) building a support network; iv) life beyond the ED; v) becoming own therapist. These themes were primarily derived from data collected via interview.

Rapid access to treatment About one-quarter of participants who provided questionnaire data identified that treatment had been provided quickly through FREED. Participants described this lack of wait positively and expressed positive attitudes towards the concept of "early intervention" more broadly.

"Early intervention is imperative. I'm at my healthy BMI now and feel great, ... just seven or eight *months from being at my lowest weight, heart rate, mental state."* (Georgia, questionnaire)

Many interviewed participants had anticipated a long wait for treatment upon referral to specialist services and described being pleasantly surprised or disbelieving when told they would shortly begin treatment. Several participants used words such as "lucky" or "fortunate" and reported feeling guilty or worried about others who did not receive treatment as quickly.

"I'm eternally grateful for [rapid access to treatment]... [it's] tinged with quite a bit of remorse I guess, for those people who weren't as fortunate." (Max, interview)

Participants reported beliefs that rapid access to treatment had been instrumental to their personal progress and/or was a positive thing more broadly, for several reasons.

Prevented behaviours becoming more engrained. Participants (~ 10%) expressed the belief that treatment had been provided at "just the right time" and believed that their difficult thoughts and behaviours would have become more engrained if they had to wait any longer for treatment.

"It's so hard to get out of that rut, but the less time you spend there in the first place the easier it is." (Georgia, questionnaire)

Several interviewed participants saw early intervention as preventing their eating difficulties becoming long-running issues.

"I'm like [to friends who are struggling] if you get help now you'll be fine, but if you wait it's going to be so hard, and you will never really be able to recover... it's something they will have to live with for the rest of their life." (Chloe, interview)

However, one interviewed participant expressed that - although they regarded the concept of early intervention positively - it did not happen early enough. At point of starting treatment, their difficult thoughts and behaviours were already engrained.

"Maybe I wasn't the best person to use it because, although it's the first time I've properly been willing to go through [treatment], ... I'd been dealing with it for quite a long time. I think that it needs quite newly-formed habits, that it might work a bit better because they're not as entrenched." (Gemma, interview)

Prevented deterioration of physical health. Participants (~ 10%) expressed the belief that their physical health would have deteriorated further if they had waited longer for treatment.

"If I had not seen my therapist as quick as I did, my bulimia would have continued, and I'd be in a much worse medical situation than I am now." (Daisy, questionnaire)

Both questionnaire and interview data indicated participants' beliefs that early intervention had been "life-saving" and believed they might not still be alive if they had not received care when they had.

"I would definitely be dead by now if I hadn't have received medical intervention." (Poppy, questionnaire)

Several participants described at interview how they had previously experienced long waiting lists for ED treatment and provided insight as to how that affected their physical health.

"There was a very long waiting period to getting help and, in the meantime, ... things were deteriorating pretty quickly.... five months is a long time to be malnourished for, so it's a big, big impact". (Max, interview)

Striking whilst the iron is hot. Several participants reported ambivalence and apprehensions about treatment when they were referred to specialist services. Participants believed rapid access to treatment had been important because they had limited time to reconsider their decision to get help.

"Initially, the denial and shame made me rethink my decision to get professional help but having early intervention meant that I was quickly in therapy and able to explore my doubts there." (Zira, questionnaire)

Indeed, one interviewed participant described her previous experience of changing their mind about engaging with treatment whilst waiting for it to be provided.

"It took a really long time.....by the time I did [get offered treatment], I kind of thought that...I was OK, and I didn't really want to go and I kind of just thought I can deal with this on my own." (Gemma, interview)

For several participants, ambivalence about receiving therapy was linked with beliefs that they were not "ill enough" to warrant treatment. Participants described that quick access to treatment validated their difficulties and facilitated the process of accepting the seriousness of their ED.

"It felt like the NHS was saying we understand that you are sick, we care, and we want to help now, you don't have to live like this, and that got me to my first appointment." (Zira, questionnaire)

Knowledgeable and concerned clinicians Several participants (10%) spoke positively of the professionals who had provided FREED treatment and identified them as an important contributor to the progress they had made.

"Please just tell [therapist name] I am eternally grateful for her help. She's a diamond." (Noah, questionnaire)

Several participants elaborated at interview that they believed that clinicians were highly knowledgeable about EDs, which made them feel safe and understood.

"I was more comfortable talking to the therapist at the eating disorder service...I think I just felt more kind of understood...I guess because they're used to talking to people...with similar problems, whereas GPs see everyone". (Sasha, interview)

Additionally, participants valued that clinicians expressed concern about the potential impact of their eating difficulties on physical health or achievement of life goals. Several participants described at interview how early appointments were characterised by a sense of urgency, emphasising that changes would need to be made early to prevent lasting damage.

"I was given an emergency meal plan, and all these vitamins and minerals to get, because I'd been underweight for quite a long time... and they were concerned about malnutrition." (Christina, interview)

These expressions of concern and the need for immediate change facilitated the process of accepting the seriousness of their condition, enhancing motivation to change.

"My therapist and the dietitian did give me a lot of information about...what malnutrition does to your brain...that did really help me to realise...I definitely don't want to be doing this to my brain." (Gaia, interview)

Building a support network Several participants described at interview how they had been encouraged throughout treatment to share resources (e.g. psychoeducational material) with family and friends and been given opportunities to include their family or friends at various stages of the treatment process (e.g. bringing a friend/family member to their assessment or a therapy session). Some participants reflected upon this emphasis on family/friend involvement as a challenging aspect of treatment, often because of fears about being a burden to others and beliefs that they should "do it themselves".

"They came to one session, but I didn't really want them to... I didn't like it." (Aaliyah, interview)

Despite it being challenging, participants identified that they had been able to increase the involvement of their family and friends over the course of treatment. They reflected that building a support network in this way had been beneficial and important to the progress they had made.

"The support provided to my family and myself was incredible and helped us all learn how to deal with my anorexia as a team." (Georgia, questionnaire)

Life beyond the eating disorder Several participants identified at interview that treatment did not focus exclusively on their eating difficulties but looked at eating difficulties within the broader context of their life. They reported that the treatment felt tailored to their age-group.

"It was really focused on... my age, the position I was in." (Annie, interview)

A minority of participants (2% of those providing questionnaire data) felt that their treatment was too focused on eating, with monitoring of weight in particular experienced as coercive and detrimental to health.

"I was forced to weigh in every week which I don't think was valid and made me even more ill." (Ruth, questionnaire)

For those participants who did feel their treatment was holistic, they identified that this focus had contributed to progress in several ways.

Life getting in the way of treatment. Several participants described at interview how instability or unpredictability in their broader life context (e.g. busy jobs with limited freedom to plan schedule, returning to the family home for summer holidays) made it more difficult to engage with treatment. Participants described how service flexibility (e.g. out-of-hours appointments; ease of rescheduling) was important to mitigate the impact of this instability on treatment.

"If one week I couldn't make it wasn't a problem, we'd just arrange for next week. That's been a real benefit, just sort of working it in around a busy job." (Max, interview)

Some participants described finishing treatment because of a residence change (e.g. moving to and from the parental home in line with university terms) and expressed beliefs that such transitions had been well-managed.

"I was transferred to services in Devon, and I was very lucky, because it came under a transfer of care, rather than a new referral." (Phoebe, interview)

However, several participants felt unclear as to how many sessions they were to receive and identified that knowing this would have been helpful for goal-setting.

"I wasn't really aware until coming towards the end of my sessions....how long [treatment] was going to be... that would be nice because obviously... [you can set] your goals a bit more specifically if you've got a time-frame." (Max, interview)

Focusing on future goals. Participants (~ 10%) described how treatment focused on future goals and getting back to life without an ED. Several participants described how clinicians explicitly discussed the detrimental impact of eating difficulties on achievement of life goals (characterised by some as a "scare-talk"), which enhanced motivation to change.

"In my first appointment, I was told that my plans to pursue a career in music and academia would be non-existent if my anorexia continued." (Hannah, questionnaire)

Many participants believed that treatment had been focused on helping them work towards goals related to life beyond their ED.

"The good thing with this treatment compared to other treatments was that this had an end-goal... we had goals about becoming more independent, dealing with change, starting university." (Eleanor, interview)

Some participants described receiving support from clinicians regarding working towards future life goals (e.g. starting university; career decisions).

"we did a lot of preparation during the summer months [for university], around forming relationships with people, eating lunch with people." (Annie, interview)

"[my therapist] was trying to help me like get back in touch with the things that I like, and the things that make me "me" ... I couldn't even decide what job I wanted to, and I managed to decide I'd like to be a paramedic." (Olivia, interview)

Becoming your own therapist Some participants identified tools that focused on helping them to monitor and self-manage their eating difficulties as beneficial (e.g. food diaries and worksheets to complete between sessions). A number of participants described how tools such as food diaries helped them to understand connections between environmental triggers and their emotions, thoughts, and behaviours, and feel more able to control their behaviour.

"The food diary idea really helps you keep a close eye on what goes on and how you can progress." (Hayley, questionnaire)

Indeed, several participants suggested at interview that more homework would be welcome.

"[I'd suggest] perhaps maybe more exercises or tasks to do in my own time, to kind of challenge how I was dealing with the things, or the new strategies that they'd given me." (Niamh, interview)

Participants described how such resources helped them feel empowered to move forward in their recovery without a therapist.

"I genuinely feel I have the tools to beat my eating disorder without a professional now." (Iris, questionnaire)

"I felt so supported all the way through, but also empowered to help myself." (Clara, questionnaire)

Discussion
Summary of findings
This is the first study to explore patients' experiences of a developmentally-informed early intervention service model for EDs. Participants were emerging adults with first-episode, recent-onset EDs who received treatment through FREED. The majority of participants had found FREED treatment helpful and reported noticeable psychological and behavioural changes. Participants identified rapid access to treatment, knowledgeable and

concerned clinicians, building a support network, focus on life beyond ED and becoming own therapist as key beneficial characteristics of the treatment received.

Psychological and behavioural change

Whilst most participants reported noticeable psychological and behavioural changes, there was variation in how such changes were conceptualised. Some participants described positive progress in terms of symptomatic improvement, whilst many participants described it in terms of being "freer" and more able to be themselves or being able to work towards goals that were not ED-related. Many participants acknowledged that they were not yet "recovered", but that treatment had made them feel empowered to work towards recovery. Importantly, a small minority of participants believed that treatment had not been associated with change, in some cases because treatment was experienced as too brief. These findings both corroborate and enrich quantitative evidence from the broader FREED-Up study, which found that FREED patients experienced significant change in ED symptoms and individualised outcomes over the course of treatment [30].

Rapid access to treatment This study found that emerging adults expressed positive attitudes about the concept of early intervention and believed it had been instrumental to improvement in their ED. This finding is consistent with previous research which has found positive attitudes towards early intervention amongst emerging adults with EDs and other diagnoses, and suggests that rapid access to treatment may be key to the improved clinical outcomes associated with FREED treatment [10, 26, 28, 39].

In particular, participants believed that rapid access to treatment had prevented their ED thoughts and behaviours becoming more engrained and their physical health from deteriorating further. This in turn made their difficulties easier to overcome. This understanding is compatible with theories of ED progression and illness stage models on which the rationale for early intervention service models for EDs are based [40]. It is also in keeping with findings within the broader FREED-Up study, with non-FREED patients more unwell at assessment than FREED patients (i.e. their condition has worsened whilst waiting for treatment) [28].

Participants reported that rapid access meant they received care before they had time to reconsider their decision to access treatment. This is a novel finding but is broadly consistent with findings within the broader FREED-Up cohort, which found that treatment uptake was higher in FREED than in non-FREED patients [29]. Findings from this study suggest that such increased treatment uptake may be due in part to the ability of

early intervention to "strike whilst the iron is hot". Indeed, previous research has identified that "motivation to change" at start of ED treatment is associated with treatment outcome [41], and it may be that increased motivation to change at start of treatment can also help to explain FREED's clinical effectiveness.

This study also found that some participants perceived that early intervention, as delivered here, was "not early enough" for them, because they already had had symptoms for some time prior to specialist referral. This is perhaps not surprising, given the evidence that emerging adults tend to come to services with a longer duration of ED than other groups [11, 12, 42, 43]. However, this finding further highlights that efforts to increase early help-seeking will be key to maximise the effectiveness of early intervention [43].

Knowledgeable and concerned clinicians Participants experienced clinicians as knowledgeable and concerned, and believed these characteristics were important facilitators of positive change. This finding aligns well with extensive evidence which suggests the important of therapeutic alliance to patient experience and treatment outcomes, particularly for younger patients and those with AN [44, 45]. It also corroborates previous research which has highlighted the importance of staff expertise to emerging adults' treatment experiences, both in EDs and more broadly [10, 39]. The perceived value of clinicians expressing concern is interesting, given that this is consistent with the FREED model's emphasis on encouraging early symptom change through psychoeducation [26]. This finding therefore provides further evidence that this core characteristic of the FREED model is valued by patients and may be a contributing factor to improved clinical outcomes.

Building a support network Efforts to recruit friends and family into a support network during treatment were viewed as beneficial by participants, and as important to the progress they had made in treatment. This is consistent with research which has demonstrated the clinical effectiveness of family-based ED treatment adapted for "transition-aged youth" (i.e. emerging adults) [46]. However, many participants were ambivalent about the inclusion of family or friends in their treatment. This corroborates previous research which has found this is often a challenging area for services working with emerging adults with EDs and other diagnoses [39, 46, 47]. It is not surprising that this is a particularly pertinent concern during emerging adulthood, given that this life-stage is characterised by ongoing autonomy development and an "in-between" (childhood / adulthood) level of independence [48, 49]. Indeed, asserting self-reliance and independence from caregivers has been previously highlighted as a particular concern for emerging adults with EDs [9, 10, 43].

Life beyond the eating disorder Many participants appreciated the focus on life beyond their ED in treatment, although a small minority believed treatment had been too focused on eating. In particular, participants reported instability in their lives, and that life sometimes "got in the way" of treatment. This is in keeping with existing evidence that emerging adulthood tends to be characterised by instability and a proliferation of life-events, which in turn have the potential to impact emerging adults' help-seeking and treatment [9, 10, 37, 48]. Importantly, participants were pleased with the flexibility FREED service showed to counteract such instability (e.g. accommodating rescheduling, supporting with transition arrangements), and believed this contributed to positive outcomes.

Additionally, participants valued that FREED treatment was focused on working towards life goals. Emerging adulthood is a key time for psychosocial development, particularly identity development in multiple life domains (e.g. relationships; vocation; ideology) [50]. Furthermore, burgeoning research has identified the important interplay between ED aetiology /treatment response and ongoing developmental context, with concurrent identity development identified as particularly relevant [9, 10, 37, 51, 52].

Becoming your own therapist Participants valued that treatment focused on them "becoming their own therapist". This is perhaps not surprising, given that emerging adulthood is a key time for autonomy development and tends to be characterised by attitudes of self-reliance [48, 49]. Making the most of such attitudes (whilst also emphasising the importance of social support) may be key to the improved clinical outcomes associated with FREED treatment [10, 26, 28]. Interestingly, this finding aligns with existing qualitative literature exploring young peoples' experiences of early intervention services for psychosis, suggesting this concept's relevance across diagnoses. A recent meta-synthesis of all such studies found that participants spoke about how treatment through early intervention services helped them realise the importance of personal agency in their recovery journey [39].

Strengths and limitations
Participants were drawn from a well-established and comprehensive cohort study. Data pertaining to key demographic and clinical characteristics were therefore available, and the sample is clearly characterized. Data were triangulated from two sources, which is likely to have increased the validity and comprehensiveness of the findings. Questionnaires allowed exploration of the experiences of a large cohort, whilst interviews offered the opportunity for experiences to be explored in greater depth.

Qualitative data regarding treatment experience were not collected from emerging adults who did not receive treatment through FREED. It is therefore not possible to make definitive statements about the extent to which the treatment experiences outlined in this paper were unique to FREED. Additionally, just 38% of eligible individuals opted to provide data for the study. Comparison of the characteristics of those who did and did not provide qualitative data indicates that these groups are broadly similar on a range of characteristics. However, the treatment completion rate was higher amongst those who provided qualitative data than amongst those who did not. It may be this sample is biased towards people who had more positive experiences of treatment.

Finally, whilst the researchers who conducted this study do not provide FREED treatment, their professional perspectives are "pro-FREED". Efforts were made to bring this bias and its impact to awareness and mitigate it as far as was possible (e.g. by considering such biases within the analytic process).

Future research
This study focused on those emerging adults who accepted the offer of and engaged with FREED treatment. Considering that 9% of emerging adults referred to FREED-UP could not be contacted after referral or did not attend their assessment appointment [29], future research might usefully consider the experiences of people who decide not to engage with treatment. Additionally, future quantitative research might focus on investigating the mechanisms of effect suggested by the present study (e.g. inclusion of measures of motivation to change, identity development).

Clinical implications
This study provides further support for wide-scale implementation of early intervention and developmentally-informed models in ED care for emerging adults. From a patient perspective the key characteristics of this model appear not just to be rapid access to treatment but also the focus on meeting developmental needs. With regard to future development, it is clear early intervention-focused approaches should be accompanied by efforts to increase early help-seeking in order to maximise their effectiveness.

Conclusion
Emerging adults with first-episode, recent-onset EDs who received treatment through FREED saw treatment as helpful and reported noticeable psychological and behavioural changes. Participants identified rapid access to treatment, knowledgeable and concerned clinicians, building a support network, focus on life beyond ED and becoming their own therapist as key beneficial characteristics of the treatment received. These findings provide further support for the value of adopting early intervention, developmentally-informed models in ED care.

Appendix
Interview Topic Guide

1. Can you tell me about your experience of treatment within the FREED service?
   Probes:
   - Impact / change
2. Was there anything you found helpful during treatment?
3. Was there anything you didn't like about treatment?
4. Do you have any suggestions for how we might improve the service?
5. Did the service feel sufficiently tailored to *your* needs?
   Probes:
   - How so?
6. What is your understanding of "early intervention"?
   Probes:
   - Importance? Why /why not?
   - Impact
7. Were your parents or friends involved in your treatment at all?
   Probes:
   - Who, how?
   - Thoughts / feelings
8. Did you have to transition to another service during your treatment?
   Probes:
   - Experience
9. You are in a time of life when you are learning to do lots of things, becoming more independent and figuring out who you are. Did treatment help with things beyond ED or was it mostly focused on your ED?
   Probes:
   - Developing identity e.g. career goals
   - Skills for independent living

Abbreviations
AEDS: Adult eating disorder services; AN: Anorexia nervosa; BED: Binge-eating disorder; BN: Bulimia nervosa; CAEDS: Child and adolescent eating disorder services; EDs: Eating disorders; FREED: First Episode Rapid Early Intervention for Eating Disorders; OSFED: Other specified feeding and eating disorders; UK: United Kingdom

Acknowledgements
The research team would like to thank the participants who generously shared their time and experience for the purposes of this project.

Authors' contributions
RP, AA, MF, KA, and US designed the study. AA and MF conducted the questionnaire-based data collection. RP conducted the semi-structured inter-views, analysed the data and wrote the manuscript, with critical revisions from US, VL, KA, AA, and MF. All authors read and approved the final manuscript prior to submission.

Funding
The FREED-Up study was supported by a scaling-up grant from the Health Foundation. RP is funded by a PhD Studentship from the National Institute for Health Research (NIHR) Biomedical Research Centre (BRC) for Mental Health, South London and Maudsley NHS Foundation Trust (SLaM) and Institute of Psychiatry, Psychology and Neuroscience, King's College London (KCL). AA is funded by a KCL International Postgraduate Research Scholarship. KA receives support from the NHS Innovation Accelerator programme. VL receives salary support from KCL. US receives salary support from the NIHR BRC for Mental Health, SLaM and KCL. US is supported by an NIHR Senior Investigator Award. This paper represents independent research funded by the NIHR BRC, SLaM and KCL. The views expressed are those of the authors and not necessarily those of the NIHR or the Department of Health and Social Care. The funders had no role in study design, data collection or analysis, decision to publish, or preparation of the manuscript.

Competing interests
The authors declare that the research was conducted in the absence of any commercial or financial relationships that could be construed as a potential conflict of interest.

Author details
[1]Institute of Psychiatry, Psychology and Neuroscience, King's College London, London, UK. [2]South London and Maudsley NHS Foundation Trust, London, UK. [3]Maudsley Health, Abu Dhabi, UAE. [4]Sussex Partnership NHS Foundation Trust, Brighton, UK. [5]Leeds and York Partnership NHS Trust, Leeds, UK. [6]Central and North West London NHS Foundation Trust, London, UK. [7]North East London NHS Foundation Trust, London, UK. [8]Division of Psychology and Language Sciences, University College London, London, UK.

References
1. Hudson JI, Hiripi E, Pope HG Jr, Kessler RC. The prevalence and correlates of eating disorders in the National Comorbidity Survey Replication. Biol Psychiatry. 2007;61(3):348–58.
2. Kessler RC, Berglund PA, Chiu WT, Deitz AC, Hudson JI, Shahly V, et al. The prevalence and correlates of binge eating disorder in the World Health Organization world mental health surveys. Biol Psychiatry. 2013;73(9):904–14.
3. Micali N, Hagberg KW, Petersen I, Treasure JL. The incidence of eating disorders in the UK in 2000–2009: findings from the general practice research database. BMJ Open. 2013;3(5):e002646.
4. Steinhausen H-C, Jensen CM. Time trends in lifetime incidence rates of first-time diagnosed anorexia nervosa and bulimia nervosa across 16 years in a danish nationwide psychiatric registry study. Int J Eat Disord. 2015;48(7): 845–50.
5. Glazer KB, Sonneville KR, Micali N, Swanson SA, Crosby R, Horton NJ, et al. The course of eating disorders involving bingeing and purging among adolescent girls: prevalence, stability, and transitions. J Adolesc Health. 2019; 64(2):165–71.
6. Eisenberg D, Nicklett EJ, Roeder K, Kirz NE. Eating disorder symptoms among college students: prevalence, persistence, correlates, and treatment-seeking. J Am Coll Heal. 2011;59(8):700–7.
7. Favaro A, Busetto P, Collantoni E, Santonastaso P. The age of onset of eating disorders. Age of Onset of Mental Disorders. Cham: Springer; 2019. p. 203–16.
8. Galmiche M, Déchelotte P, Lambert G, Tavolacci MP. Prevalence of eating disorders over the 2000–2018 period: a systematic literature review. Am J Clin Nutr. 2019;109(5):1402–13.

9. Potterton R, Richards K, Allen K, Schmidt U. Eating Disorders During Emerging Adulthood: A Systematic Scoping Review. Front Psychol. 2020; 10(3062). https://doi.org/10.3389/fpsyg.2019.03062.

10. Mitrofan O, Petkova H, Janssens A, Kelly J, Edwards E, Nicholls D, et al. Care experiences of young people with eating disorders and their parents: qualitative study. BJPsych Open. 2019;5(1). https://doi.org/10.1192/bjo.2018.78.

11. Weigel A, Rossi M, Wendt H, Neubauer K, von Rad K, Daubmann A, et al. Duration of untreated illness and predictors of late treatment initiation in anorexia nervosa. J Public Health. 2014;22(6):519–27.

12. McClelland J. Prodromal eating disorders in adolescents and young adults: King's College London; 2019.

13. Sánchez-Ortiz V, Munro C, Stahl D, House J, Startup H, Treasure J, et al. A randomized controlled trial of internet-based cognitive-behavioural therapy for bulimia nervosa or related disorders in a student population. Psychol Med. 2011;41(2):407–17.

14. Treasure J, Schmidt U, Hugo P. Mind the gap: service transition and interface problems for patients with eating disorders. Br J Psychiatry. 2005; 187(5):398–400.

15. Arcelus J, Bouman WP, Morgan JF. Treating young people with eating disorders: transition from child mental health to specialist adult eating disorder services. Eur Eat Disord Rev. 2008;16(1):30–6.

16. McClelland J, Simic M, Schmidt U, Koskina A, Stewart C. Defining and predicting service utilisation in young adulthood following childhood treatment of an eating disorder. BJPsych Open. 2020;6(3). https://doi.org/10.1192/bjo.2020.13.

17. England N. Access and Waiting Time Standards for Children and Young People with an Eating Disorder 2015. https://www.england.nhs.uk/wp-content/uploads/2015/07/cyp-eating-disorders-access-waiting-time-standard-comm-guid.pdf.

18. Beat. Delaying for Years, Denied for Months. 2018 https://www.beateatingdisorders.org.uk/uploads/documents/2017/11/delaying-for-years-denied-for-months.pdf.

19. Psychiatrists RCo. Position Statement on Early Intervention for Eating Disorders 2019. https://www.rcpsych.ac.uk/docs/default-source/improving-care/better-mh-policy/position-statements/ps03_19.pdf?sfvrsn=b1283556_2.

20. Lindgren E, Söderberg S, Skär L. Swedish young adults' experiences of psychiatric care during transition to adulthood. Issues Ment Health Nursi. 2015;36(3):182–9.

21. Loos S, Walia N, Becker T, Puschner B. Lost in transition? Perceptions of health care among young people with mental health problems in Germany: a qualitative study. Child Adolesc Psychiatry Ment Health. 2018;12(1):41.

22. McGorry PD, Goldstone SD, Parker AG, Rickwood DJ, Hickie IB. Cultures for mental health care of young people: an Australian blueprint for reform. Lancet Psychiatry. 2014;1(7):559–68.

23. Winston AP, Paul M, Juanola-Borrat Y. The same but different? Treatment of anorexia nervosa in adolescents and adults. Eur Eat Disord Rev. 2012;20(2):89–93.

24. Schmidt U, Brown A, McClelland J, Glennon D, Mountford VA. Will a comprehensive, person-centered, team-based early intervention approach to first episode illness improve outcomes in eating disorders? Int J Eat Disord. 2016;49(4):374–47.

25. Allen KL, Mountford V, Brown A, Richards K, Grant N, Austin A, et al. First episode rapid early intervention for eating disorders (FREED): From research to routine clinical practice. Early Interv Psychiatry. 2020;14(5):625–30.

26. Fukutomi A, Austin A, McClelland J, Brown A, Glennon D, Mountford V, et al. First episode rapid early intervention for eating disorders: A two-year follow-up. Early Interv Psychiatry. 2020;14(1):137–41.

27. Brown A, McClelland J, Boysen E, Mountford V, Glennon D, Schmidt U. The FREED project (first episode and rapid early intervention in eating disorders): service model, feasibility and acceptability. Early Interv Psychiatry. 2018;12(2):250–7.

28. McClelland J, Hodsoll J, Brown A, Lang K, Boysen E, Flynn M, et al. A pilot evaluation of a novel first episode and rapid early intervention service for eating disorders (FREED). Eur Eat Disord Rev. 2018;26(2):129–40.

29. Flynn M, Austin A, Lang K, Allen K, Bassi R, Brady G, et al. Assessing the impact of First Episode Rapid Early Intervention for Eating Disorders on duration of untreated eating disorder: A multi-centre quasi-experimental study. Eur Eat Disord Rev. 2020. https://doi.org/10.1002/erv.2797.

30. Austin A, Flynn, M., Shearer, J., Allen, K., Mountford, V., Glennon, D., Grant, N., Brown, A., Franklin-Smith, M., Schelhase, M., Rhys-Jones, W., Brady, G., Nunes, N., Connan, F., Mahony, K., Serpell, L & Schmidt, U. The First Episode Rapid Early Intervention for Eating Disorders – Upscaled (FREED-Up) study. In preparation.

31. Chenail RJ. How to conduct clinical qualitative research on the Patient's experience. Qual Rep. 2011;16(4):1173–90.

32. Moore GF, Audrey S, Barker M, Bond L, Bonell C, Hardeman W, et al. Process evaluation of complex interventions: Medical Research Council guidance. BMJ. 2015;350:h1258. https://doi.org/10.1136/bmj.h1258.

33. Fletcher AJ. Applying critical realism in qualitative research: methodology meets method. Int J Soc Res Methodol. 2017;20(2):181–94.

34. Bhaskar R. Enlightened common sense: the philosophy of critical realism. Oxford: Routledge; 2016.

35. Patton MQ. Enhancing the quality and credibility of qualitative analysis. Health Serv Res. 1999;34(5 Pt 2):1189.

36. Etikan I, Musa SA, Alkassim RS. Comparison of convenience sampling and purposive sampling. Am J Theor Appl Stat. 2016;5(1):1–4.

37. Goldschen L, Lundblad W, Fertig AM, Auster LS, Schwarzbach HL, Chang JC. Navigating the university transition among women who self-report an eating disorder: a qualitative study. Int J Eat Disord. 2019;52(7):795–800.

38. Braun V, Clarke V. Using thematic analysis in psychology. Qual Res Psychol. 2006;3(2):77–101.

39. Hansen H, Stige SH, Davidson L, Moltu C, Veseth M. How do people experience early intervention Services for Psychosis? A Meta-Synthesis. Qual Health Res. 2018;28(2):259–72.

40. Currin L, Schmidt U. A critical analysis of the utility of an early intervention approach in the eating disorders. J Ment Health. 2005;14(6):611–24.

41. Vall E, Wade TD. Predictors of treatment outcome in individuals with eating disorders: a systematic review and meta-analysis. Int J Eat Disord. 2015;48(7):946–71.

42. Austin A, Flynn M, Richards K, Hodsoll J, Duarte TA, Robinson P, Kelly J, Schmidt U. Duration of untreated eating disorder and relationship to outcomes: a systematic review of the literature. Eur Eat Disord Rev. 2020. https://doi.org/10.1002/erv.2745.

43. Potterton R, Austin A, Allen K, Lawrence V, Schmidt U. "I'm not a teenager, I'm 22. Why can't I snap out of it?": a qualitative exploration of seeking help for a first-episode eating disorder during emerging adulthood. J Eat Disord. 2020;8(1):46.

44. Zaitsoff S, Pullmer R, Cyr M, Aime H. The role of the therapeutic alliance in eating disorder treatment outcomes: a systematic review. Eat Disord. 2015; 23(2):99–114.

45. Graves TA, Tabri N, Thompson-Brenner H, Franko DL, Eddy KT, Bourion-Bedes S, et al. A meta-analysis of the relation between therapeutic alliance and treatment outcome in eating disorders. Int J Eat Disord. 2017;50(4):323–40.

46. Dimitropoulos G, Landers AL, Freeman V, Novick J, Garber A, Le Grange D. Open trial of family-based treatment of anorexia nervosa for transition age youth. J Can Acad Child Adolesc Psychiatry. 2018;27(1):50.

47. Dimitropoulos G, Tran AF, Agarwal P, Sheffield B, Woodside B. Challenges in making the transition between pediatric and adult eating disorder programs: a qualitative study from the perspective of service providers. Eat Disord. 2013;21(1):1–15.

48. Arnett JJ. Emerging adulthood: a theory of development from the late teens through the twenties. Am Psychol. 2000;55(5):469–80.

49. Inguglia C, Ingoglia S, Liga F, Coco AL, Cricchio MGL. Autonomy and relatedness in adolescence and emerging adulthood: relationships with parental support and psychological distress. J Adult Dev. 2015;22(1):1–13.

50. Schwartz SJ, Zamboanga BL, Luyckx K, Meca A, Ritchie RA. Identity in emerging adulthood: reviewing the field and looking forward. Emerg Adulthood. 2013;1(2):96–113.

51. Verschueren M, Claes L, Bogaerts A, Palmeroni N, Gandhi A, Moons P, et al. Eating disorder symptomatology and identity formation in adolescence: a cross-lagged longitudinal approach. Front Psychol. 2018;9:816.

52. Koskina A, Schmidt U. Who am I without anorexia? Identity exploration in the treatment of early stage anorexia nervosa during emerging adulthood: a case study. Cognit Behav Ther. 2019;12.

Permissions

The contributors of this book come from diverse backgrounds, making this book a truly international effort. This book will bring forth new frontiers with its revolutionizing research information and detailed analysis of the nascent developments around the world.

We would like to thank all the contributing authors for lending their expertise to make the book truly unique. They have played a crucial role in the development of this book. Without their invaluable contributions this book wouldn't have been possible. They have made vital efforts to compile up to date information on the varied aspects of this subject to make this book a valuable addition to the collection of many professionals and students.

This book was conceptualized with the vision of imparting up-to-date information and advanced data in this field. To ensure the same, a matchless editorial board was set up. Every individual on the board went through rigorous rounds of assessment to prove their worth. After which they invested a large part of their time researching and compiling the most relevant data for our readers.

The editorial board has been involved in producing this book since its inception. They have spent rigorous hours researching and exploring the diverse topics which have resulted in the successful publishing of this book. They have passed on their knowledge of decades through this book. To expedite this challenging task, the publisher supported the team at every step. A small team of assistant editors was also appointed to further simplify the editing procedure and attain best results for the readers.

Apart from the editorial board, the designing team has also invested a significant amount of their time in understanding the subject and creating the most relevant covers. They scrutinized every image to scout for the most suitable representation of the subject and create an appropriate cover for the book.

The publishing team has been an ardent support to the editorial, designing and production team. Their endless efforts to recruit the best for this project, has resulted in the accomplishment of this book. They are a veteran in the field of academics and their pool of knowledge is as vast as their experience in printing. Their expertise and guidance has proved useful at every step. Their uncompromising quality standards have made this book an exceptional effort. Their encouragement from time to time has been an inspiration for everyone.

The publisher and the editorial board hope that this book will prove to be a valuable piece of knowledge for researchers, students, practitioners and scholars across the globe.

List of Contributors

Marit Nilsen Albertsen
Department of Global Health and Primary Care, University of Bergen, Bergen, Norway
Department of Eating Disorders, Division of Psychiatry, Haukeland University Hospital, Institute of Psychological Counselling, Bergen, Norway

Eli Natvik
Department of Health and Caring Sciences, Western Norway University of Applied Sciences, Førde, Norway

Målfrid Råheim
Department of Global Health and Primary Care, University of Bergen, Bergen, Norway

Rouba Karen Zeidan
Faculty of Public Health, Lebanese University, Fanar, Lebanon
INSPECT-LB: Institut National de Santé Publique, Epidemiologie Clinique et Toxicologie, Beirut, Lebanon
CERIPH: Center for Research in Public Health, Pharmacoepidemiology Surveillance Unit, Faculty of Public Health, Lebanese University, Fanar, Lebanon

Chadia Haddad
Psychiatric Hospital of the Cross, Jall-Eddib, Lebanon
Univ. Limoges, UMR 1094, Neuroépidémiologie Tropicale, Institut d'Epidémiologie et de Neurologie Tropicale, GEIST, 87000 Limoges, France

Rabih Hallit, Karl Honein and Maria Akiki
Faculty of Medicine and Medical Sciences, Holy Spirit University of Kaslik (USEK), Jounieh, Lebanon

Souheil Hallit
INSPECT-LB: Institut National de Santé Publique, Epidemiologie Clinique et Toxicologie, Beirut, Lebanon
6Faculty of Medicine and Medical Sciences, Holy Spirit University of Kaslik (USEK), Jounieh, Lebanon

Marwan Akel
INSPECT-LB: Institut National de Santé Publique, Epidemiologie Clinique et Toxicologie, Beirut, Lebanon
School of Pharmacy, Lebanese International University, Beirut, Lebanon

Nelly Kheir
Faculty of Pedagogy, Holy Family University, Batroun 5534, Lebanon

Sahar Obeid
INSPECT-LB: Institut National de Santé Publique, Epidemiologie Clinique et Toxicologie, Beirut, Lebanon
Psychiatric Hospital of the Cross, Jall-Eddib, Lebanon
Faculty of Arts and Sciences, Holy Spirit University (USEK), Jounieh, Lebanon

Laura A. Berner and Robyn Sysko
Department of Psychiatry, Icahn School of Medicine at Mount Sinai, New York, NY, USA

Tahilia J. Rebello and Kathleen M. Pike
Department of Psychiatry, Columbia University Irving Medical Center, New York, NY, USA

Christina A. Roberto
Department of Medical Ethics and Health Policy, Perelman School of Medicine, University of Pennsylvania, Philadelphia, PA, USA

Kevin Glisenti, Esben Strodl and Robert King
School of Psychology and Counselling, Queensland University of Technology, Faculty of Health, Brisbane, Queensland, Australia

Leslie Greenberg
Department of Psychology, York University, Faculty of Health, Toronto, Canada

Matteo Aloi, Marianna Rania, Elvira Anna Carbone, Mariarita Caroleo and Giuseppina Calabrò
Outpatient Unit for Clinical Research and Treatment of Eating Disorders, University Hospital "Mater Domini", Catanzaro, Italy
Department of Health Sciences, University "Magna Graecia" of Catanzaro, Catanzaro, Italy

Carlo Cosentino and Paolo Zaffino
Department of Experimental and Clinical Medicine, School of Computer and Biomedical Engineering, University "Magna Graecia" of Catanzaro, Catanzaro, Italy

Giuseppe Nicolò and Antonino Carcione
Third Centre of Cognitive Psychotherapy – Italian School of Cognitive Psychotherapy (SICC), Rome, Italy

Gianluca Lo Coco
Department of Psychology, Educational Science and Human Movement, University of Palermo, Palermo, Italy

Cristina Segura-Garcia
Outpatient Unit for Clinical Research and Treatment of Eating Disorders, University Hospital "Mater Domini", Catanzaro, Italy
Department of Medical and Surgical Sciences, University "Magna Graecia" of Catanzaro, Catanzaro, Italy

Salomé Adelia Wilfred
Department of Psychology, University of Missouri-Kansas City, Kansas City, MO, USA

Carolyn Black Becker
Department of Psychology, Trinity University, San Antonio, TX, USA

Kathryn E. Kanzler
ReACH Center, UT Health San Antonio, San Antonio, TX, USA

Nicolas Musi and Sara E. Espinoza
Barshop Institute, UT Health San Antonio, San Antonio, TX, USA
South Texas VA Health System, Audie Murphy Veterans Hospital, San Antonio, TX, USA

Lisa Smith Kilpela
Barshop Institute, UT Health San Antonio, San Antonio, TX, USA
South Texas VA Health System, Audie Murphy Veterans Hospital, San Antonio, TX, USA

Ashley A. Moskovich, Michael A. Babyak, Patrick J. Smith, Lisa K. Honeycutt, Jan Mooney and Rhonda M. Merwin
Duke University Medical Center, DUMC, Durham, NC 27712, USA

Natalia O. Dmitrieva
Northern Arizona University, Flagstaff, AZ, USA

Amy L. Burton and Maree J. Abbott
School of Psychology, The University of Sydney, Camperdown, NSW, Australia

Marcelo Papelbaum and José Carlos Appolinario
State Institute Diabetes and Endocrinology, Rio de Janeiro, Brazil
Group of Obesity and Eating Disorders, Institute of Psychiatry of the Federal University of Rio de Janeiro and State Institute Diabetes and Endocrinology, Avenida Ataulfo de Paiva 204, 707, Leblon, Rio de Janeiro 22440-033, Brazil

Rodrigo de Oliveira Moreira, Walmir Ferreira Coutinho, Rosane Kupfer and Silvia Freitas
State Institute Diabetes and Endocrinology, Rio de Janeiro, Brazil

Ronir Raggio Luz
Institute for Studies in Public Health, Federal University of Rio de Janeiro, Rio de Janeiro, Brazil

Manal M. Badrasawi and Souzan J. Zidan
Department of Nutrition and Food technology, Faculty of Agriculture and Veterinary Medicine, An-Najah National University, Tulkarm West Bank, Palestine

Elin Monell and Andreas Birgegård
Centre for Psychiatry Research, Department of Clinical Neuroscience, Karolinska Institute, and Stockholm Health Care Services, Stockholm County Council, Norra Stationsgatan 69, SE-11364 Stockholm, Sweden
Department of Medical Epidemiology and Biostatistics, Karolinska Institutet, Stockholm, Sweden

David Clinton
Centre for Psychiatry Research, Department of Clinical Neuroscience, Karolinska Institute, and Stockholm Health Care Services, Stockholm County Council, Norra Stationsgatan 69, SE-11364 Stockholm, Sweden
Department of Medical Epidemiology and Biostatistics, Karolinska Institutet, Stockholm, Sweden
Institute for Eating Disorders, Oslo, Sweden

Mirjam W. Lammers and Maartje S. Vroling
Amarum, Expertise Centre for Eating Disorders, GGNet Network for Mental Health Care, Den Elterweg 75, 7207 AE Zutphen, The Netherlands
Radboud University, Behavioural Science Institute, Montessorilaan 3, 6525 HR Nijmegen, The Netherlands

Tatjana van Strien
Radboud University, Behavioural Science Institute, Montessorilaan 3, 6525 HR Nijmegen, The Netherlands

Ross D. Crosby
Sanford Center for Biobehavioral Research, Fargo, North Dakota, USA
University of North Dakota School of Medicine and Health Sciences, Fargo, North Dakota, USA

Jiwon Yang
Department of Nursing, Kyungil University, Gyeongsan-si, South Korea

Kuem Sun Han
Department of Nursing, Korea University, Seoul, South Korea

Başak İnce
Department of Psychology, Haliç University, Istanbul, Turkey

Johanna Schlatter
Department of Psychosomatic Medicine and Psychotherapy, University Hospital Tübingen, Osianderstraße 5, 72076 Tübingen, Germany

Sebastian Max and Christian Plewnia
Department of Psychiatry and Psychotherapy, Neurophysiology & Interventional Neuropsychiatry, University of Tübingen, Tübingen, Germany

Stephan Zipfel, Katrin Elisabeth Giel and Kathrin Schag
Department of Psychosomatic Medicine and Psychotherapy, University Hospital Tübingen, Osianderstraße 5, 72076 Tübingen, Germany
Competence Center of Eating Disorders Tübingen (KOMET), Tübingen, Germany

Laura S. Silverstein and Lattice Sams
Department of Pediatric Dentistry, Children's Hospital Colorado, 1575 N Wheeling Street, Aurora, CO 80045, USA

Carol Haggerty
Division of Comprehensive Oral Health, University of North Carolina Adams School of Dentistry, Chapel Hill, NC 27599-7450, USA

Ceib Phillips
Division of Craniofacial and Surgical Sciences, University of North Carolina Adams School of Dentistry, Chapel Hill, NC 27599-7450, USA

Michael W. Roberts
Division of Pediatric and Public Health, University of North Carolina Adams School of Dentistry, 228 Brauer Hall CB #7450, Chapel Hill, NC 27599-7450, USA

Tiffany Patterson-Norrie
Centre for Oral Health Outcomes & Research Translation (COHORT), School of Nursing and Midwifery , Western Sydney University/South Western Sydney Local Health District/Ingham Institute for Applied Medical Research, Liverpool BC, Locked Bag 7103, Sydney, NSW 1871, Australia

Lucie Ramjan
School of Nursing and Midwifery, Western Sydney University, Centre for Oral Health Outcomes & Research Translation (COHORT), Sydney, Australia

Mariana S. Sousa
IMPACCT, Faculty of Health, University of Technology Sydney, Sydney, Australia

Lindy Sank
Sydney Dental Hospital, Oral Health Services, SLHD, Sydney, Australia

Ajesh George
Centre for Oral Health Outcomes & Research Translation (COHORT), Western Sydney University/South Western Sydney Local Health District/University of Sydney/Ingham Institute for Applied Medical Research, Sydney, Australia

Malin Bäck
Department of Behavioural Sciences and Learning, Linköping University, Linköping, Sweden
Futurum: Academy for Health and Care, Jönköping, Region Jönköping County, Sweden

Fredrik Falkenström and Rolf Holmqvist
Department of Behavioural Sciences and Learning, Linköping University, Linköping, Sweden

Sanna Aila Gustafsson
Faculty of Medicine and Health, University Health Care Research Center, Örebro University, Örebro, Sweden

Gerhard Andersson
Department of Behavioural Sciences and Learning, Linköping University, Linköping, Sweden
Department of Clinical Neuroscience, Karolinska Institute, Stockholm, Sweden

Katie Grogan, Diarmuid MacGarry, Jessica Bramham and Amanda Fitzgerald
School of Psychology, University College Dublin, Dublin, Ireland

Mary Scriven and Caroline Maher
Elm Mount Unit, St. Vincent's University Hospital, Dublin, Ireland

Rachel Potterton, Amelia Austin, Michaela Flynn and Vanessa Lawrence
Institute of Psychiatry, Psychology and Neuroscience, King's College London, London, UK

Karina Allen and Ulrike Schmidt
Institute of Psychiatry, Psychology and Neuroscience, King's College London, London, UK
South London and Maudsley NHS Foundation Trust, London, UK

Victoria Mountford
Institute of Psychiatry, Psychology and Neuroscience, King's College London, London, UK
South London and Maudsley NHS Foundation Trust, London, UK
Maudsley Health, Abu Dhabi, UAE

Danielle Glennon and Nina Grant
South London and Maudsley NHS Foundation Trust, London, UK

Amy Brown
South London and Maudsley NHS Foundation Trust, London, UK
Sussex Partnership NHS Foundation Trust, Brighton, UK

Mary Franklin-Smith, Monique Schelhase and William Rhys Jones
Leeds and York Partnership NHS Trust, Leeds, UK

Gabrielle Brady, Nicole Nunes and Frances Connan
Central and North West London NHS Foundation Trust, London, UK

Kate Mahony
North East London NHS Foundation Trust, London, UK

Lucy Serpell
North East London NHS Foundation Trust, London, UK
Division of Psychology and Language Sciences, University College London, London, UK

Index

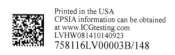

Printed in the USA
CPSIA information can be obtained
at www.ICGtesting.com
LVHW081410140923
758116LV00003B/148